# Keep the Legs You Stand On

Dr. Mark Hinkes

©2009

Nightengale Press

A Nightengale Media LLC Company

KEEP THE LEGS YOU STAND ON
Copyright ©2009 by Dr. Mark Hinkes
Cover design ©2009 by Nightengale Press

For information about Nightengale Press please
Visit our website at www.nightengalepress.nom.
Email: publisher@nightengalepress.com
Or send a letter to:
Nightengale Press
10936 N. Port Washington Road. Suite 206
Mequon, WI 53092

Library of Congress cataloging-in-publication data

Hinkes, Dr. Mark,
Keep the Legs You Stand On/ Dr. Mark Hinkes
ISBN:1-933449-71-3
ISBN 13: 978-1933449-71-5
Medical

Copyright Registered: 2009

First published by Nightengale Press in the USA

March 2009

10 9 8 7 6 5 4 3 2 1

Printed in the USA and the UK

# Disclaimer

*Keep The Legs You Stand On* is intended as a guide to assist with clinical and educational information on amputation prevention; it is for informational purposes only. The content is not intended to be a substitute for professional medical advice, diagnosis, or treatment.

Never disregard professional medical advice because of something you have read in this book. If you think you may have a medical emergency, call your doctor or 911 immediately. The author and publisher are not responsible or liable for any damage or loss resulting from any medical evaluations, recommendations, or medical treatments listed in this book. Your reliance on the information found in this book, without consultation with a qualified medical professional is at your own risk. Always consult with your medical professional for individual patient evaluation, treatment, or recommendations.

# Endorsements

"Every thirty seconds someone with diabetes loses their leg somewhere in the world. Most of these amputations are preventable. It's through books like *Keep the Legs You Stand On* that educate the patient that make a difference. This educational effort will keep more legs on more bodies."
—David G. Armstrong, DPM, PhD, Professor of Surgery University of Arizona College of Medicine Director, Southern Arizona Limb Salvage Alliance (SALSA), Tucson, Arizona

"Dr. Hinkes has built an outstanding easy to read "owner's manual for diabetic patients and loved ones that want to help prevent limb loss". As a physician and researcher who is a also a diabetic and treats diabetes, I am grateful that this book has been written for folks across the globe who seek this knowledge and deserves to be guided through this often complex issue. I will not only use this book in my clinical practice, but I will be sure to get a copy for my family members! BRAVO, for Dr Hinkes!"
—Vickie R Driver, MS DPM FACFAS, Director, Clinical Research Foot Care, Endovascular and Vascular Services Associate Professor of Surgery Boston Medical Center and Boston University School of Medicine, Boston, Massachusetts

"Bravo to Dr. Mark Hinkes on his monumental accomplishment in publishing the first of its kind, *Keep the Legs You Stand On*. His poignant perspective and practical introspection is unprecedented in a field of highly technical texts. I highly recommend this book to all involved in the care of diabetes, diabetic feet, and the issues surrounding this complex disease process. This is a thoughtful, well-written book that is a joy to read!"

—Cynthia Fleck, RN, BSN, MBA, ET/WOCN, CWS, DNC, FACCWS, President and Chairman of the Board, The American Academy of Wound Management (AAWM), St. Louis, Missouri

"*Keep The Legs You Stand On* is a must-read text for podiatry students, residents, and clinicians alike. It's an insightful and personal look at the high-risk diabetic patient we see in our offices or clinics, and a reminder of what we can do to help keep them be healthy, active, and on their feet. Mark's personal experiences make him an expert in this area and we can all definitely learn from his insight and approach. While there is a tendency to fall into the realm of "a routine" with our patients, this book helps us remember and realize that these patients need unique direction and care, and that as podiatrists we are the ones best trained to provide this specialized treatment for them. An easy read, an excellent review, and first-rate insight!"

—Howard Green, DPM, DABPS, FACFAS, Head, Department of Podiatry and Director of Podiatry Residency Training, Vancouver General Hospital / University of British Columbia, Vancover, BC

"I highly recommend Dr. Hinkes' book *Keep the Legs You Stand On* for everyone with diabetes and their family members. Education is the key to preventive medicine and this book has a wealth of information. Although quite long, the style is easy to read with interesting stories and case studies to illustrate all aspects of foot health and disease from anatomy to treatment methods and including sections on cultural and financial considerations. The photographs throughout the book are fascinating. Dr. Hinkes has shared the highlights of over 30-years of an exciting career as a podiatrist. All I can say is, Dr. Hinkes, thank you for sharing!"

—Linda Halperin MD, Assistant Chief of Physical Medicine, Tennessee Valley Healthcare System, Nashville, Tennessee

"What a wonderful, monumental work!"
—Laura F. Jacobs, MD PhD, Physical Medicine and
Rehabilitation, President
and CEO NormaTec PCD, Newton Center, MA

"It is estimated by the American Diabetes Association that over 90,000 patients with diabetes will have a leg amputated this year. Once someone with diabetes loses one leg, the chance that they will be living in five years from now is only 50 percent. This survival rate is worse than most of the common forms of cancer. Yet, unlike cancer, many of the complications of diabetes are firmly within your control. By understanding the disease, how it affects your foot and what you can do to prevent this from occurring it has been proven time and time again that the number of foot and leg amputations, and subsequent deaths, can be dramatically reduced. With this book, Dr. Hinkes has given you, the patient with diabetes, all of the tools you need to understand how to save your foot, leg and life. But, as thorough as this book is, unless you are fortunate enough to be a veteran in the Nashville area who has Dr. Hinkes as a podiatrist, Dr. Hinkes can only "lead you to water." It is up to you to *drink it!*"
—Warren S. Joseph, DPM, FIDSA, Consultant, Lower
Extremity Infectious Diseases, Huntingdon Valley, PA

"Dr. Hinkes has produced a tremendous resource for patients with diabetes and for those lay people who act as their caregivers. We, as podiatrists, understand the catastrophic sequelae that can develop from a diabetic foot infection. We also are very much aware of the opportunities for limb preservation with appropriate education for our patients and for those who help care for them. There is no doubt that an "educated" diabetic individual is better off than the person who doesn't understand the disease. Oftentimes, being able to recognize the "problem signs" can mean the difference in preserving a foot or leg.

I am not aware of a more comprehensive text on diabetes, written in a manner, that a lay person could easily read and understand. This book should be a "must" in all diabetic households and at all diabetic education centers. My hat goes off to Dr. Hinkes for a job very well done!"

—Jay D. Lifshen, DPM, FACFAS, President, Southwest Podiatry, LLP Dallas, Texas

"My goal as a certified diabetes educator is to help people with diabetes achieve the best possible blood glucose control and avoid chronic long-term complications associated with diabetes. Amputation is a complication of diabetes that can be prevented with appropriate and timely self-care practices. *Keep the Legs You Stand On* is an important resource for people with diabetes. It provides practical guidelines for basic foot care and prevention of foot injury, as well as direction on what to do when foot problems are identified. Adoption of the foot care practices discussed in this book will reduce the incidence of amputation for individuals with diabetes."

—Elaine McLeod, MSN, APN, BC-ADM, ACNS-BC, CDE, Tennessee Valley Healthcare System, Nashville, Tennessee

"As an individual recently diagnosed with type 2 diabetes and with serious hereditary foot issues, I am reading the book with an eye toward ongoing preventive measures that will allow me to avoid serious complications, and understand what needs to be done to deal with the horrible tragedy of preventable amputations in the US and abroad. Kathleen and I are very pleased to give you our whole hearted endorsement of *Keep the Legs You Stand On* and are extremely proud to have known you as you were working so hard to complete this very valuable endeavor. This book has the potential of impacting the lives of many thousands of at-risk individuals."

—Michael J. Philps, President and Kathleen Philps, Vice President, MJ Philps & Associates LLC, Upland, California

"Dr. Hinkes has provided a much-needed resource for patients with diabetes and for people who love someone with diabetes. With both amputation rates and death rates on the rise we must all stand up and take responsibility for our own health. Doctors and nurses can only do so much and it is up to each and every one of us to be in charge of the things that are within our control. Regarding diabetes, that's a lot. Dr. Hinkes has successfully woven fact and recommendation into an easy to read resource that should empower people to not only take control of their lives but also to negotiate the sometimes confusing and complicated healthcare system here in the United States. Make no mistake about it, the United States has the finest healthcare providers in the world; however, negotiating the system is a different matter. Use this book as a blueprint for personal health and put an end to unnecessary amputation and disability."

—, Jeffrey Robbins, DPM, ABPOPPM - ABPH. Fellow - American College of Foot and Ankle Orthopedics and Medicine, Director Veterans Administration Headquarters, Podiatry Services Chief Podiatry Section, Louis Stokes Cleveland VA Medical Center Cleveland, Ohio.

"I believe *Keep The Legs You Stand On* will prove to be an invaluable reference for all those who work and live with the diabetic foot. There is a tremendous amount of information in these pages that will no doubt help prevent those preventable amputations. Dr. Hinkes has done a wonderful job in a caring and informative manner."

—Laura Roehrick RN, Certified Foot Care Nurse, Santa Rosa, California

"Mark, your book is outstanding and it is exactly what we need. I think every DPM should have it in their office for sale; better yet, every insurance company should give it to their patients with diabetes."

—Lee C. Rogers, CLEAR Fellow 2006-2007, Director Amputation Prevention Center Broadlawns Medical Center Des Moines, Iowa.

"As a layperson and medical writer who is also a caregiver to a diabetic patient, I found Dr. Hinkes' book to be extremely valuable in bringing me up-to-date on the latest developments in diabetes. I would wholeheartedly recommend it to anyone, either professional or lay person, who wants an easy to read book written by a knowledgeable caregiver. Congratulations, Dr. Hinkes and thank you for all of the hard work that went into helping diabetics, their families and caregivers, and a wide range of medical professionals. You have done a great service to us all."

—Sari Staver, Medical Writer, San Francisco CA

"This book can provide a greater degree of education than what any doctor can provide in a 15-minute office visit. Reading it at leisure can arm patients with enough good information that they can make better decisions and navigate the system."

—James Wrobel, DPM, MS, ABPOPPM, Associate Professor of Medicine, Associate Professor of Surgery Director, Center for Lower Extremity Ambulatory Research Center (CLEAR), North Chicago, Illinois

# Contents

# Foreword

*Stop it at the start it's late for medicine to be prepared when disease has grown strong through long delays.* ~ Ovid (Remedia Amoris, line 91)

Diabetes is an epidemic disease, seen on every continent and in every country. It affects nearly 24 million people in the United States, with another 57 million people estimated to have pre-diabetes. Worldwide it is projected that the prevalence of diabetes will reach 333 million people in the year 2025. People with diabetes are at increased risk of developing the long-term complications of cardiovascular disease, kidney disease, eye disease and nerve disease. For many people affected by diabetes the two most feared complications are blindness and lower limb amputations. However, these are not inevitable outcomes and can be prevented or delayed with proper education and diabetes care. Diabetes self-management education is the cornerstone of care for people with diabetes. This essential component of care has been proven to improve health outcomes and quality of life.

Two years ago, Dr. Mark Hinkes called me to discuss his concept for a book on preventive foot care for people with diabetes. He was passionate in his conviction that patient education together with comprehensive podiatric care would make a difference in the quality of life for his patients. His objectives were simple, to provide people with diabetes with a better understanding of their disease and its complications as well as the importance of foot health and early recognition of warning signs. When Mark first discussed this project with me, I thought that his goals were ambitious; however I am happy to say that he has far exceeded my expectations and he has hit a home run with this book. His discussion of the subject is comprehensive, practical and entertaining. His case stories are instructive and help to provide the reader with the necessary knowledge to recognize the early warning signs of diabetic foot disease and the importance of early recognition and treatment. Dr. Hinkes provides references for further reading and sources for products. He discusses the role of footwear and orthotics as well as how to determine if you are eligible for therapeutic shoes under Medicare.

*Keep the Legs You Stand On* is recommended reading for all people with diabetes, their families and caregivers. In addition, I believe that this book provides medical students, interns, residents and nurses with important insight regarding the evaluation, risk assessment and management of the diabetic foot. In the words of my friend and distinguished colleague Dr. Lawrence Harkless, "You see what you look for and recognize what you know."

I heartily congratulate Dr. Hinkes, on behalf of the many people with diabetes and their care givers who will be helped by this splendid book.

Lee J. Sanders, DPM
Past President, Health Care and Education
The American Diabetes Association

# Acknowledgements

Andrew Boulton, MD, internationally recognized and highly-respected researcher, author and clinician, who teaches at Manchester University in England and at the University of Miami in Florida, U.S.A. With focus on the foot, his work in the area of diabetic neuropathy and how it affects patients with diabetes has provided a basis of understanding that guides the care of every diabetic patient today.

Bijan Najafi, Ph.D. Member of the CLEAR group. Assistant Professor and Director Human Performance Lab, Dr. William M. Scholl College of Podiatric Medicine. Specialist on biomechanics, gait, balance, and falling.

Bob Goldfarb, my friend who encouraged me to pursue my dreams and write this book.

David Smith, DPM, of Thunder Bay, Ontario, Canada. He works with native Inuit Canadian Indians and provided me insights about them.

Dennie Terry, RN, the nurse from North Carolina who loved her father so much and taught me a life lesson about patients and amputation prevention.

Douglas Balfour, DPM of Green Bay, Wisconsin, who was kind enough to permit me to extern in his office.

Gary McAuliffe, a pharmaceutical sales representative who offered me my first opportunity to lecture and share information with my colleagues about issues in podiatry and the diabetic foot.

Jan Freeman, "the wizard," who taught me about data and databases and how to use them for analysis of the PACT Program. She taught me how to think in "computer" and the advantages of using data bases to understand preventive foot health.

Marc Lennet, DPM, and Michael Sherman, DPM, Program Directors Podiatric Externship at Lutheran Hospital of Maryland, Baltimore, Maryland. Thank you for the opportunity to participate in an outstanding program that was a pivotal experience in my podiatric education and training.

K.R. Suresh, MD. Director and consultant vascular surgeon at Jain Institute of Vascular Sciences in Bangalore, India. He is currently working with stem cells to heal diabetic foot wounds and shared with me issues of the diabetic foot in India.

Karel Bakker, MD. Chair, IDF Consultative Section of the Diabetic Foot, and International Working Group on the Diabetic Foot in Heemstede, Netherlands.

Keith Kashuk, DPM and the podiatric medical staff at Westchester General Hospital in Miami, Florida. My thanks to all the members of the podiatric medical staff who helped me develop my medical and surgical skills and to those who graciously opened their offices to me and taught me about my profession.

Lawrence B. Harkless, DPM. a clinician, researcher, teacher, educator, and author. A mentor and leader of the podiatric medical profession. Founding Dean, Western University of Health Sciences in Pomona California. While he was the Chief of Podiatry, he received the Louis T. Bogy Professor of Podiatric Medicine and Surgery—the first fully-funded endowment professorship for the Podiatry Division at the University of Texas Health Science Center at San Antonio.

Lee C. Rogers, DPM, Director of Amputation Prevention Center in Des Moines Iowa. Dr. Rogers represents the newest generation of young podiatric medical practitioners who specialize in care of the diabetic foot.

Lee J. Sanders, DPM. Chief of Podiatry Section, Acute Care/Specialty Services at Veterans Administration Medical

Center in Lebanon, Pennsylvania. Former National President for Health Care and Education of American Diabetes Association (1998–2000) Co-author of *A Practical Manual of Diabetic Foot Care*. Dr. Sanders received the second fully-funded endowment professorship for the Podiatry Division at the University of Texas Health Science Center at San Antonio: The Lee J. Sanders Professorship in Lower Extremity Amputation Prevention.

Luca Dalla Paola, MD, endocrinologist and surgeon, who is a Professor and Chief of the Diabetic Foot Department at Bologna, Italy University School of Medicine.

Members of the PACT Programs in both the Salem, Virginia and Nashville, Tennessee Veteran Affairs Hospitals who have worked with me in the goal of saving limbs and lives.

Renee Stiles, PhD. for her kind help in the statistical analysis of the PACT data.

Ron Rubin, my friend who supported and encouraged me to write this book.

Sam Hollander, my friend who encouraged me to try harder and work smarter. He gave me support, brought good cheer, and encouraged me to write this book.

Sheldon Langer, DPM. a mentor, educator, and friend who helped me to be a better podiatrist by understanding podiatric biomechanics and the use of foot orthotics.

Steven Weinberg, DPM, Buffalo Grove, Illinois who was kind enough to permit me to extern in his office.

Tom Freidman, whose work has influenced me to think globally and understand the power of communications, especially via the Internet, for the benefit of patients with diabetes and foot care issues around the world.

Tony Robbins, who opened my eyes to so many fundamental issues in life and from whom I learned the concept of being outstanding.

Zhang-Rong XU, MD. Member of the IWGDF who is an advocate of care of the diabetic foot in China.

## Special Thanks

To my parents, Jules and Esther, for their love and support and for providing me with a philosophical basis of life and the encouragement to pursue my medical career.

My wife, Susan, and my children, Drew and Laura, who have encouraged and supported my work even though I have left them alone more than I should have.

My brother, Kenny Hinkes, who more than anyone else encouraged and motivated me to write this book. My sister, Susan Warren, for proofreading support of the book.

Claudia Reynolds, who helped me in generating the initial development of the manuscript that resulted in this book.

Yvonne Perry, Editor and Owner of Writers in the Sky Creative Writing Services (WITS), who provided developmental and copy editing for this book. Thanks to WITS team member Sarah Moore, who transcribed hours of audio recordings for this book.

To the following people for allowing me to personally interview them for this book:

Bob Frykberg, DPM, Chief of Podiatry at Carl T. Hayden VA Medical Center in Phoenix.

Chongbin Zhu, OMD, PhD, Licensed holistic acupuncturist and oriental medicine practicing in Nashville, Tennessee.

Christopher Attinger, MD, Medical Director of Wound Healing Clinic, and Professor of Plastic Surgery at Georgetown University Hospital, Washington DC.

Cynthia Fleck, RN, BSN, MBA, ET/WOCN, CWS, DNC, FACCWS, President and Chairman of the Board for the American Academy of Wound Management; Director of the Association for the Advancement of Wound Care (AAWC); President of CAF; Clinical Consultant and Vice President of Clinical Marketing for Medline Advanced Wound and Skin Care.

David G. Armstrong, DPM, Professor of Surgery at the University of Arizona. He is also Founder and Co-Director with renowned Vascular Surgeon Professor Joseph Mills of the Southern Arizona Limb Salvage Alliance (SALSA) at the University of Arizona and the Southern Arizona VA Health Care System.

Dennis J. Janisse, Certified Pedorthist and Owner of National Pedorthic Services, Inc. headquartered in Milwaukee, Wisconsin. Dennis is the Past President of the Pedorthic Footwear Association, Director of Pedorthic Education for PW Minor, and current director with American Board for Certification in Orthotics, Prosthetics, and Pedorthics.

Howard Green, DPM, Director of the Podiatry Surgical Residency Program at Vancouver General Hospital in Vancouver, Canada.

James Powers, MD, Associate Professor of Medicine at Vanderbilt University and Medical Director of the Senior Care Service, and Chief of Geriatrics at the VA Hospital in Nashville, Tennessee.

James Wrobel, DPM, MS, Director of CLEAR and Associate Professor of Medicine, Director of Outcomes Research at Dr. William M. Scholl College of Podiatric Medicine, North Chicago, Illinois.

Jeffrey Robbins, DPM, my classmate, mentor, and friend who taught me about prevention and the diabetic foot and encouraged me to participate in the PACT Program.

John Steinberg, DPM, Assistant Professor of the Department of Plastic Surgery Georgetown University. A clinician, researcher, teacher, educator, and patient advocate who has brought podiatric medicine and surgery to become a legitimate member of the limb salvage team at Georgetown University.

Laura Roehrick, RN, CFCN, a nurse and educator with a vision of worldwide diabetic foot care that knows no boundaries.

Lawrence Lavery, DPM, MPH, Professor of Surgery at Scott & White Hospital, Texas A&M Health Science Center College of Medicine in College Station Texas, and Editor-in-Chief of *Foot and Ankle Quarterly*.

Linda Halperin, MD, Associate Chief of Physical Medicine and Rehabilitation and my associate in the VA At-Risk Foot Clinic in Nashville, Tennessee.

Margaret "Elaine" McLeod, Certified Diabetes Educator and my associate in the VA At-Risk Foot Clinic in Nashville, Tennessee.

Ruben Zamorano, President of Diabetica Solutions in San Antonio, Texas—an inventor of products for diagnosing diabetic foot problems.

Vickie Driver, DPM, Director of Clinical Research Foot Care, Endovascular and Vascular Services Associate Professor of Surgery, Boston Medical Center and Boston University School of Medicine. In addition, she is chair of the APMA Clinical Practice Advisory Committee (CPAC).

# Dedication

To my patients who have given me the opportunity to serve them and learn from them.

# Introduction

Imagine that a 747 airplane, filled to capacity, lands in your local airport every day of the year and all the passengers get off the plane, into their cars, and drive straight to the local hospital to have a leg amputated. That is the approximate number of people with diabetes who have amputations every day in the United States.

In 2003, patients and insurance companies spent $5 billion on approximately 82,000 lower limb amputations due to diabetes. The Center for Disease Control estimates that up to 85 percent of all non-accident-related lower limb amputations occur in patients with diabetes. The CDC estimates that up to 80 percent of these amputations can be prevented. Changing these statistics, as well as giving some common sense tips for common foot problems with diabetes, is the focus of this book.

There is a huge need for this book and the information it provides to people who are at risk of losing a limb due to diabetes. This book is also aimed to help the parents of children with diabetes as well as the caregivers and professionals who treat and care for "at-risk" people. Children with diabetes typically do not suffer the comorbidities that are common with adults who have had diabetes for many years. However, if the preventative behaviors addressed in this book become a normal part of a diabetic child's life, they may very well prevent the young one from suffering with life and limb issues later on. The value of proactive prevention cannot be over emphasized when it comes to keeping the legs you stand on.

Diabetes is a disaster of a disease. It affects every organ and organ system of the body: the eyes, kidneys, circulatory system, neurological system, brain, heart, skin, muscles, bones and joints, soft tissues, nails, and of course the foot. Most patients are ill-equipped to deal with the multiple complications of the disease because they lack education about their medical condition. For example, they don't know what a hemoglobin A1c test is and what it tells the doctor about the patient's blood glucose levels. Many patients don't know or understand the risks of diabetes or, at best, are in denial. They're diabetic and don't have a clue as to why their grandmother lost a limb. They don't realize that certain foods cause blood sugar levels to elevate and they are ignorant of the consequences that chronically elevated blood glucose levels have on their bodies. They don't understand the concept of prevention and preventive behaviors, and they do not know about the benefits that preventative treatment offers.

I have been a foot care professional for the past thirty years. In the last ten years, my eyes have been opened to the issues relative to patients with diabetes who are at risk for the loss of their lower extremities. In my experience and talking with patients, more often than not, patients lack the basic understanding of diabetes, what it is, how it affects their body, and how to deal with it and the many complications that commonly accompany it. In his article in the *Wall Street Journal*, Michael J. McCarthy says, "The problem is generally one of ignorance. Simple foot wounds that are left untreated or that don't respond to treatment may be a sign of serious circulatory trouble...many people don't realize a serious infection is setting in, so they don't seek help...And even when a problem is correctly diagnosed, doctors aren't always aware of available preventive measures."[1]

In the early 1970s when I was deciding on a career, I learned about the profession of podiatry. The future seemed bright for this small struggling group of medical and surgical specialists. I visited several of the schools of podiatric medicine and learned even more about a career in this under-utilized healthcare service. Classmates who had attended podiatry schools shared with me the fantastic things they were doing for people and their foot health. Since the profession offered a challenge to my personal growth and development of surgical skills, I felt that I would enjoy working in this area of medicine to help people resolve their foot problems.

Podiatry gave me the opportunity to practice both as a physician and as a surgeon. I was very interested in the surgical aspect of this profession. However, I soon realized that not all patients can have surgery because some are not in satisfactory physical condition to tolerate surgery; others do not have the insurance or the money to afford it. Some don't have the time away from work to recuperate from surgery and others are plainly phobic about foot surgery. While the emphasis in podiatric medical training has traditionally been surgical, there are treatments other than surgery that can be provided by podiatrists to help people with their foot problems.

Podiatric Biomechanical theory, which is the science that explains how the bone structure affects foot function, has strongly influenced me in terms of how I evaluate and manage patients. I have found podiatric biomechanics to be the secret science that sets podiatry apart from other fields of medicine. We not only understand physiology and anatomy, we also understand the functioning of the foot and the human gait cycle. This gives podiatry a tremendous advantage in terms of our ability to understand why a patient may develop an ulcer or a callus, a bunion, or a hammer toe, and heel or fore foot pain. It can also help us to understand if a person's foot pain is actually coming from their back or other non-foot structures. It also gives us the ability to resolve those issues by understanding how the patient functions in the 3-D world.

I frequently see patients with diabetes also having cardiovascular disease, end-stage renal disease, neuropathy, smoking addiction, obesity, malnutrition, and other serious conditions. The common thread is that these patients suffer from a lack of knowledge about their diabetes and from not practicing preventive behaviors. They do not understand their disease or how important it is to maintain blood sugar in the proper range. They do not realize that painless or silent trauma is a trigger that leads to a cascade of events resulting in an amputation.

During the first twenty years of my career when I was in a private practice that offered elective surgery, biomechanics, sports medicine, and primary podiatric care, most of the patients I saw were women and children. It was a shock to enter the Veterans Affairs (VA) system where more mature problems affecting mostly men were the norm. When I first went to the VA facility in Salem, Virginia, I walked into the reception area and was totally shocked and overwhelmed by what I saw. In a room half the size of a football field it seemed to me that there were more people without legs than with legs. That was scary for me even as a physician and surgeon. I learned firsthand the intensity of this problem, the number of people involved, and the affect it had on their lives. I also began to understand my ability to help these patients.

Those who had two legs and were at risk of losing one of them became a priority in my practice because I realized I could help them by teaching them about prevention behavior to arrest an existing problem. Those who had only one leg and were at risk of losing the other leg became a super-priority. I wanted to make sure they kept that leg. The energy expenditure necessary to walk rises 30 percent when there is a below-the-knee amputation. In an above-the-knee amputation it rises close to 60 percent. Ask any amputee and many will tell you they feel a sense of loss of personal liberty after losing a leg. These issues were very touching to me.

While working in Virginia, I had a patient—an older gentleman with diabetes, who had been a tobacco farmer. His daughter brought him from a little town near Durham, North Carolina to see me in Salem, Virginia. He had an ulcer on his toe. While they lived close to Duke University, the VA Hospital, and other private hospitals there, the only treatment plan his physician could come up with was an amputation of his toe. I didn't understand why his daughter was willing to drive such a distance on two-lane twisting mountain roads every week to help heal her father's ulcer, but she was diligent. She brought a notebook with her to each visit and wrote down every word I said about how we would manage her father's treatment. She followed my instructions without fail and together we did in fact heal his ulcer and avoided an amputation.

When her father passed away, I attended his funeral. His daughter told me that he always had a wish that when he passed away, he would still have all of his body parts. That was why she was willing to drive for hours to see me and explicitly follow my instructions. Her dedication to her father opened my eyes and my heart to the issues relative to diabetes—especially people's feet—and what lengths people were willing to go to if they could find someone who could save that toe or foot. More than any patient in my lifetime, this one man and his daughter made me realize how important my work is. This experience is one of the main reasons why I pursued my gifts, talents, and abilities to work with these special patients and provide care that was perhaps not available in any other place. It is also good reason for writing this book.

I am a podiatrist and have studied and practiced my field of expertise for my entire thirty-year career. The results have been my ability to be outstanding at what I do and have earned lots of wonderful letters after my name. I have medical and surgical training and am board certified in foot surgery. I have the wisdom of years where I have seen all kinds of patients with all kinds of foot problems. While some were outside the scope of what I was able to provide care for, many of them were amenable to the care we were able to provide. My experience in working with these patients has given me a rare opportunity to provide insights into patients with diabetes and why they have problems. If they don't heal a wound, I can help them understand why they don't heal and what solutions might work in terms of evaluating their circulation, neurological status, biomechanics of gait, and footgear to help them heal a wound. I can also identify the subtleties that affect the patient's life including current medical conditions, previous surgery to their feet, medications, social behaviors, and their support system. Every one of these issues contributes in one way or another to the health and well being of the patient. As a practicing clinician, it has been my honor and privilege to treat patients.

As I moved into the VA system in the last ten years of my professional career, I have happily accepted the appointment as chairman of PACT (Preservation, Amputation, Care and Treatment) Program. This government program is mandated, but unfunded. It seeks to have us identify patients who are at risk of losing a leg. We are to categorize and put them into risk management groups and provide care to prevent amputations. Through chairing this committee, I have learned about the issues relative to patients with diabetes, the administrative issues, issues of policy making, cost for services and treatment, quality of patient lives, and opportunities for prevention. The success of managing the PACT program in two VA Hospitals—one in Salem, Virginia and the other in the Nashville, Tennessee—has given me more energy and provided me with constant motivation. I not only see the issues of these patients from a clinical perspective, but also from an administrative point of view. We've been able to improve the quality of life for patients and also identify the tremendous cost benefits of proactive care through the PACT Program.

When I first became involved in the PACT Program in 1999 at the Veterans Affairs Medical Center in Salem, Virginia, I became acutely aware that either patients or doctors did not realize the serious nature of the diabetic foot and how a minor injury can lead to amputation. Unfortunately, during my thirty-year career, I have come across a few doctors whom I felt just didn't take the necessary time and energy to really help patients who came in with a contaminated foot or a smelly, ugly infection moving up the leg. Conservative wound care is time consuming for both the physician and caregiver and requires a cooperative, interdisciplinary medical approach. Lower limb amputation resolves the issue more quickly, but at a higher price for the patient. My approach is to attempt everything possible to see if a foot or leg can be saved. I believe it is sinful to rob a person of a limb when there is any chance at all of saving it.

My experiences motivated me to gather a group of like-minded healthcare workers from different disciplines—an interdisciplinary team who would determine what each of us could do to identify and care for patients who were at risk for a lower limb amputation. Identifying at-risk patients before it is too late and they are facing the loss of part of their foot or their leg is the key. Within two years of starting the program, we had achieved a surprising success rate. The hospital in Salem, Virginia had a cost savings of over $1 million, and more importantly, there was a 27 percent decrease in the lower limb amputation rate. I was pleased for the patients and for the cost savings, but I wondered whether this was a fluke or truly a powerful preventive care strategy.

Then, an opportunity to relocate to the Veterans Affairs Medical Center in Nashville, Tennessee came my way. I sought the position of Chairman of the PACT Program again because I wanted to see whether the Virginia results could be duplicated or bettered. In the first year of the program, the cost savings were just under $1 million, and the amputation rate significantly decreased. In the second year, the cost savings were over $1 million, and the amputation rate decreased to just less than 1 percent per thousand patients. Outside the VA, the rate is 6 percent per thousand patients. The cost savings came from decreased spending in the areas of pharmaceuticals, laboratory costs, and in-patient hospital bed days. As a result of the prevention program, instead of losing a foot or a leg, patients might only lose a toe. We credited this to the early identification of at-risk patients and providing them with preventive care and education. We had hit a home run. Although I didn't know all of the patients, it was a great feeling to know that we did something for at-risk people that increased the quality of their lives and, oh, by the way, saved Uncle Sam almost a million dollars.

Our interdisciplinary team offers a valuable service to patients with diabetes by providing preventive care and trying to rescue whatever is left of a patient's leg making it viable and biomechanically functional. However, I cannot help enough patients quickly enough. If I have a patient in my treatment chair, I have an opportunity to educate and respond to questions from that one individual. If I am lucky enough to have Vanderbilt residents at a lunchtime conference or at our "foot at-risk clinic" or podiatry clinic, then I have the opportunity to educate four to six budding young doctors who will then be able to take this knowledge and use it to the benefit of hundreds or even thousands of patients in their lifetimes. But, even at that rate, I still felt that I was not doing enough. In an effort to give patients an opportunity to have an equal chance against their disease, I feel it is extremely important to identify the issues that affect patients and provide them with an educational experience at their level. In this book, I will not use big, fancy words without explaining them. I will use everyday language that the average person can understand.

The goal of this book is to prevent patients with diabetes from losing their legs and to affect a better quality of life. Many patients are afflicted with diabetes, peripheral vascular disease, or peripheral neuropathy. Some patients cannot use their hands to treat or care for themselves due to arthritis. Those who are legally blind or have low vision are not able to see their foot, and others may be physically or mentally unable to care for themselves.

My priority is to make the lives of patients with diabetes better and to prevent unnecessary amputation. My plan is to start a revolution with the slogan, "Let them have healthy feet!" And in this revolution our mission is to keep all of our body parts intact and functioning, unlike Marie Antoinette, who is now missing her head! The royal subjects we are particularly interested in are those at the highest risk of foot problems—the patient with diabetes. At the rate in which diabetes is spreading throughout "kingdoms" across the globe, it is likely that you or someone you know will face this disease, whether you are royalty or commoner, unless we change the current practices in detection and treatment. My goal for this book is to help you *Keep the Legs You Stand On*.

# Preface

An ounce of prevention is worth a pound of cure
~ *Benjamin Franklin*

The best medicine ever known to man is prevention. While hereditary diseases, including diabetes, may not be completely preventable, the risks associated with the illness can be greatly reduced and many symptoms can be diminished by exercising proper self-care and following the expert advice given by your medical professionals. Taking the responsibility for your health is the key to any wellness plan. Your doctor cannot do it all for you. Neither can your spouse or other caregiver. Your health is up to you. That includes educating yourself about your illness and understanding the complications that go along with it. Knowing what you can do to self-manage your diabetes and foot health and when to get professional care can go a long way in helping you avoid amputation. Prevention is especially important when healthcare is not readily available or made affordable to everyone.

This book is intended for people everywhere who suffer with diabetes. The book will take you all over the world and show what is going on in different countries—from the latest treatments available to the limitations on healthcare in other nations. I have not only called upon my own personal thirty-year experience as a podiatrist, I have gathered information from national and international experts in order to help you better understand what you are up against and what hope there might be for a future cure of this horrible disease.

The need for better treatment for diabetes and its comorbidities of vascular and neurological disease are the same everywhere, but the treatment youmay receive and your ability to practice preventative behavior may differ. That's because the treatment you may expect for diabetes is dependent upon your latitude and longitude. For example, if you live in India where there is little available treatment for diabetes and you walk the streets in ill-fitting shoes or open sandals, your risk for trauma leading to infection and amputation is far greater than in the United States. If in your community people are not allowed to wear shoes inside the house due to religious beliefs, you increase the risk of cutting or hurting your foot—especially if you have no feeling in your foot to let you know you have injured it. If you live in European countries the level of care that podiatrists can provide is very limited in comparison to the United States. Podiatrists can provide care for superficial foot problems that includes corns, calluses, nails, and biomechanical problems, but are not able to do surgery in the deep tissues of the foot. If you need that type of foot surgery such as for bone or soft tissue infections, a podiatrist may not be able to care for your foot problem, and it may be a challenge to find a physician or surgeon who can help you.

Even if you are fortunate enough to live where healthcare is available, you may not be able to afford it. Therefore, I hope the message of this book will reach the political arena as well as the business decision makers in the healthcare industry, and motivate people to stand up and lobby for universal healthcare benefits and better treatment facilities. Although the care for diabetes in the United States is better than in most countries, there is still a great need for improvement when it comes to cooperation between primary care physicians (PCP), diabetes specialists, podiatrists or foot surgeons, pharmacists, nurses, insurance companies, and caregivers. There needs to be a one-stop system where the goal is to treat the whole patient and not just the symptoms present during that particular visit. This requires each healthcare professional to know what the other players on your team are up to.

At the end of each chapter in this book you will find "Foot Notes." These are not traditional references where cited information is found. Works cited and research sources will be documented in the bibliography and at the end of the book as "end notes." The Foot Notes at the end of each chapter are for *you*. They contain healthy foot habits, facts, quizzes, prevention exercises, and tips to help you better care for your feet. I encourage you to use these notes and share them with others on your healthcare team.

Throughout the book, I will use patient's stories to help illustrate the point being made. I believe these stories will be entertaining, educational, and perhaps somewhat shocking to the casual reader. All stories are used with permission from the patients. The names of some have been changed to protect their identity. The same is true for the photographs used.

Chapter 1 will define diabetes and how it relates to foot health. We will give a brief but interesting history of diabetes and show who is most at risk for getting diabetes. Since denial is one of the biggest obstacles to overcome when taking responsibility for one's diabetic condition, we will give tips for staying on target with the choices needed to care for the condition.

In Chapter 2, we will use demographic statistics to show who is at risk for amputation. You will be better informed and able to know your individual risks.

Chapter 3 asks "Who takes care of your feet?" We look at the history of podiatry and what it can do for you today. Then, you'll learn when to seek medical exams by a podiatric physician and when it is okay to use self-care. Did you know that a pedicure at a nail salon could lead to a foot infection or something even worse?

Chapter 4 will touch on the role of a caregiver and wrap up the chapter with a footnote that provides a checklist of things a caregiver needs to know.

Chapter 5 teaches Foot Anatomy 101 and presents how balance, falling, and peripheral neuropathy are related to diabetes. We will give information about gait cycle interruptus and how motor or sensory neuropathy affects stability and causes falling.

In Chapter 6, we will take a look at the cause of common foot problem such as bone, nail, and soft tissue deformities, and give best treatment options and tips for seeking the right professional care.

Chapter 7 deals with the loss of protective sensation in the feet and gives facts about diabetic peripheral neuropathy that includes the three sub categories of sensory, motor, and autonomic neuropathy. Alcoholic neuropathy will be discussed as well as Charcot foot (neurogenic arthropathy), and nerve entrapment. Test your circulation, and learn the real issues about dry skin in patients with diabetes.

Understanding vascular disease and the circulatory system that includes, arterial, venous, and lymphatic systems is the premise of Chapter 8. Here, we present what you should know about varicose veins, venous insufficiency, venous stasis dermatitis, edema, ischemia, and ABI testing, and interpreting the results.

In Chapter 9, you will receive a thorough understanding of the foot ulcer, and know the causes as well as where ulcers may be found and why they occur in that spot. It gives remedies for healing foot and heel ulcers and preventing their reoccurrence.

This is followed by Chapter 10 where we study wound care, types of dressings to treat bacterial, viral, mold, yeast, and fungus infections, and present material by a wound care expert, Cynthia Fleck, RN.

In Chapter 11, we will explore immunopathy, inflammation, infection, the immune system and its toolbox, and discuss how a wound heals.

Chapter 12 deals with finding and wearing appropriate socks. Learn what to look for and what to stay away from. Learn about the use of compression stockings.

Chapter 13 has tips for buying prescription footwear for the patient with diabetes, and discusses foot orthotics, types of shoes and inserts. Take the shoe quiz to tell whether or not your shoes fit properly. An interview with pedorthist, Dennis Janisee, C.Ped gives insight into different types of shoes and orthotics.

Chapter 14 is all about depression and how diabetes affects the emotional and psychological aspects of patients who struggle with diabetes. Foot Notes will help you manage the psychological aspect of diabetes.

In Chapter 15, we take a broader look at diabetes around the world. Who does this disease affect most and why? What treatments are available and where? We will hear from several international experts and get a glimpse at their work.

What does diabetes cost us as a society? Chapter 16 deals with the cost of amputation, hospitalization, rehabilitation, prosthetics, and home healthcare. Learn about the personal, financial, psychological, and social aspects of amputation.

Tools for hope are given in Chapter 17, which addresses complementary therapies and medicines such as acupuncture, hyperbaric oxygen therapy, alpha lipoic acid, and discusses the role of proper nutrition and exercise in the prevention and treatment of diabetes.

Chapter 18 not only discusses preventive foot care to reduce the number of lower extremity ulcers and amputations, but also what to do if amputation is unavoidable. Do you know how to tell when amputation is truly necessary? We delve into healthcare reform and why it is beneficial for insurance companies to start paying for preventative care. Learn what needs to be done in order to give everyone equal access to the treatment they need.

The appendices and supplemental sections at the end of the book give resources such as my online survey (www. amputationprevention.com) for patients with diabetes, for the medical practitioner, new ways to quit smoking, recommended reading, and an index to help you locate and define terms used in the book.

Ignorance is not *bliss*. Many patients with diabetes do not see a podiatrist, yet taking care of your feet is one of the most important things a person with diabetes can do to avoid amputation of a lower extremity. Perhaps you are not familiar with podiatry and the benefits it has for patients with diabetes and the prevention of amputation. We will highlight those issues in Chapter 1. Let's begin by exploring the history of the disease we call diabetes.

Keep the Legs You Stand On

# Chapter One

## What Does Diabetes Have to Do with My Feet?

> *The greatest wealth is health.* ~Virgil

Diabetes mellitus is the Hurricane Katrina of the medical world and the human body! Diabetes-related problems to the neurological and circulatory systems are among the most devastating of all diseases as they affect the feet and legs. Diabetes is the sixth leading cause of death[1] and is reaching an epidemic proportion. According to U. S. Government estimates on June 24, 2008, 24 million people in America have type 2 diabetes caused by poor diet and lack of exercise. That is an increase of more than 3 million in two years, which means that nearly 8 percent of the U.S. population has been diagnosed with this disease. When you include the 57 million who have pre-diabetes and those who do not know they have diabetes, you realize the severity of the situation.[2] And the numbers keep changing with more and more people being diagnosed all the time. All throughout the writing and editing process, we researched the Internet using the words "diabetes and amputation prevention." While we are trying to provide accurate information, these figures seem to shift constantly and are always on the rise. Don't be surprised if you find numbers that are actually higher than the ones we quote.

> *Diabetes is a terrible disease that affects just about every part of your body.* ~ Lee J. Sanders, DPM

In 2003, the International Diabetes Federation estimated that almost 200 million people around the world had diabetes. That's almost 5.1 percent of the adult population! IDF estimates that this figure will rise to 333 million by 2025 as a consequence of longer life expectancy, sedentary lifestyle and changing dietary patterns.[3] The World Health Organization predicts that the number of adults with diabetes in the world will rise to 370 million by the year 2030.[4]

That equates to approximately one in every fourteen people, which means that more than likely you or someone you know has diabetes. Many more are at risk for developing this life-threatening disease. And, the worst part is while medical science is working on it, there is currently no cure for diabetes.

But this book is not only about statistics. It is about caring, educating, and helping the people we love. Having diabetes means a total life change for the patient and those who care for them. However, many people do not understand the disease, what causes it, or how to keep their blood sugar (glucose), blood pressure, and blood fat levels as close to normal as possible.

Normal blood glucose levels should be between 70 and 110 and a normal hemoglobin A1c test is below 7 percent (ADA) and below 6.5 percent in Europe.

Diabetes is a chronic, debilitating, and often deadly disease that occurs when the pancreas does not produce enough insulin or when the body cannot effectively use the insulin it does produce. Insulin is a hormone made by the pancreas that helps sugar (also known as glucose) exit the blood and enter the cells of the body where it may be used as fuel. There are two types of diabetes. When a person has type 1 diabetes, their pancreas does not produce the insulin they need. In type 2 diabetes, their body cannot make effective use of the insulin they produce.

The symptoms of uncontrolled type 1 diabetes are:
- Excessive thirst
- Frequent urination
- Sudden weight loss
- Extreme fatigue
- Blurred vision.

People with type 2 diabetes may have the same symptoms, but they may be less apparent.

There is another type of diabetes known as gestational diabetes, which affects about 4 percent of pregnant women. There are about 135,000 cases of gestational diabetes in the United States each year. These women do not have diabetes but they develop high blood sugar levels during pregnancy due to hormones that block the action of the mother's insulin in her body. This insulin resistance makes it difficult for the mother's body to use insulin. Therefore, she may need up to three times as much insulin during pregnancy. Once the pregnancy is ended, the hormone causing insulin resistance diminishes; however, 30 percent of these women will have a problem with type 2 diabetes later on in life.

Diabetes is not a communicable disease. You don't catch it from someone or pass it to another person. It is a personal disease that usually shows no outward physical signs until late in the disease when serious complications such as kidney failure, blindness, cardiovascular disease, or neuropathy have occurred. That's because over time, high blood sugar levels can damage the blood vessels and nerves in your body. If you don't have enough blood pumping to your legs, you may not be able to heal an ulcer; and if you have a burning pain or loss of feeling in your feet or legs, you might have diabetic neuropathy.

I think of diabetes as a home disease. As such, it is between the patient and how they take care of their body that ultimately affects how they will live out their lives. Every action or health-related decision of the patient with diabetes has consequences. Most of these consequences will happen later in the patient's life. Some patients are aware of the long-term effects of the health decisions they make today and some are not. Too many patients with diabetes are not educated enough about their disease to understand the consequences they may face later in their lives if they fail to take good care of themselves today. That is why education is the main focus of this book.

A person's failure to be vigilant about their diabetes may eventually place them in a terrible situation. For example, a patient may develop a problem like an infected ulcer on their foot. While the foot needs local wound care, the health of the total patient needs attention as well. The situation can become even more complex with multiple systems being affected and each needing the attention of a specialist. Medical conditions like peripheral arterial disease (PAD), or immunopathy may be too far advanced for someone like me to provide any meaningful care to prevent an amputation.

Due to a sedentary lifestyle and a diet filled with sweetened drinks and sugary, refined foods, the United States ranks in third place in the world as the country with the highest number of people having diabetes. Over three million people die each year due to diabetes-related causes. The good news is that meticulous blood sugar control can enable a person to delay or even prevent the progression of diabetes and its many long-term complications. The rising prevalence of diabetes all over the world has brought with it an increase in the number of lower limb amputations performed as a result of the disease. Epidemiological reports indicate that over one million amputations are performed worldwide on people with diabetes each year. This amounts to a leg being lost to diabetes somewhere in the world every thirty seconds. The sad thing about this is that up to 85 percent of these amputations are preventable with proper care and treatment. This is where a podiatrist can be a vital part of a diabetic person's foot- or leg-saving posse.

## Who Is at Risk of Getting Diabetes?

My brother had the right idea about risk. He flies small single-engine airplanes and my mom and dad were usually a bit concerned about his safety. He always said that you might as well do your thing lest you get hit by a "pie wagon" and have your life ended prematurely. I personally was not too worried about this, as I have not seen a pie wagon in my neighborhood for a long, long time. I suppose anyone can wake up, fall out of bed, and break his neck. I have never met anyone that this has happened to, but the fact remains that it *could* happen.

The concept of risk continues to be a very individual thing. What the patient perceives as risk and what the physician perceives as risk can be and usually are two different things. On a daily basis, doctors are communicating to patients about the risks of diabetes, but it seems that they never really communicate the real reason this disease is so rampant—our poor diet and lack of exercise. Couch potatoes and "junk food junkies" have the biggest chance of ending up with diabetes. That risk is compounded if someone in your gene pool has a history of hereditary diabetes.

About 40 percent (41 million) of adults between the ages of forty and seventy-four have pre-diabetes. This is a condition where blood glucose levels are higher than normal, but not yet high enough for a diagnosis of diabetes. Pre-diabetes raises a person's risk of developing type 2 diabetes, heart disease, and stroke. According to the U.S. Department of Health and Human Services, racial and ethnic minorities, especially the elderly, are at an even greater risk. For example, if you are African-American, you are about twice as likely to get type 2 diabetes than a Caucasian-American. The highest incident of diabetes in African Americans occurs between 65-75 years of age. Women are more affected than men. If you are Hispanic, you are 1.9 times more likely to have diabetes than non-Hispanics. More than 10 percent of Hispanic-Americans already have diabetes. Native Hawaiians are 5.7 times as likely as Caucasians living in Hawaii to die from diabetes.[5] People with diabetes are two to four times more likely to have heart disease or suffer a stroke than non-diabetic persons due to peripheral arterial disease (PAD). Fortunately, there is something you can do to lower your risk:

1. Monitor and keep your blood glucose (sugar), blood pressure, and cholesterol levels in the target range: blood glucose hemoglobin A1c test should be less than 7 percent, blood pressure should be less than 130/80 mmHg, cholesterol (LDL) should be less than 100 mg/dl;

2. Eat healthy foods, avoid sugary and alcoholic beverages, limit fat and calorie intake;

3. Physically exercise on a regular basis (thirty minutes a day at least five days a week);

4. Educate yourself about this disease and practice preventative behaviors. A patient is more likely to practice preventive foot behaviors if they first had a diabetes education class.

## History of Diabetes

Here is a brief synopsis regarding the history of diabetes. You may find it interesting to know that this is not a "new" illness nor was it ever exclusive to one ethnic group or country.

In 1552 BCE, Egyptian physician, Hesy-Ra of the Third Dynasty, made the first known mention of diabetes. It was found on the Ebers Papyrus and lists remedies to combat the "passing of too much urine."

In 120 CE, Greek physician, Aretaeus of Cappodocia, gave the first complete medical description of diabetes, which he likens to "the melting down of flesh and limbs into urine."

In 1797, Scottish physician, John Rollo, created the first medical therapy to treat diabetes. He prescribed an "animal diet" for his patients of "plain blood puddings" and "fat and rancid meat" to manage the disease with foods their bodies could assimilate. We know now that this was not a good remedy. A diet high in animal fat raises cholesterol levels, which puts a person at risk for heart disease.

In 1869, a German medical student named Paul Langerhans discovered the islet cells of the pancreas but was unable to explain their function. The finding is called the "Islets of Langerhans."

The book would be remiss if we failed to mention one of the earliest pioneers of diabetic medical care. Born in Oxford, Massachusetts in 1899, Elliott Joslin, MD, (also known as EPJ) is considered a pioneer in diabetes. He was the first doctor in the U.S. to specialize in diabetes at a time when little was known about the disease or how to treat it. While Dr. Joslin was attending Yale University and Harvard Medical School, his aunt Helen was diagnosed with diabetes. Not too long after that, his mother was also diagnosed. He studied the disease as he treated patients and documented the results, thus compiling a listing of his patients complete with all the facts, progress and outcomes. This listing became the first diabetes registry in the world. Comparing his data with public statistics, the field of diabetes epidemiology (study of factors affecting the health and illness of populations) was launched. His data was the largest collection of clinical data on diabetes in the world. It was so complete that the Metropolitan Life Insurance Company used Dr. Joslin's statistics for their actuarial tables. He later assembled 1,000 of his own cases and created the first diabetes textbook, *The Treatment of Diabetes Mellitus.*

EPJ had a theory about how diabetes should be managed: diagnose diabetes early, manage tight control of diet by limiting carbohydrates, getting regular exercise, and constantly testing blood glucose levels. He published his theory in the first diabetes patient handbook known as the *Diabetic Manual for the Doctor and Patient*. This book resulted in significant progress in educating patients about diabetes and helping people feel empowered instead of victimized by the disease. Thanks to EPJ, diabetes became recognized as a serious public health issue when he informed the U.S. Surgeon General of the diabetic epidemic that was taking place right after World War II. As a result, the U.S. government began a 20-year study that proved Dr. Joslin's theory to be correct.

To this day, the Joslin approach and the goals of JoslinCare practiced in Joslin Clinics are helping people live a healthy and happy life while managing a chronic disease. When insulin was discovered in 1923, Dr. Joslin's practice grew and he began working with other diabetes specialists such as Leo Krall, MD, Howard Root, MD, and Priscilla White, MD who all followed the Joslin way of treating the patient using a team approach. Dr. Joslin encouraged nurses to become educators who would go out into the community to teach people with diabetes about insulin management, diet, and exercise. Today, these nurses are called certified diabetes educators. Dr. Joslin's posse was the first team assembled to treat any illness, and even now an interdisciplinary team is still the best way to treat diabetes.

EPJ created Troika—a three-horse chariot motif that symbolized insulin, diet, and exercise as the three components needed to achieve "victory" over diabetes. In 1953, the figure became part of the signage for the Diabetes Foundation, Inc. Less than ten years later (1962) EPJ died at the age of 92.

In 1901 during his work at Johns Hopkins University in Baltimore, an American pathologist named Eugene Opie established a connection between the failure of the Islets of Langerhans in the pancreas and the occurrence of diabetes.

In 1919, Dr. Frederick Allen of the Rockefeller Institute (New York) published his work known as *Total Dietary Regulations in the Treatment of Diabetes*. It suggests a therapy of strict dieting or a "starvation treatment" as a way to manage diabetes.

Frederick Banting, born in 1891 near Alliston, Ontario, conceived of the idea of insulin after reading an article by Moses Barron titled "The Relation of Islets of Langerhans to Diabetes with Special Reference to Cases of Pancreatic Lithiasis." In late 1920, Banting moved to Toronto to continue his research with the support of Professor Macleod of the University of Toronto, and the assistance of graduate student Charles Best, and chemist, James Collip.

Using a variety of different extracts on depancreatized dogs, in 1921, Banting's work led to the discovery of insulin. Banting and Best discovered a plentiful, inexpensive source for insulin from cattle (fetal pancreas) that lowers blood sugar levels of depancreatized dogs. The first human to receive an injection of insulin to treat diabetes was 14-year-old Leonard Thompson at the Toronto General Hospital in January 1922. This led to the public use of the word "insulin" when Professor Macleod presents a paper titled "The Effect Produced on Diabetes by the Extracts of Pancreas" to the Association of American Physicians annual meeting in Washington, D.C. on May 3, 1922.

On May 30, 1922, Indianapolis-based pharmaceutical manufacturer Eli Lilly & Co. and the University of Toronto enter a deal for the mass production of insulin, which became commercially available in the United States and Canada in October 1923. This was the same month that Banting and Macleod were awarded the Nobel Prize in Physiology and Medicine. Banting shared his award with Best, while Macleod shared his with Dr. James Bertram Collip, a biochemist from the University of Alberta, who joined the Banting-Best team in December 1921.

In 1936, Sir Harold Himsworth of the University College Hospital in London presented a series of research papers stating that diabetes falls into two types based on insulin insensitivity. This discovery led to the diabetes classifications of type 1 diabetes (insulin dependent) and type 2 diabetes (non-insulin dependent) in 1959. Also in 1936, founder of Novo Nordisk, Hans Christian Hagedorn, discovered that adding protamine (a weak anticoagulant) to insulin prolongs the active duration of the medication.

The standard insulin syringe was introduced in 1944 to make diabetes management more uniform. The first pancreas transplant was performed at the University of Manitoba in 1966.

The first patent for a portable blood glucose meter called the Ames Reflectance Meter was issued to Anton Hubert Clemens in the fall of 1971. Dr. Richard K. Bernstein, an insulin-dependent physician, used the meter to monitor his blood glucose at home, and then published a report on his experiences.

In 1982, Eli Lilly & Co. developed the first biosynthetic human insulin using recombinant DNA technology. This product, known as Humulin®, is identical in chemical structure to human insulin and can be mass-produced.

In 1991, the International Diabetes Federation (IDF) started World Diabetes Day to bring about awareness of the devastating effects of the disease and to offer education for prevention. Preventive treatment was recognized in 1993 when after ten years of clinical study, a report published by the Diabetes Control and Complications Trial (DCCT) clearly demonstrated that intensive therapy delays the onset and progression of long-term complications in individuals with type 1 diabetes.

On Dec. 20, 2006 in honor of Frederick Banting's birthday, The United Nations recognizes diabetes as a global threat and designates November 14 as World Diabetes Day, to be observed every year starting in 2007.[6]

## Comorbidities

While this is a descriptive chapter about diabetes, please remember that the disease is limited to how the body handles glucose metabolism. Comorbidities are the secondary illnesses resulting from the primary illness. Patients with diabetes need to know the comorbidities of diabetes, especially how the neurological and vascular systems are affected by faulty glucose metabolism. It is the comorbidities of diabetes that do the real damage to patients. I will briefly mention these now, but I'll give in-depth information about each of these in the upcoming chapters.

1. Cardiovascular disease. Patients with diabetes are two to four times more likely to develop cardiovascular disease than people without diabetes. Cardiovascular disease has multiple effects on function of the kidney, liver, brain, and heart. Vision can be affected by cardiovascular disease resulting in blindness. It can damage blood vessels and result in stroke or heart attack as well as cause a delay or inability to heal a wound on the foot or leg.

2. Diabetic neuropathy is damage to the nerves affecting the legs and feet. Foot ulcers—one of the triggers for amputation—are commonly seen in patients with diabetes. Seventy percent of all diabetic amputations are related to diabetes.

3. Diabetic nephropathy or kidney disease can result in total kidney failure and may necessitate kidney transplant or renal dialysis treatment. Diabetes causes 35 to 40 percent of new cases of end stage renal disease each year.

4. Diabetic retinopathy is damage to the retina of the eye leading to vision loss. The incidence of blindness is twenty-five times higher in people with diabetes than in the general population.

5. Neurological diseases can affect function in the kidney, liver, and intestines. They can cause numbness in the feet and legs resulting in painless trauma that can lead to foot infections, ulcers, and amputations. Pain, burning, tingling, and/or numbness are other affects to the nervous system. Lack of balance may cause falling and the associated fears of concussion or hip fracture.

6. Uncontrolled blood glucose levels affect the body physically, physiologically, and psycho-socially. Depression is commonly seen in patients with diabetes and many patients with diabetes have difficulty in social situations due to psychological issues.

7. The comorbidity of diabetes that perhaps has the ultimate effect on patients is the inability to work or provide for family combined with the loss of personal freedom and reliance on others after an amputation.

## Denial and Resignation ~ Two Ends of a Gray Rainbow

The most dangerous culprit of diabetes is not the illness; it is the denial of it! This psychological state causes a person to feel exempt from reality and think, "Not me. This can't be happening. There must be some mistake. I don't believe it." A patient might say, "My uncle had gangrene, but that's not going to happen to me," and this is exactly the guy who's going to end up with a gangrenous leg. This type of reaction is so common that some doctors think it's part of the process of accepting the news when someone is first diagnosed with diabetes.

Humans tend to deny old age, obesity, business failure, ignorance, military defeat, even the end of a relationship, and there are many reasons why. People want to think of themselves as being well. Like gray hair and wrinkles, the demands of diabetes remind the sufferer that he is not eternal. Some folks don't want to think about it, so they tune it out. But if you have diabetes, denial used as an excuse to not practice good self-management is as harmful as drinking arsenic—it is a slow poison.

Sometimes denial serves a purpose. It is a way of coping with bad news. It can keep you from getting overwhelmed and depressed. It lets you accept bad news little by little, as you are ready. Denial also lets your family and friends pretend that nothing is wrong. But prolonged denial keeps a person from practicing behavior that could prevent comorbidities of vascular and neurological disease. It shields you from the fact that diabetes is a lifelong, chronic illness, which, if left untreated, can result in serious, and for some patients, life threatening complications.

Doctors who do not specialize in diabetes care may fuel your denial. They may talk about a "mild" case of diabetes or say there is "just a touch of sugar" in your blood. Though well-meaning, these terms send the wrong message. What you believe is, "I don't need to worry. My diabetes is not serious." Truth told, any form of diabetes *is* serious.

Some people get mad when they find they have diabetes. In our culture, there is still the strong belief that afflictions are visited upon those who deserve them; that disease comes from moral defect, or is punishment for sin. For one who believes this, to admit diabetes is to admit character defect. We know that diabetes is not a character defect, but for many, this ancient guilt-laden belief system is still quite real. Someone knows he or she has lived a decent life, and yet winds up having to lose weight, exercise, watch their diet, test their blood, and inject insulin may find it hard to understand and may question, "Why me?"

Some folks have a psychological need to be "in control." All their lives, these people have resisted authority, public opinion, and social pressures to conform. They may be effective salesmen and negotiators, but diabetes cannot be cheated at the bargaining table. Lacking the emotional skills to deal with a disease they cannot overcome, and unable to confront it in their traditional fashion, these folks are lost at sea.

If you were told about your risk for lower extremity amputation, you might think twice about eating that piece of chocolate cake, skipping your medicine, or ignoring any of the other steps to foot health that we will be discussing. For example, I tell my patients who smoke, "You can have your cigarettes or you can have your legs but you probably won't get to keep both." For my overweight patients, I suggest, "Now that we have your feet in good shape, you need small victories. I'd like you to start a walking program—walk a half a mile a day. Your goal is to lose one pound this month."

On the other end of the psychological spectrum is resignation. As opposed to denial, people who are resigned to losing a leg feel that no matter what they do, they cannot avoid losing a limb. Their thinking is my father, my brother and my uncle all lost their legs to diabetes and there is just no way I am going to avoid this in my own life. It is meant to be.

## Home Blood Glucose Testing and Hemoglobin A1c Lab Test

Testing your blood sugar (glucose) level at home is an important part of a preventive routine for those who have diabetes. When you have a spike in glucose, you can look at what you have eaten recently and adjust your next food choice, medication, insulin dosage, or physical activity accordingly.

Blood glucose levels are usually tested at home by pricking a fingertip with a lancing device and applying a drop of blood to a glucose meter, which reads the value. Some folks test before and after meals and at bedtime. Some meters currently on the market are: Accu-Check Advantage, Freestyle, One Touch Ultra, and Sure Step. Some devices give readings faster than others; some

- Average glucose before a meal is 80-120 mg/dl.

- Two hours after a meal should be below 140 mg/dl.

- Bedtime range is 100-140 mg/dl.

require less blood to sample; some have a larger screen to make reading easier for the visually impaired.

The goal is to keep the blood glucose levels near the normal range of 80 to 120 mg/dl before meals and under 140 mg/dl at two hours after eating. The traditional unit for measuring blood glucose is mg/dl (milligrams/deciliter); however, most scientific journals are starting to use mmol/L exclusively. Some journals are using the universal measurement as the primary unit, but they also quote mg/dl in parentheses to assist healthcare providers, researchers, and patients who are already familiar with mg/dl. Since this book is intended for a global readership, I'll show both readings in the chart below.

| mg/dl | mmol/L | What this reading means |
|-------|--------|-------------------------|
| 35 | 2.0 | Extremely low, danger of unconsciousness |
| 55 | 3.0 | Low, try to eat something |
| 75 | 4.0 | A little low, may be feeling lethargic |
| 100 | 5.5 | Minimum for non-diabetic before a meal |
| 90-110 | 5 to 6 | Normal for non-diabetics before a meal |
| 150 | 8.0 | Normal for non-diabetics after a meal |
| 180 | 10.0 | Maximum for non-diabetics after a meal |
| 200 | 11.0 | A little too high |
| 270 | 15.0 | High |
| 300 | 16.5 | Very high |
| 360 | 20.0 | Way up there |
| 400 | 22.0 | Danger level. This is as high as some meters and strips will read |
| 600 | 33.0 | High danger of severe electrolyte imbalance |

You can't depend entirely upon these meters to accurately reflect the blood sugar level because the values can fluctuate. That's why your doctor uses a Hemoglobin A1c test to get an idea of the overall effectiveness of blood glucose control over a three-month period of time.

Hemoglobin is the oxygen-carrying pigment that gives blood its red color and is the predominant protein in red blood cells. Hemoglobin A1c is a specialized component of hemoglobin to which glucose is bound. For more than twenty years, the gold standard measurement of chronically elevated blood sugar levels has been the glycilated hemoglobin (A1c). Hemoglobin A1c measures the average concentration of glucose in the blood for the *prior* twelve weeks. It is a look backward to see how well blood glucose has been controlled in the recent past.

If you've ever spilled syrup on your counter top, you know it can be difficult to remove the sticky substance after it dries. The blood sugar in your body is the same way. The sugar in your blood sticks to proteins in your red blood cells. The longer it has been attached to your cells, the harder it is to get it off. These cells live about three months so the A1c test shows us your average blood sugar level for the past three months. The normal range for a patient without diabetes is 4 to 5.9 percent. The American Diabetes Association currently recommends that a person with diabetes should try to keep their A1c level below 7.0 percent. If your A1c is higher than 8.0 percent, you need to get a better handle on controlling your sugar levels.

| A1c Reading | Blood Sugar (mg/dl) | Blood Sugar (mmol/l) |
|---|---|---|
| 6% | 135 | 7.5 |
| 7% | 170 | 9.4 |
| 8% | 205 | 11.4 |
| 9% | 240 | 13.3 |
| 10% | 275 | 15.3 |
| 11% | 310 | 17.2 |
| 12% | 345 | 19.2 |
| | | |

You decrease your relative risk by 10 percent for every 1 percent reduction in your A1c reading. So, if you lower your A1c reading by two percent, you also lower your risk for microvascular complications by almost 20 percent. Even though you still aren't within target range, you are making improvement.

## Foot Notes: Tips for Staying in Touch With Reality About Diabetes

To get the most out of this book, you will need to recognize when or if you are in denial and use that knowledge to live as healthy a life as possible in spite of this disease. Denial has a few catch phrases. If you hear yourself thinking or saying anything similar to these listed below, you are probably avoiding some part of your diabetes care.

- One bite of this candy won't hurt.

- This sore will heal by itself.
- I'll go to the doctor later.
- I don't have time to check my blood sugar levels.
- My diabetes isn't serious. I only have to take a pill, not shots.

> Amputation prevention is not just treating the foot; it's treating the whole patient because the loss of a foot is the manifestation, or result of other conditions that must be addressed.
> ~ Howard Green, DPM

Because denial sabotages your healthcare and can creep into any aspect of diabetes self-care, it can be dangerous. Yet, it is bound to crop up from time to time. When it does, you can recognize what's going on and fight back. Here are a few tips for recognizing when you are in denial:

*Ignoring your meal plan.* Changing eating habits and food choices is tough. When your doctor told you to see a dietitian, follow a meal plan, and change your eating habits, maybe you thought to yourself:

- It's too expensive to see a registered dietitian.
- I can't ask my family to change what they eat. I don't want to eat alone or fix two meals.
- There's no place to buy healthy food where I work.
- It's too hard to bring my lunch.

Eating right may not be as difficult as you think. A dietitian can help you put together a plan that meets your personal needs.

*Forgetting your feet.* You know you should check your feet each day, but it takes too much time, or you forget, or you have limited mobility and it's too hard. Washing and checking your feet for signs of trouble every day is essential to avoid serious injury. Ask someone to help you with this task.

*Smoking* for ten minutes can decrease the tissue oxygen concentration and blood flow in the body for up to one hour. If you smoke regularly throughout the day, your body is consistently denied the oxygen needed to assist a wound that is trying to heal. If you are in denial, you might tell yourself, "I'll only take a few puffs. Smoking keeps me from eating too much. If I quit, I'll gain weight." Smoking and diabetes are a deadly duo because smoking increases your risk for complications. Quitting is one of the best things you can do for your health.

*Not bothering to check your blood glucose* regularly. You may decide you "know" what your blood glucose is by how you feel. But a meter is a much better measure of blood glucose than feelings.

The demands of diabetes self-management are merciless. Today, tomorrow, and every day after, you must perform the tasks that will keep your blood sugars as close to non-diabetic normal as possible. There is no vacation; and there is little forgiveness for departure from that almighty schedule. Some folks do well for a time, and then lose patience with the necessary discipline. They depart from good self-management, and their health suffers. Here are some tips from the American Diabetes Association[7] for staying on track:

1. Write down your diabetes care plan and your healthcare goals. Accept that it will take time to reach your goals. If you find you are denying some

parts of your diabetes care, ask your diabetes educator for help. If you have trouble with your food plan, talk to a registered dietitian. Together you can come up with solutions.

2. Tell your friends and family how they can help. Let them know that encouraging you to go off your plan is not a kindness. Inform them about how you take care of your diabetes; they might even want to adopt some of your healthy habits.

3. Educate Yourself. Because fact cures fiction, the best response to denial is education. Education shows the consequences of departure from good self-management, but it also shows the rewards of tight blood glucose control. It shows what we need to do to keep going, but it also shows how that task has become easier. Education helps know what foods are helpful to live a long, full, and in-the-mainstream life. Education shows the undeniable truth about diabetes and that is what this book is all about.[8]

Beware, many medical practitioners rely on the latest information when giving advice to their patients with diabetes, but some of them haven't cracked a diabetes journal or a current textbook in years. Twenty-five years ago, the outlook for a life with diabetes was not what it is today! There have been great changes in what we know about this condition, and in how it is best treated. Research has given us new medications, better glucose monitors, less-painful syringes, new ways to schedule testing and medication, more convenient meal-planning techniques, and the real hope of a cure. Make sure your diabetes advisor is up to date. Treating a patient for amputation prevention not only involves the foot, but the whole person. The physical, social, and psychological aspects should all be considered and managed.

# Chapter Two

## Who Is at Risk for Amputation

> *One of the challenges that we have as we move forward in the early part of the twenty-first century is to understand how we can help people make the right choices to understand that they have real control of a lot of the health risks in their lives.* ~ James Allen, New Zealander Statesman Minister of Defense (1912-20)

Diabetes is a serious disease that has reached epidemic proportions globally, and is worse than most cancers. There are 57 million people suffering from pre-diabetes with no idea about their condition because these people have yet to develop any symptoms. In 2006, the CDC and *Prevention* magazine estimated that one in every three children born in the last five years can expect to become diabetic, and Latinos can expect half of their children to develop diabetes. This is to be expected as our population continues to become overweight, eat a diet high in refined sugar and carbohydrates, and does not exercise. Parents must intervene to help children change their eating and exercise habits!

The consequences of having diabetes can be major, even life threatening, and the comorbidities can kill you if ignored. Those who have diabetes and do not keep their blood sugar levels under control are very likely to require amputation if they get a foot ulcer or infection that will not heal. In fact, 15 percent of diabetics are expected to have lower limb amputations. That's over three million people, and enough to fill a 25,000-seat football stadium 120 times. Approximately 85 percent of diabetes-related lower extremity amputations can be prevented with proper identification by the medical community of patients who are at risk for a lower limb amputation and by providing them with preventive, proactive care. I have witnessed this decrease in lower limb amputations and proven cost savings in the PACT Programs in Virginia and Tennessee.

Combined with statistics from CDC (Center for Disease Control),[1] and IDF (International Diabetes Federation),[2] and VA Podiatry.com,[3] here are some facts and figures about amputation:

- Approximately 80 percent of amputees are people over the age of fifty.

- The rate of lower-extremity amputation is 2.6 higher in men than in women.

- There are three million amputees in North America, and leg amputations make up 90 percent of them. It is estimated that by the year 2025 there will be almost 260,000 diabetic lower extremity amputations in the United States. Since the U.S. has almost 10 percent of the worldwide population of diabetics, we can extrapolate this data to infer that on a worldwide basis, the number of diabetic lower extremity amputations will be well over 2 million.

- Up to 70 percent of all leg amputations happen to people with diabetes. In fact, people with diabetes are twenty-five times more likely to lose a leg than people without the disease.

- A foot ulcer is the cause for more than 85 percent of all amputations. One in six people who have diabetes will have an ulcer during their lifetime.

- Patients with diabetes with foot infections have 154 times the risk for amputations. Foot ulcers can be prevented with suitable healthcare and informed self-care.

- Thirty percent of patients with diabetes who experience amputations will lose their other leg within three years. Forty-seven percent of these patients will die within five years of having had that first amputation.

## People with a Diabetic Foot

The diabetic foot is one of the most common yet neglected long-term complications of diabetes mellitus. The diabetic foot is a term used to describe foot problems in patients with diabetes. These problems are caused by abnormalities such as neuropathy (tingling, burning, pain) and/or ironically a loss of protective sensation, which prevents patients from feeling pain in their foot or that their foot has been injured. This inability of patients to sense their physical surroundings because of numbness in their foot may contribute to falling and injury. Infections are common in the diabetic foot and are difficult to heal. If you have an infection that will not heal because of poor blood flow, you are at risk for developing gangrene—the death of tissue. To keep an infection or gangrene from spreading and becoming life threatening, a surgeon may have to remove a toe, part or all of the foot, or part of a leg.

## Patients with Diabetes and Peripheral Arterial Disease (PAD)

Peripheral arterial disease (PAD) is caused by the accumulation of fatty deposits known as plaque in the arteries that restrict blood flow to the extremities and organ systems. PAD is one of the main complications of diabetes that lead to foot ulcers that can result in amputation. We will discuss PAD and the ankle-brachial index used to test for it in chapter eight, but for now, let's look at the demographics for those who are most at risk for lower extremity amputation (LEA) due to diabetes.

## Risk by Demographics

Diabetic foot complications are a major cause of hospital admissions and are more common in ethnic minority groups. Naturally, it follows that LEAs are also common in diabetic minority patients.

Demographics of ethnicity, sex, and geography show that the people losing legs to diabetes at the highest rate in the

United States are the Pima Indians in the Gila River Indian Community in Arizona, who also have the highest rate of diabetes in the world. They are followed in descending order by Hispanic females, which are the fastest growing group in the United States, Hispanic males, African-American females, African-American males, Anglo females, and Anglo males. Regarding geography, the southern United States is considered the Diabetes Belt. A simple breakdown of the percentage of minority populations in the United States reveals that Hispanics (15 percent), Blacks (13.4 percent), Asians (5 percent), and Native Americans (5 percent) have the highest risk of LEA due to diabetes.

## Hispanics

If you are Hispanic, you are 1.9 times more likely to have diabetes than non-Hispanics. More than 10 percent of Hispanic Americans already have diabetes. The disease is hereditary, but Hispanics are affected more by the "improving" economy of Central America that has brought changes in diet and lifestyle in recent decades. As countries become more Americanized, their new lifestyle tends to discourage people from exercise and traditional diet. This high-calorie diet and lack of physical activity increases the risks for obesity, diabetes, and cardiovascular disease.

Dr. Jaime Sepulveda, the coordinator of Mexico's National Institutes of Health, sees diabetes as one of the most complicated diseases to prevent. "It's not like giving a vaccination where even in a country with many poor, isolated regions, you can still reach every one," said Dr. Sepulveda. "With diabetes and obesity, we're dealing with a major cultural change, and we're fighting against globalization and urbanization. This disease has momentum that is huge."[4]

## African-Americans

African-Americans are almost three times as likely to suffer from a lower limb amputation as Caucasian-Americans. Many do not have health insurance and therefore tend not to seek medical care for a foot problem. These patients usually receive care only when the problem becomes serious enough for hospitalization. In November 2007, the American Podiatric Medical Association conducted a national survey that found nearly 10 percent of the 3.2 million African-Americans with diabetes are uninsured. Of those, 75 percent have *not* seen a podiatric physician for diabetes treatments reportedly due to lack of health coverage compared with 45 percent of those with insurance who do seek coverage.

*American Journal of Preventive Medicine* published a national study of more than 15,000 adults, which found that African-Americans are more prone to having problems with circulation in their legs due to hardening of the arteries. Arterial leg disease (tested by ankle-brachial index) was diagnosed in 4.4 percent of Black women, 3.1 percent of black men, compared to 2.3 percent of white men in the study.[5]

## Native Americans

American Indians and Alaska natives are 2.3 times as likely to have diabetes as non-Hispanic Whites of similar ages. About 15.1 percent of American Indians and Alaska natives twenty years or older who receive care from the Indian Health Services have diabetes. Of First Nations people, diabetes is least common among Alaska Natives (8.1 percent) and most common among American Indians in the southern United States (26.7 percent).

On average, type 2 diabetes affects six percent of Native American people. The majority of those affected are elders. They have a difficult time understanding what is happening to them and how lifestyle directly affects the advancement of the disease. Due to difficulty healthcare providers have in effectively communicating with the elders, many of them die rather than change their eating habits and level of exercise. Sadly, the experience following diagnosis is captured in this quotation I found in an article titled "Talking with Elders about Diabetes" by Ruth Ann Cyr, RN, M. Ed:

> *"Most of my people are shocked, scared, or angered when they are told they have diabetes. The facts about the disease, and the exercise, and meal plans that should be followed are overwhelming to them. They do not understand what is happening to them and often they deny that diabetes exists and just ignore instructions. They are scheduled into classes and put on treatment without the time to accept the diagnosis or to ask questions."*[6]

## Asians and Pacific Islanders

Generally speaking, Asians have the same rate of diabetes as non-Hispanic Whites; however, Asians are 20 percent less likely to die from diabetes. According to the Office of Minority

Health, native Hawaiians are almost two times more likely than Caucasians living in Hawaii to have diabetes, but only 5.7 times more likely to die from the disease. A national health interview survey shows that Filipinos living in Hawaii have more than three times the death rate as Caucasians living in Hawaii.[7]

There are more demographical statistics on a Web site operated by Podiatry Associates of Virginia: http://www.vapodiatry.com/Medical_info.html.

## The Financially Poor

Another category not traditionally noted as a minority is the financially poor. Ultimately, the frequency of amputations increases in people from disadvantaged socio-economic groups. They often do not have access to care or education and may not fully understand the effects of diabetes and the behaviors that will help prevent the loss of a leg.

According the U.S. Census Bureau, the percentage and the number of people without health insurance increased to 15.8 percent in 2006, which is up from 15.3 percent in 2005. The number of uninsured increased from 44.8 million to 47.0 million.[8]

## The Elderly

August 23, 1992 was a turning point in my life. Hurricane Andrew hit Miami and changed my life forever. After living in a nice middle-class home in the suburbs of Miami with a very successful podiatry practice, I lost it all in one night. Our roof was ripped off, the windows were blown out, and our family room furniture landed in the swimming pool. My family and

I were lucky to survive the storm. We essentially lost all our material possessions. Above that, I also lost most of my patient base.

As a result of the storm my practice was not able to survive financially. A thriving podiatry practice of eighteen years was lost.

This event moved me from Miami to the Blue Ridge Mountains in Salem, Virginia where I took a position as Chief of Podiatry at the Veterans Affairs Medical Center. That change opened the door for me to become involved with elderly and aged people. I learned to better appreciate the geriatric population and the value they bring to society as well as understanding how vulnerable and fragile these folks are. This led me to a path of focusing on these at-risk patient with diabetes and neuropathy. I was given the opportunity to see and treat these patients and help assure a good quality of life for them. Statistics show that 80 percent of amputees are people over the age of fifty. The CDC reports that almost 25 percent of the population sixty years and older had diabetes in 2007.[9]

## Who You Gonna Call?

Let's say you are a patient with diabetes who is unaware of any current foot health problems, but you want to be proactive about your health, especially about your foot health, and you want to know if you are at risk for an amputation. It would be smarter to be evaluated *before* you develop a problem, but who would you call? This is a perplexing question, and most patients with diabetes do not know the answer.

If your health insurance policy does not require a referral by your primary care provider, you might start by calling your local hospital's patient referral service to ask about their medical staff, the staff's areas of specialization, and what services are provided. For instance, do they have diabetes educators or diabetes education classes? Do they offer nutrition classes? Do they have capabilities to perform diagnostic testing such as an MRI, MRA, or CT (computerized tomography) testing? Do they have a vascular lab where an ABI and other vascular testing can be done? Are they equipped to do vascular surgery and do any of the surgeons at that hospital practice endovascular surgery? Do they have a wound clinic? Do they have an orthotics and prosthetic department? Do they have podiatrists on their staff?

You could call the county, state, or national medical associations or societies to get information on the names of physicians and especially podiatrists who are practicing in your area. Learn about their scope of services in various specialties and ask for referrals. You could also seek hospitals with limb preservation programs. Always look for a physician who is board certified, which is an indication of a higher level of knowledge and experience and can be very valuable in complex or more difficult cases.

If your situation is not urgent, say you don't have an open wound, and you want to know where you stand in terms of your risk for an amputation, information can be gathered by a simple screening exam. This exam should include an evaluation of your neurological status for autonomic, sensory, and motor neuropathy with emphasis on identification of loss of protective sensation. It should also identify any bone, soft tissue, or nail deformities you may have in your feet. This information combined with a circulatory evaluation will identify your risk level for an amputation. With this information, a treatment plan can be formulated for your specific foot health situation to prevent an amputation.

## Diabetic Foot Risk Classification System

The International Working Group on the Diabetic Foot (IWGDF) is a worldwide organization whose initial goal was to establish internationally accepted guidelines on the management and prevention of the diabetic foot. The international consensus on the diabetic foot and the practical guidelines were published in 1999, and have since been translated and published in twenty-five languages. The table below is the Diabetic Foot Risk Classification System established by IWGDF. It lists risk categories and makes recommendations for treatment options and ongoing care activities based on each patient's individual risk factors. The crucial portion of the exam that identifies patients who are at risk for amputation uses the monofilament testing device to establish whether the patient has loss of protective sensation due to peripheral sensory neuropathy caused by diabetes.

In each category below, there are numbers that represent the odds of a patient developing an ulcer. For example, the odds of developing an ulcer in category 0 are 0. In category 1, a patient is 1.7 times more likely to develop an ulcer; in category 2, a patient is 12 times more likely, and the worst chances of developing a ulcer is in category 3 where a patient is 36.4 times more likely. These numbers need to be respected.

## Risk Category 0

The lowest-risk patient with diabetes has protective sensation and can feel the monofilament testing device. There is no history of a foot ulcer and no foot deformity. We offer them education on diabetes with a detailed handout on preventive foot care, and as long as they can take care of their own feet, we only have to see them once a year for reevaluation.

Next are categories 1, 2, and 3. Patients in these categories do not have protective sensation (we call this Loss of Protective Sensation or LOPS) and are vulnerable to painless trauma

**Risk Category 1**

These low-risk patients have lost protective sensation, but have no deformities or history of ulcers to their feet. We see them at least once a year and provide them with patient education and diabetic shoes. We encourage them not to walk barefooted, sock footed or in house shoes, and we may recommend a preventive, cushioned insole for their shoes for shock absorption and protection from shearing forces against the foot.

**Risk Category 2**

These medium-risk patients have not only lost protective sensation, but they also have a foot deformity of the bones, soft tissues, or nails. We provide them with education on preventive foot behaviors and professional foot care several times a year, and, if needed, we will recommend insoles or custom-made biomechanical orthotics and/or special diabetic shoes to relieve pressure or to accommodate a deformed foot.

If they need to have a callus, corn, or nail trimmed, we trim them. We know that these special patients may have bad vision and maybe even worse hand-eye coordination. The instruments they use may not be appropriate or sterile, so they may injure themselves and cause an infection. We want to take away every diabetic or at-risk patient's bathroom surgeon's license.

Patients in category 2 and 3 have more serious foot conditions that may require "ongoing" foot care, and return visits are an excellent opportunity for healthcare practitioners to educate patients.

### Risk Category 3

Patients in category 3 are at the highest risk for amputation. Not only have they lost protective sensation, they also typically have a history of a previous ulcer, bone infection, amputation, Charcot Foot, rest pain (pain in the legs at night while lying in bed), intermittent claudication (characterized by exercise, pain, rest, relief cycle in the leg muscles), gangrene, or a diagnosis of end-stage renal disease with renal dialysis. We see them every two months or sooner, depending on their needs. In their on-going foot care and education about the pedal manifestations of their disease, we emphasize prevention and protection and evaluate them for insoles, shoes, braces, or the appropriate treatment for their medical needs.

This strategy is used worldwide and is considered to be the best system for evaluating and managing the foot of the patient with diabetes or "at risk" foot. To complete the process, it is essential that an appropriate foot health history is taken and each patient's specific foot problems of the bones, soft tissue, and nails be identified, treated, and hopefully resolved. This type of care has worked well for many of my patients. It's simple, cost effective, and it uses treatment methods that have been proven effective by evidence-based medicine research studies.

## At Risk Foot Questionnaire
Circle "Yes" or No" as you answer each question.

| | | | |
|---|---|---|---|
| 1. | My toenails are discolored, streaked, or thickened. | Yes | No |
| 2. | The sides of my toenails dig into the skin and may hurt. | Yes | No |
| 3. | I have a large bony prominence or bump behind my big toe on the inside of my foot. | Yes | No |
| 4. | I have a large bony prominence or bump behind my small toe on the outside of the foot. | Yes | No |
| 5. | I get an extremely painful cramp in the area of my third and fourth toes, especially when wearing shoes. | Yes | No |
| 6. | My toes are not straight; they are cocked up or bent. | Yes | No |
| 7. | I have painful or painless calluses on the ball of my foot. | Yes | No |
| 8. | I have corns on my toes no matter what shoe I wear. | Yes | No |
| 9. | The inside of my arch and bottom of my heel hurts, but it's most sore when I step out of bed in the morning. | Yes | No |
| 10. | Sometime I lose my balance or fall because I cannot feel the floor. | Yes | No |
| 11. | I have cramps in my legs when I walk. | Yes | No |
| 12. | My ankles are swollen all the time. | Yes | No |
| 13. | My feet are always dry and scaly. Sometimes they itch. | Yes | No |
| 14. | My feet and legs hurt all over when I stand or walk a lot. | Yes | No |
| 15. | I have numbness in my feet. | Yes | No |

| | | | |
|---|---|---|---|
| 16. | I have burning in my feet. | Yes | No |
| 17. | I have persistent pain in my feet or legs. | Yes | No |
| 18. | I have a skin rash on my feet or legs. | Yes | No |
| 19. | I have an open wound on my foot or leg. | Yes | No |

If you answered yes to *any* of these questions, see your doctor or podiatrist *now*!

## When Is Amputation Absolutely Necessary?

Ischemia is the term that describes the loss of blood flow that can be seen in any portion of the body, but for our discussions we will limit it to the legs and feet. When a patient has critical limb ischemia (CLI), sometimes vascular surgery will improve blood flow and amputation may be avoided. This should be considered as a first option before considering amputation.

Dr. Lee Rogers, a podiatrist at the Broadlawns Medical Center in Des Moines, Iowa, points out that many non-research oriented clinicians may not be aware of ongoing research trials on promising treatments that may prevent amputation. He recommends that before patients consent to an amputation they consult www.clinicaltrials.com to learn about the most up to date clinical trials on the subject.

In his presentation at the 8th Annual New Cardiovascular Horizons and Management of the Diabetic Foot & Wound Healing Conference in New Orleans in September 2007, David Allie, MD, Director of Cardiothoracic and Endovascular Surgery at the Cardiovascular Institute of the South in Lafayette, Louisiana, cited the Euro Intervention Study in 2005 which revealed that 67 percent of patients who had lower extremity amputations did not have any vascular studies before amputation. Thirty-five percent had an ABI Exam and 8 percent had an arteriogram.

However, if surgical intervention doesn't work and your vascular surgeon cannot restore vascular function, amputation may be the only solution to rid your body of infection. In any case, thorough testing should be conducted to see where adequate blood flow is available to heal the wound. Removing a toe or part of the foot or leg below that point practically insures that you will need another amputation later on because where there is not sufficient blood flow, a wound cannot heal.

The feet of patients with diabetes are subject to all the same physical forces, stresses, and resulting deformities that would affect any patient. It is because the body of the patient with diabetes responds differently to these problems that they are at higher risk to develop complications.

It is vital that you become a partner with your physicians in the care plan for resolving your foot problems. You have a significant responsibility for your overall health, and that includes your foot health. You control whether you eat properly, take your medicine, stop smoking, exercise, wear foot gear at all times, visually inspect your feet daily, or seek medical care in an appropriate time frame when you have a foot problem.

Here are some of the warning signs to identify the foot at risk:

- Swelling of the foot or ankle

- Cold feet or legs

- Color changes in skin

- Pain in legs

- Open sores (even small ones)

- Non-healing wounds

- In-grown toenails
- Corns and calluses
- No hair growing on foot

## Foot Notes: Healthy Foot Habits

In too many cases, patients who are at risk for amputation fail to understand their vulnerability, and their behaviors reflect this attitude. They set themselves up just as surely as a 1920s gangster would set up a "hit."

Patients with diabetes must be part of the solution of their own foot health, or they will unwittingly become part of the problem. To be part of the solution, they must develop healthy foot habits. This includes:

- Inspecting feet daily. If you have difficulty seeing your feet, use a mirror or have another person look at your feet. Examine around nails, between the toes, and the bottoms of the feet. If any corns, calluses redness, increase in local temperature, pus, swelling, sores, or cracks in the skin are noted, or if you have pain, immediately consult your doctor.

- Washing feet with soap and lukewarm water and rinsing thoroughly, especially between the toes. Do not soak sore feet.

- Drying feet thoroughly especially between the toes before putting on socks and shoes. Never rub the feet vigorously.

- Massaging with lanolin-based or urea-based lotion or cream. Avoid putting lotion between the toes or around toenails.

- Applying a mild foot powder or baby powder after washing and drying carefully. Prescription medications are available for non-responsive cases of foot perspiration.

- Wearing shoes or slippers at all times—no sandals or open-toed shoes. Shoes should cover, support, and protect your feet and allow room for your toes to be in their natural position. Consult your podiatrist or pedorthist to make sure your shoes are fitting correctly.

- Spraying your shoes with Lysol™ each night and allowing them to dry before wearing again. It is best to have several pairs of well-fitting shoes that you can rotate wearing.

- Checking inside the shoes daily for foreign objects like coins, keys, small stones, or other debris before putting on the shoe.

- Keeping overlapping toes separated with lamb's wool or silicone pads.

- Keeping feet at room temperature. Wear two pairs of seamless socks if your feet are cold, but do not use artificial heat sources such as a heating pad, hot water bottle, heated bricks, open fires, fireplaces, or radiators in an attempt to warm up cold feet.

- Avoiding cutting or picking at loose skin, warts, corns, or calluses on your feet nor pop open any blisters. Do not use over-the-counter medicines such as ingrown toenail remover, corn, callus, or wart remover, or medicated foot pads that contain salicylic acid. These treatments are dangerous because they use a chemical that destroys tissue painlessly.

- Using a good light to cut nails straight across and file away rough ends. Leave the corners (sides) of the nails slightly longer than the middle so they do not push into the skin as they grow. It's best to trim nails after bathing when they are softer. If your nails are too thick or tend to split or crack when trimming, have your podiatrist cut them for you.

- Controlling blood sugars and blood pressure.

- Ceasing smoking.

- Exercising on a regular basis. Walking and swimming are best. Wear swim sneaks or old tennis shoes to protect your feet from painless injury at the beach or pool.

- Not crossing legs or ankles while sitting. If you must sit for a long period of time, use range of motion exercises to aid circulation.

- Getting a foot exam on a regular basis that utilizes a monofilament testing device—an essential diagnostic tool to identify loss of protective sensation.

- Having an annual dilated eye exam to detect vascular disease in the eye that leads to retinopathy and blindness.

- Having an annual dental exam to detect tooth and gum disease, a common cause of infections.

- Immediately seeking medical attention if your foot develops an amputation trigger like an open wound, a crack in the skin between the toes, or a red, swollen, or locally warm area. Many patients with diabetes with neuropathy fail to do this, usually because they do not feel pain in their feet and believe their problem is not of any consequence, as it does not hurt. This leads them to big trouble. There are some patients who are either mentally or physically unable to provide self-care. For instance, some people cannot reach their feet. Social service agencies can provide home healthcare or nursing support for individual foot care needs.

# Chapter Three

## Who Takes Care of Your Feet?

> *Whether or not you have an amputation is a function of who you get sent to.* ~ Economist Dr. Ho

Foot care is one of the most neglected areas of health in the general population, and especially in the diabetic population. Most people would probably say that controlling blood sugar levels and watching their diet are the most important things to do. Yes, these are important, but foot care should be just as high a priority in the overall strategy of diabetic health. People who could benefit the most from professional care often rely on folk remedies, like what their Aunt Blanch always did for that problem or use over-the-counter products, perhaps looking for a quick fix to their problem. Some patients are so vulnerable they can be injured simply by having their sock double over on itself, causing enough of an increase in pressure to create an ulcer. We know that a number of people's feet cannot tolerate temperature extremes, rough tissue handling, or the application of abrasive creams or exfoliants. Some patients are in a fragile and risky condition.

Who takes care of your feet? I have lost count of how many times I have asked patients this question, but it seems like I must have asked it at least a million times. Some patients report that they use the services of a podiatrist. That always pleases me because I know that these patients are receiving an appropriate diagnosis and professional care in a safe, clean environment. Unfortunately, the number of patients who receive professional care represents only a small percentage of the total population of people with some type of foot problem.

Other than receiving professional foot care, throughout the years, I have heard four basic answers when I ask who takes care of your feet:

- nobody does it;
- my family does it for me;
- I do it myself, (I have seen patients who do not bathe their feet, and as you might expect, their feet have skin and nail infections that include fungus, mold, yeast, or bacteria. I have seen patients that use every manner of instrument from a pocket knife to a razor blade, and it is not unusual for a patient to come to my office due to a self-inflicted laceration (see the case study below).

Some patients report a distressing fourth answer: they receive foot care services at nail salons, beauty spas, and pedicure parlors—a service that is less expensive, more accessible, and seemingly less threatening. These aesthetic services include not only trimming of the nails, but also debridement of keratosis (hardened tissue such as corns and calluses) on the feet. At first, it would seem that this should be a commonly accepted form of foot care, but a closer look may reveal why it's not such a good idea—especially for someone with diabetes.

## Death by Pedicure

I have never met a person who said they wanted to lose a leg, yet many patients with diabetes unwittingly put themselves at risk for fungus, yeast, or bacterial infection, and possibly a laceration of the skin that could lead to an infection all because they use the pedicure services of a nail salon. Some nail boutiques are extremely conscientious about sterilization of instruments and sanitary practices, but unfortunately many are not. Regardless of the sanitation issue, a pedicure exposes you to risk because it disturbs the skin and cuticle, which serve as a protective seal around nails.

The level of foot care that is provided in a nail salon may be soothing, but instruments that are able to draw blood also carry the danger of transferring bacterial organisms. Since sharp, cutting instruments like nail clippers and "potato peeling-type" gadgets are used to trim nails and calluses in every manicure and pedicure parlor in the world, you might want to ask yourself these questions:

- Are technicians appropriately trained to use these instruments?
- Are technicians trained to identify the risk factors their clients may have?
- Do technicians modify their care to be consistent with that risk?
- Are the instruments sterile?

- If I get cut while having my pedicure, am I leaving myself vulnerable to AIDS, HIV, or hepatitis during my brief spa visit?
- If I have a problem with my feet will my pedicurist recognize it and recommend professional care?

Several years ago, I visited a school of cosmetology where pedicure services were taught. I was shocked by the low level of education these students received concerning the medical or health issues that related to their client's feet and legs. The emphasis was on the aesthetics as one might expect, but these students had only the most rudimentary knowledge concerning diabetes, peripheral vascular disease, skin and nail infections, and the concept of sterility of the instruments used to care for their clients. When it came to medications, they knew little about the how Coumadin™, Heparin™, or aspirin and other drugs affect the bleeding and clotting characteristics of their clients. I began to have serious concerns about the environment that at-risk patients might put themselves in while at a pedicure.

In an effort to learn more about the issues, I visited several pedicure salons and asked the technicians how they sterilized their instruments. Each salon performed this task differently. One proudly showed me a container of blue solution they soaked their instruments in; another showed me a "toaster oven-type" contraption that the instruments were cooked in. I have since come to learn that there is apparently very lax supervision of these businesses and apparently no legal standards and negligent inspections of these places. In fact, I recently read that a woman died from an infection she acquired from a pedicure.

Several podiatrists have made statements in the national media to alert consumers about the risks they take by seeking foot care at such establishments. And there is a book titled *Death by Pedicure The Dirty Secret of Nail Salons* written by Dr. Robert Spalding, DPM, a podiatrist in Chattanooga, Tennessee. *Death by Pedicure* gives a sobering look at health code violations in nail salons, and the catastrophic and sometimes lethal consequences. I recommend this book for anyone in the nail care industry—especially nail technicians who would like to learn more about detecting foot problems and suggesting that clients see a podiatrist for further care.

The most important issue about salon pedicures is that this type of care robs people of the opportunity to receive a legitimate diagnosis, recognition of their risk factors, education concerning prevention, and legitimate treatment. I'd rather my patients avoid pedicures in a non-professional environment. I would prefer they see a podiatrist who is specially trained for diabetic foot care. If you know you have risk factors like neuropathy or PAD, and you insist on going to a nail salon, reduce your risks of contracting diseases by bringing your own instruments. You can always sterilize your instruments at home by soaking them in a diluted bleach solution or by boiling them in water.

## Case Study ~ Improper Self-care

Mr. E came to my clinic as a referral from the hospital diabetes educator. Margaret is my coworker in the At-Risk Foot Clinic. In the past several years, we have evaluated close to 250 patients per year and we have seen pathology that most healthcare providers only hear stories about or see pictures of in books. Margaret has a vast knowledge of diabetes and has authored several book chapters on diabetes-related subjects. Every time we discuss a case or evaluate a patient, I learn something new about diabetes and management of the disease and the patients.

One Wednesday morning she stopped by my clinic, poked her head in the door, and with a sly smile on her face asked if I had time to see a patient that she felt needed a debridement for a foot wound. On most days my clinic is booked solid and usually I end up seeing a few more patients than were scheduled in the clinic because the demand for podiatry services far exceeds my ability to provide the care. I know that Margaret would not ask me to see a patient on a same-day basis unless it was truly medically necessary. Without hesitation I told her to bring the patient to the clinic and I would be happy to see him. This is an example of how our inter-disciplinary team or entourage can work for the benefit of quality patient care; all the providers needed are in one location and accessible in a timely fashion.

During her evaluation of Mr. E, Margaret noted that he had been admitted to the hospital because of a serious infection to his right great toe. Although he was receiving intravenous antibiotics, his foot wound had not yet been debrided. She thought the patient would benefit from a debridement. He also needed his nails to be trimmed because they were long and thick and she was concerned that he might lacerate one of his toes with his own nails.

Mr. E was a 57-year-old male who was diabetic, type 1 (insulin-dependent) whose blood sugar levels ranged from the low 200s all the way to the low 500s. It was clear to me that he was in a select group of the most non-compliant patients I had ever seen. When Mr. E arrived in my treatment chair, I knew right away that he had a terrible infection. I could smell it as I approached to introduce myself.

Mr. E was wearing sandals and there was no dressing on his foot wound. The skin of the first toe was thickened in some places and flaking in others. A portion of the toenail remained attached but was lifted up from the nail bed and the tissue underneath was whitish in color and was the source of the foul odor from the wound. This indicated that his wound had been festering for more than a few days. There was a hole in the tip of his toe the size of a quarter and the ulcer site had gummy yellow to grayish black infected tissue present. I reviewed his X-ray and noted the classic moth-eaten appearance of the smallest bone in the big toe that is under the toenail called the distal phalanx. This helped confirm my suspicion; he had a bone infection.

Mr. E told me that he tried to trim his toenail with a razor blade, the most convenient instrument he had in his bathroom. Instead of trimming the toenail, he cut the end of his toe off and felt nothing. Mr. E was legally blind, and had a history of non-compliance concerning the control of his blood sugars and diet. Whether he had not been educated about his diabetes, or did not understand or care about the long-term complications, he had allowed his diabetes to remain uncontrolled for many years.

Debriding the toenails was a straightforward procedure but debriding the infected ulcer was a bit trickier. First, I removed the remaining portion of the toenail and then started on the soft tissues. At first, there was significant callused tissue at the end of the toe, which surrounded the ulcer. That came off with ease, but the gummy tissue on the ulcer bed was different. The tissues had become a mass of fibrin (fibrinous tissue) that could not be trimmed with conventional tissue forceps. I switched tactics and used a #15 scalpel blade to remove the infected tissue until I got to normal tissue that bled when I trimmed it. Probing the wound with a sterile instrument, I was able to touch the bone and calculated that the infection had reached the bone. The X-ray confirmed my clinical evaluation. The best option we had was to remove the bone, fearing that if we didn't, the infection would spread and he would lose his leg or worse.

Mr. E underwent a successful digital amputation of his great toe. After the procedure, we provided him with diabetes education, nutritional counseling and consultations with an endocrinologist and a prosthetist. Being cognizant of the other problems that may be brewing due to pathology in the vascular system, we also referred him to a cardiologist and ophthalmologist to evaluate his cardiovascular system and his eyesight. We fabricated a custom-molded biomechanical orthotic with a plug for the missing toe and provided him with diabetic shoes. I continued to see him for ongoing foot care and he has not had another significant incident since he got an entourage to help him control his diabetes.

What can we learn from Mr. E's case?

The most important lesson was that controlling blood sugars is paramount for patients with diabetes. We also need to learn that educating patients with diabetes and following up with continuing education is critical. Why was this patient able to ignore taking his medications while no one kept an eye on him? At-risk patients need to have professional foot care. Through a care strategy that combines prevention, multi-disciplinary treatment of foot ulcers, close monitoring, and the education of healthcare professionals and patients with diabetes, it is estimated that amputation rates can be reduced by as much as 85 percent.

There was a remarkably revealing survey done by the American Podiatric Medical Association titled, "How Americans 18 Years of Age or Older Treated Selected Foot Problems During the Past Twelve Months, 2000." The survey identified thirteen specific foot problems and how patients chose to manage them. It had a breakdown of the type of provider dispensing care and what percentage of the overall care they allotted for each problem. An analysis in the next paragraph is quite telling about foot care in the United States.

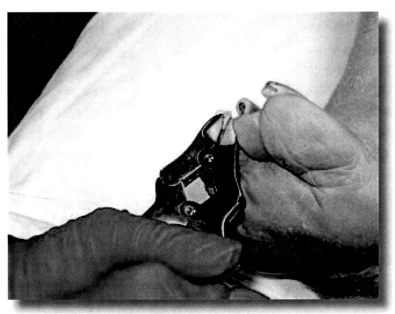

**Nails Trimmed by Podiatrist**

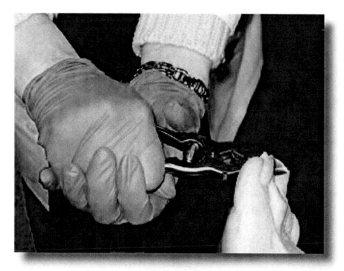

**Two Hands Required**

Podiatrists were rated the highest for care of bone spurs followed by bunions, infections, and warts. Family physicians were rated highest for arthritis of the toes and were strong in foot injuries, warts, infections, and bone spurs. Orthopedists were rated highest for hammertoes and were used for foot injuries and bone spurs. The category of "unsure what to do" had its highest rating in the section on thickened and deformed nails, followed by bone spurs, heel pain, and flat or fallen arches. The most distressing results came in the remaining two categories: "self-treated" and "other." The highest percentage (62 percent) of patients self-treated for foot problems such as athlete's foot, followed by ingrown toenails and infections. I wonder how many of those who self-treated were diabetic? I am deeply concerned about the category of "other." In this category, the problems were hammertoes, thickened and deformed nails, and bunions.

## What Is Podiatry?

We've talked a lot about foot care and that it should be performed only by a professional, licensed physician who is best qualified to provide such care. So, let's talk about those foot specialists who are best qualified to treat the foot—especially the diabetic foot—a podiatrist.

The medical profession known as podiatry was once called chiropody. It started with the itinerant corn and callus cutters who roamed the country during the eighteenth and nineteenth centuries. Podiatry emerged because local town or country doctors didn't deal with issues related to the foot. Although folks didn't know much about foot care at that time, when a problem arose with their feet, they sought the person with the reputation for knowing the most about feet. They'd go to the chiropodist to have their nails cut, corns or calluses trimmed, or feet taped or padded for comfort.

After a century of gathering knowledge wherever they could, a group of physicians led by Dr. Maurice J. Lewi, a physician and educator then serving as secretary to the New York State Board of Examiners, founded the New York School of Chiropody in 1911. Lewi also suggested the change of the name of this young profession from chiropody to podiatry. Today, there are approximately 14,000 podiatric physicians and surgeons in the United States. This yields a physician-to-patient ratio of 1:20,000. There are nine schools of podiatry in the United States, and most are affiliated with universities:

1. Barry University School of Graduate Medical Sciences in Miami, Florida

2. College of Podiatric Medicine at Rosalind Franklin University of Medicine and Science in North Chicago, Illinois
3. College of Podiatric Medicine and Surgery at Des Moines University in Des Moines, Iowa
4. Arizona Podiatric Medical Program at Midwestern University in Glendale, Arizona
5. New York College of Podiatric Medicine in New York, New York
6. Ohio College of Podiatric Medicine in Cleveland, Ohio
7. California School of Podiatric Medicine at Samuel Merritt College in Oakland, California
8. Temple University in Philadelphia, Pennsylvania
9. College of Podiatry Western University of Health Sciences in St. Pomona, California

There are also schools of podiatric medicine and surgery in Australia, the United Kingdom, South Africa, New Zealand, Canada, and Spain. The practice has risen from humble beginnings to become an internationally accepted medical specialty.

The education for doctors of podiatric medicine (DPM) is similar to that for allopathic, or medical doctors (MD) and doctors of osteopathy (DO), also known as osteopathic physicians. In many podiatry schools affiliated with other medical schools, all medical students, regardless of specialization, study together for the first two years taking the same courses and exams. In fact, prospective students for podiatric medical schools take the Medical College Admission Test or MCAT test required for entrance to all medical schools in the United States. At the end of the first two years, when the allopathic and osteopathic students move into the study of general medicine, podiatrists go into the intensive study of the lower extremities with courses that include anatomy, physiology, and biomechanics.

Because of the high level of education, training, and how the laws are written in the United States, podiatrists have the ability to perform surgery on the deepest structures of the foot including the bones and soft tissues. In most other countries, podiatrists can provide care for the superficial tissues and cannot do any surgery that involves structures deeper in the foot. This limits them to caring for skin, soft tissue, nails, problems of gait and ambulation, and the use of biomechanical orthotics. This ability to provide care for all of the structures on the foot makes the podiatrist in the United States the most qualified physician and surgeon of the foot anywhere on the planet.

In 1976, when I graduated from podiatry school, only one out of every three people who applied for a hospital-based residency program was selected. This meant that two out of every three candidates looked to alternative forms of post-graduate education. Many chose a preceptor program working with an established podiatrist in their office. Not only did these young practitioners learn about the profession in a real world setting to help them further develop their skills as foot surgeons and healers, their education also included office layout, practice management, billing, and understanding medical insurance practice, marketing, human relations, and time management. Now, in the United States every practitioner who graduates from a podiatric medical school has an opportunity for at least a two-year hospital-based residency. Then, they can take a third year as a fellowship, which can be in advanced or specialized surgery, sports medicine, diabetes, or arthritis.

Today, there are 213 residency-training programs in the U.S. approved by the Council on Podiatric Medical Education. Every podiatrist has the opportunity for multi-year residency training that includes rotations in specialties such as general, vascular, and neurological surgery, anesthesia, emergency medicine, pediatrics, endocrinology, radiology, dermatology, orthopedics, and primary care. Today's graduating residency-trained podiatrist is the best trained and most prepared to handle any foot problem since M.J. Lewi's time.

As podiatric medical education has become globalized, so has postgraduate training as American podiatrists attend schools and learn the latest techniques in Switzerland, Russia, Israel, and England. The highlight of these programs is learning advanced and specialized techniques in foot care that have been developed at facilities outside the United States for treatment of pathology of the foot and lower leg. In the arena of fracture care, the newest techniques are being developed outside the U.S. These techniques include both internal fixation using screws and plates and now external fixation where the mechanism that holds the mending portions of the bone together is actually on the outside the body. Like structural scaffolding on the outside of a building, these external fixation devices can be adjusted as necessary to aid in the healing process, especially in limb salvage cases.

Podiatric training teaches the essentials of diagnosing all types of foot problems and how to provide a wide range of services to resolve these problems. As a result, podiatrists can provide the most basic elements of foot care, including palliative care, the debridement (removal) of corns and calluses, and nail care. We also provide the most sophisticated twenty-first century cutting-edge care to relieve patients of pain and functional disability including the use of lasers, artificial joints, stem cells, and sophisticated computers.

Podiatry focuses on an area that other medical specialties and traditional medicine have failed to treat. A medical doctor can treat any part of your body, but you probably would not go to him for care of your teeth because that is not his specialty. He doesn't have the education, specialized training, or tools to help you the way a dentist can. It's the same with podiatrists. We have the specialized education, training, and tools to treat the foot—especially the diabetic foot—better than most other providers. However, podiatry is still the least known and understood of the medical professions. Sometimes confused with pediatrics, which deals with the development, care, and diseases of children, podiatry specializes in the conditions and function of the human foot. It includes examinations, diagnoses, and treatments by medical, surgical, and biomechanical methods.

Americans spend a great deal of time on their feet and the aging baby boomer segment of the population is going to need foot care to help them maintain a healthy lifestyle. As the nation ages and remains active across all age groups, the need for foot care will become increasingly important.

## What Does a Podiatrist Do?

The human foot is a complex structure. It permits us to translate a vertical force from our legs into a horizontal force in our feet. This process allows us to move in three dimensions—to walk, run, jump, dance, and move. Most of us take our feet for granted until something happens that stops our normal function. Each foot contains twenty-six bones plus a complex series of structures including muscles, tendons, nerves, ligaments, blood vessels, and specialized skin on the bottom. The foot is designed to support our weight and to provide balance and mobility. The fifty-two bones in your feet make up about one-fourth of all the bones in your body. The foot may be the first area to show signs of serious conditions such as arthritis, diabetes, and cardiovascular disease. When it comes to the lower leg and foot, podiatrists have a better working knowledge in all of the systems that can develop problems including orthopedic, vascular, neurological, dermatological, and problems of gait and ambulation involved in walking called biomechanics than any other medical practitioner who may treat problems of foot structure and function.

Podiatrists diagnose and treat disorders, diseases, and injuries of the foot and lower leg to keep this part of the body working properly. We treat a variety of foot problems such as:

- Ankle and foot bone fractures, sprains, strains, and foot injuries
- Arthritis and joint diseases
- Benign and malignant tumors
- Bone spurs, hammer toe, mallet toe, claw toe, and bunions
- Corns and calluses
- Warts or plugged up sweat gland ducts that result in thickening of the skin on the bottom of the foot

- Diseased or ingrown toenails
- Foot complaints associated with diabetes, gout, ulcers, and PAD
- Heel spurs/heel pain and arch problems
- Flat feet
- Nerve pain (pinched nerves)
- Problems of gait and ambulation in adults who have difficulty walking or who trip or fall, as well as 'growing pains' syndrome in children's legs
- Bacterial or fungal skin infections
- Limb length inequalities caused by implant surgery of the knee or hip

These conditions may result from birth defects, heredity, trauma, improper shoes, abnormal gait, and muscle and joint imbalances. To diagnose a foot problem, a podiatrist may order imaging tests like X-rays, CT Scans, MRIs, and other lab tests. To treat these problems, podiatrists can use local anesthetics, prescribe drugs, order physical therapy, set fractures, and perform surgery. Podiatrists can also fit corrective shoe inserts called orthotics, apply plaster casts and strappings or pads to accommodate and treat foot deformities, and prescribe custom-made shoes.

The great thing about podiatry is that what we do is straightforward. Short of medical emergencies, like trauma, we can pretty much give patients relief from pain and make them comfortable on the first visit, and that includes treating more than 300 possible diagnosable problems. Podiatrists are licensed by all fifty states, have Drug Enforcement Agency (DEA) numbers and can prescribe medications from narcotics to antibiotics; we are accepted in almost every hospital in the country. Podiatrists practice in a variety of settings including solo practice, associates groups, orthopedic, and multi-disciplinary groups with other medical specialists. Many podiatrists are limited in their practices anatomically to the foot but can treat all problems of the systems affecting the foot. State laws vary on this, and some podiatrist practices may extend to the ankle or lower leg. For instance, in Tennessee, a podiatrist can treat diseases of the foot and leg up to the ankle. In Florida, podiatrists can treat problems up to the knee.

## Jeffrey Robbins, DPM

When I look at all the people involved in the field of diabetic foot care, some people stand out as giants in the field. My mentor, classmate, and teacher, Dr. Jeffrey Robbins is one of them. Few people have had the leverage and the ability to affect change the way he has.

As a podiatrist, Jeff came from humble beginnings. He was set to embark on a career in private practice and podiatric surgery, but he had a turning point in his career in 1982 when he suffered an injury that left him permanently partially disabled. He was forced to redirect his career toward things like the diabetic foot, public health, primary care, geriatrics, residency training, and administration. In having to face this life-changing event, he embarked upon a brand new career, which led him to a whole new group of issues and problems present at the time. Those issues were predicatively going to get significantly worse without some type of major paradigm shift or policy change within the profession of podiatry and public health—

especially in the American public. Unfortunately, many of those predictions have come true. As a society we are more obese, more diabetic, and part of a population that is the oldest and largest single generation to ever exist. As baby boomers, we have moved paradigms, thoughts, and trends since we were in college and we continue to do so. Within that, there has come an increase in poor health and unreasonable expectations. As a vegetarian who exercises on a regular basis, Jeff cares about what he eats and puts in his body. He keeps his stress level low, and cares for his mental and emotional health. Jeff refers to himself as a health-nut, which I suppose makes the rest of the population, who embrace disease as a way of life, normal.

In terms of the diabetic foot, when Jeff graduated his residency program in the 1970s, the medical field was first beginning to see remarkable new medications such as human-derived insulin, Humulin®, Glipizide®, and other new medications for diabetes. This misled some people to believe that diabetes would become a very minor disease in ten to fifteen years instead of the plague it is now. Jeff foresaw that the diabetic foot with its morbid complications was going to continue and become even more of a problem. Seeing this, he took a career path in academia that led him to the Department of Veterans Affairs where he had the opportunity to participate and ultimately run the VA's amputation prevention program (PACT) for the entire United States. PACT is a model public health program in that it seeks to be preventative in nature by identifying those patients at risk for amputation (those having diabetes, end-stage renal disease and peripheral vascular disease) and then establishing a screening program so that every single patient is screened for risk factors that can lead to foot ulceration, wound, infection, gangrene, and ultimately amputation. From the evaluation, a risk score is assigned and a care algorithm defines how they should be cared for on a long-term basis to not only to prevent amputation, but to prevent ulcers, wounds, and infections and to keep patients walking and functioning at a maximum potential. Not all amputations can be limited or prevented because patients do not always cooperate, nor are they always willing to change their diet and lifestyle. However, the inroads made by PACT in the fight to keep limbs attached to the body has been remarkable. It is the benchmark in amputation prevention in the United States. Since accepting the unique position as national program director for podiatry services for the Department of Veterans Affairs, Jeff has written policy, developed programs, and provided oversight for those programs. Due to his exemplary leadership over the past eleven years, the amputation rate for all patients in the VA system is 1.5 percent, and the amputation rate nationally for patients with diabetes is in the three to four percent range. Jeff's work is part of a growing army of folks who are creating awareness and attempting to treat the diabetic foot. There are 350 podiatrists in the VA system. There are 125-130 hospitals that have podiatrists on staff. As the director of one of the world's largest residency training programs, Jeff brings nearly 200 new practitioners per year into the field of podiatry. Even with the success of this program and the rate of amputation being almost half that of the rest of the country, Jeff says that far too many limbs are still being amputated in the VA system and especially in the general population.

When a person suffers an amputation, their life span is greatly decreased. They have a five-year survival rate at

KEEP THE LEGS YOU STAND ON — Dr. Mark Hinkes

about fifty percent, which means that within five years, half of them will have died—usually from cardiovascular disease. Cardiovascular disease is a natural consequence of diabetes and is almost a certainty. The degree and severity of their cardiovascular disease depends upon how well they control their diabetes and blood glucose levels. If controlled, they can live usually live a fairly long and relatively healthy life.

Jeff is doing research concerning the gravity of diabetes as compared to other diseases. Data shows that the five-year survival rates for ischemic ulcers and amputations is far worse than Hodgkin's disease, and colon, prostate and breast cancer. Only lung and pancreatic cancers have a worse five-year survival rate than patients with ischemic ulcers and amputations. Diabetes should be viewed as a malignant metastatic disease so patients will muster the same kind of dedication to fighting it as they would if they received a diagnosis of cancer.

With the amount of resources and research being focused on the diabetic foot and with the energies and leadership of other podiatrists including David Armstrong, Larry Lavery, Lee Sanders, Larry Harkless, Vickie Driver, Bob Frykberg, and Warren Joseph, Jeff believes we will see some inroads on the care of the diabetic foot within the next twenty-five years. That will require the encouragement of a change in the paradigm, how we look at this disease, and how we treat it. Diabetes is not going away. We can affect it if we are vigilant and can convince patients to do the right thing. While we need to continue to treat patients who already have diabetes, the most important thing is to prevent type 2 diabetes before it starts. The obesity epidemic in children and young adults is frightening, and we need to make them aware of the risk factors and teach them to exercise, eat properly, and keep their feet in good shape. We need to teach them to be a health nut rather than a disease nut.

Smoking, poor diet, and lack of exercise are the three behaviors that cause almost 35 percent of deaths in the United States. No wonder 80 percent of Americans over the age of sixty-five have at least one chronic disease. If people adopt healthier lifestyles, they will not develop chronic diseases such as diabetes, cancer, and heart disease. Just think of the cost savings in healthcare treatment alone!

## A Visit to the At-Risk Foot Clinic

The At-Risk Foot Clinic at the VA Hospital in Nashville, Tennessee is staffed by an inter-disciplinary group which includes Linda Halperin, MD (associate chief of physical medicine and rehabilitation), and Margaret "Elaine" McLeod (certified diabetes educator), and me. According to Dr. Halperin, we accept referrals of patients with diabetes from primary care physicians or family doctors to evaluate the risks for amputation. Our job is to evaluate and manage these patient's lower extremities and decide if and what type of preventive foot care should be implemented for each patient based on our exam and the PACT program criteria. Many times we find patients who are borderline from one category to another and we will take a time out to debate the merits of one category versus another and decide on specific treatments or care that would be best for the patient. In the end, we usually err on the side of being conservative; as this provides the patient the most benefit in terms of what supplies, shoes, insoles, or braces from the prosthetics department would be best for their condition.

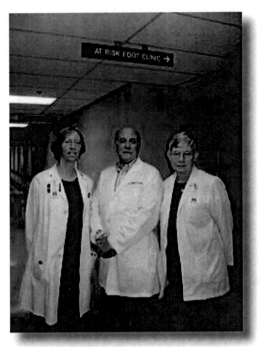

**Nashville At-Risk Foot Clinic Staff**

People having no overt foot problems may have been examined by their PCP, who used the monofilament testing device and realized that the patient did not have protective sensation. Those patients at high risk for ulcers, infections, and perhaps amputation are referred to our clinic where we do a thorough assessment and offer detailed education on how to take care of their feet to prevent amputation. We almost always grant appointments within thirty days depending upon how many referrals we have at the time.

Our exams identify people who have foot deformities, vascular, neurological or biomechanical problems that can be helped with proper treatment. Our real mission remains the educating of people who are at high risk for ulcer, infection, or amputation. There are statistics that show our education efforts are having a positive impact, but most importantly patients say we make a difference in the quality of their lives. Some of our patients are obviously non-compliant, and we know that is going to bring our numbers down. No one can help someone who will not help themselves.

We give each patient a print-out stating the specifics of what our exam showed and what the patient needs to do to improve his preventive behaviors. It's extremely unusual for us to see a patient more than once, so this personalized paper that reads, "You are category 2, and that means..." is even more helpful than just verbally telling them.

We usually see six to eight patients in a morning, and we all feel very good about our individual contributions to the process. Some patients are so happy to have someone pay attention to them and listen to their complaints; they are thrilled to share every nuance of their medical history and life with us. A day at the VA might be the social highlight of their week or perhaps month.

Our exam evaluates not only the physical patient but looks to their social support system and other issues including vision, use of hands, and ability to reach and self-care for their feet. We evaluate the patient's vascular, neurological, and musculoskeletal systems as well as identify bone, soft tissue, and nail deformities. I was once asked about the issue of being a podiatrist and having to deal with smelly feet. I always answer, "That is a layman's concern." But, in truth I must admit that I have met some folks whose foot odor could have been used as a secret weapon.

Each of us has specialized duties in the at-risk foot clinic. Elaine performs the monofilament test and is available to answer questions regarding diabetes education, medications and blood glucose control. I perform the lower extremity and foot physical exam. As the assistant service chief, Linda is more involved in the medical history and tends to look at things from an amputation perspective since she also runs the amputation clinic. She has been at the Nashville VA Hospital since February 1999. Linda deals with a lot of patients who are debilitated and have musculoskeletal issues, and victims of neurological-stroke, head injury, spinal cord injury, and of course, amputees. She prescribes prosthetics, power wheelchairs, or whatever type of equipment is most appropriate for them. The VA is unique; we actually provide the equipment needed, which greatly expedites the process. In the outside world, if you need a power wheelchair, your doctor writes a prescription, and then it's up to you (and your insurance or Medicare) to get it and pay for it. But in the VA, if we say you need it, we give it to you.

In the private sector a doctor may write a prescription whenever he or she thinks there's a chance a patient may need an item, but since they're not actually paying for the items, they may not do a complete evaluation to determine necessity. The VA looks at a patient's needs over the long haul; private insurance usually does not. They may not have as much emphasis on the insensate foot and preventing amputation because they probably won't be the patient's insurance company five years down the road. The person may have an amputation by then, but in the VA, we know the patient is ours for life, so we are a lot more concerned about prevention. I may have a lot of frustrations about the VA system, but I think there is a lot more good about it than there is bad.

Because the VA is paying for it and giving them this equipment, we have to be certain this is what they need. From a cost standpoint, we want to give them the right thing the first time that will allow them to be functional and independent.

On the first and third Tuesdays, we have amputee clinic. If you want to have a sad but enlightening experience, spend some time in this clinic. This is the place where we see those poor souls who were not lucky enough to have prevented their amputations and who are being evaluated for a prosthetic leg. Most of the folks have the same story, "I did not know I was at risk for losing my leg." And at that point, they usually begin to talk about how the loss has changed their lives. Sometimes the emotionally involved patients will cry. I always thought that these patients should have consultations for "adjustment disorder," but few do. It is a sad, sad place, and I usually leave the room depressed for the patients and glad I still have both my legs.

### What Can Podiatry Do for You?

My wife has found a terrific little restaurant named Bronte's inside the Davis Kidd Book Store here in Nashville. What makes this venue unique is that it is within the confines of a bookstore and therefore is pretty quiet. For a bonus, there is no smoking permitted, there are no loud noises like dishes crashing in the kitchen, and not even any elevator music to compete for the "ear time" of a private conversation.

One night, our waitress was a lady named Donna, who had a beautiful voice, sparking eyes, and a limp. Only a foot doctor might have noticed the limp because it was so slight. After seeing her walk a bit, and at an opportune time, I asked her if her heel was bothering her. At that moment, before Donna could answer, my wife spoke up saying, "He is a foot doctor; that's why he noticed your foot."

With a face that revealed more than her voice did, she replied, "I have rheumatoid arthritis and thankfully the only problem I have right now is with my ankle." She continued, "They operated on it and fused all the bones. It still hurts, but at least I can walk."

After coffee and dessert, we had a chance to talk further. "My rheumatologist tells me I am lucky that only my ankle hurts." Through our conversation I learned that she was not aware of podiatry and had not visited a podiatrist to see if there were any services that could improve her quality of life. Apparently, her rheumatologist did not consider referring her to a podiatrist. We discussed the options such as shoe modifications, recommendations for special shoes, and a prescription for custom-made insoles that provide the most efficient function and might help in reducing foot and ankle pain. Other treatments might include steroid injections or physical therapy treatments.

Donna was very pleased to learn about podiatry and the services that may be helpful for her condition and mentioned she would investigate podiatry and speak to her doctor about it. On the way home, I thought again about Donna and her foot condition. It was a shame for a young woman to be limping. I started wondering how many patients with diabetes there are who don't know about podiatry and the services they can take advantage of for a better quality of life.

## Multi-disciplinary Team

With the issues of cost containment and patient quality of life being the measures of quality care, more and more podiatrists have gravitated to the area of prevention and are taking their place in multi-disciplinary groups. Through this new focus, we are beginning to see new hospital-based limb salvage programs specializing in preserving limbs instead of amputating them. There is a void in this area, and podiatrists are best qualified to treat the foot manifestations of peripheral vascular disease (PVD) and neuropathy in the foot.

The podiatrist's inclusion in the multi-disciplinary team reflects the education, training, and specialized skills of the podiatrist and is an acknowledgement that the podiatrist is a critical member of any diabetic patient's health team.

Vickie Driver, DPM, had a successful career in business and a family, but wanted to also be in service to her fellow man. She thought about allopathic medicine as a career choice, but when she learned about podiatry, she decided that was where she needed to be. Being a patient with diabetes herself, she realized she could do more for other patients with diabetes through podiatry than by any other medical specialty. Vickie started her podiatry career in Tacoma, Washington at Madigan Army Base in a specialized program of limb salvage taking care of military personnel on the west coast and from the Pacific Rim as well as their family members. She has taught residents and fellows and is a researcher and policy advisor to Medicare. She now works in the limb salvage program at Boston University. I once heard her say, "A limb salvage program without a podiatrist on board is not a fully-staffed limb salvage program." I couldn't agree more. A dedicated diabetic foot care team must include a podiatrist.

What other experts should you expect to participate on a multi-disciplinary team? Here is what Christopher Attinger, MD, medical director of the wound healing clinic and professor of plastic surgery at Georgetown University Hospital, Washington D.C. says:

*Number one, you need a vascular surgeon, an orthopedist or podiatrist who's qualified to do limited amputations that are biomechanically stable. You also need to have someone who can do very good below- and above-knee amputations if the process goes awry or the leg is non-salvageable. Next, you need a podiatrist or orthopedist (or both) who is able to repair or remove heel wounds and infected Charcots.*

*Number three, you need someone who's adequate at soft tissue management to close wounds. That may be a vascular surgeon or a podiatrist, an orthopedist, who knows all the different techniques to close tissue. You occasionally need a micro-surgeon to close a wound that can't be closed with normal techniques. If you can get a plastic surgeon, it would be a miracle.*

*In terms of medical folks, what you need is an infectious disease expert on every case because complications from antibiotics are huge and if you can eliminate the patient's exposure to antibiotics by giving appropriate short-term antibiotics, they do much better, so that's number one. We have a hospitalist who manages the patients in-*

*house because their sugars are wacky. Some have congestive heart failures or are on dialysis. These conditions have to be managed by someone who knows and understands the medications used to treat them. We need a diabetologist to help the patient keep their sugar levels in the 100–150 range so they will heal better and decrease the risk of infection. You sometimes need to have a psychiatrist on board to help the patient better cope with a limb loss. Those are the key people we have internally.*

*And then, there's a whole bunch of ancillary folks you need. You need a pedorthist who makes orthotics, you need a prosthetist who makes prostheses, you need a physical therapist who can apply outpatient wound techniques. You need nurse practitioners who not only take care of pre-op patients to make sure they can go through surgery, but also manage their discharge and some other medical problems when they're on the floor. You obviously need nurses who are competent at wound techniques, casting, etc.*

## What Your Doctor Doesn't Know Can Harm You

While younger physicians may now train with podiatrists and are more aware of our DPM expertise and routinely refer their patients to us, I have found that many older medical doctors my age (sixty) and older have a very ignorant, and strongly negative connotation of podiatrists in general. They never trained side-by-side with a podiatry student or resident.

DPMs my age were trained in small hospitals since it was rare for large hospitals to have a podiatric residency program in the mid to late 1970s.

Unfortunately, most doctors are not trained to know what to look for regarding the feet. In a routine visit, most doctors do not ask to see your feet. The feet tell an amazing story and should be part of every physical exam. Here's an example:

JP, a 75-year-old type 2 diabetic male with a history of rheumatoid arthritis, came to the office with complaints of chronic pain in his feet. The onset of the pain was several years previous, but he had received limited treatment. He reported his pain was of a burning nature at level 10 out of 10; he had difficulty moving his toes and walking. When he took his shoes off, the pain worsened. He was not sure if his pain was due to his diabetes or his arthritis. He had used at least three different types of insoles in his shoes at the same time in an attempt to relieve his pain. He sat in my treatment chair with his arms crossed across his rather large stomach and had an angry, frustrated look on his face.

Without really looking at me, he stuck out his hand and showed me an amber-colored plastic bottle, said, "This is what my doctor gave me and it didn't work." The medication his doctor had prescribed was Neurontin™ and he was to take one 300 mg capsule three times a day totaling 900 mg per day. I told JP that to be effective, the dosage of this medication may have to be increased over a period of time and that some patients take as much as 3,600 mg per day in order to get relief of their neuropathy symptoms.

JP incredulously responded, "My doctor never told me that. I expected to take the pills and be better." JP's history showed that his internal medicine doctor never asked JP to take off his shoes to examine his feet. He assumed that JP's pain was due to peripheral neuropathy since he had a history of diabetes. Further questioning revealed that JP's pain was mostly in his forefoot and radiated into the toes and back up the foot toward his ankle. However, the bottom of the foot was not affected. Furthermore, his pain was episodic in nature and not constant.

The physical exam revealed deformed toes that were painful with movement and a loss of the normal protective fat pad that covers and protects the bottom of the front of the foot. There was pain when I pressed on the area between the toes. This sharp or burning pain is most often caused by an irritated nerve known as a trigger point or nerve entrapment. This is a very common foot problem and is not caused by diabetic sensory neuropathy.

*When the patients finally arrived at my office after having their feet treated by primary care MDs, I was appalled at the lack of knowledge displayed by these doctors. They diagnosed corns as dermatophytosis and vice versa. Ingrown toe nails were diagnoses as gangrene, etc. I wondered at times if these doctors had ever seen a human foot in their entire clinical careers.*

—Elliot Udell, DPM, Hicksville, NY

JP could not feel the monofilament testing device, indicating that he did have sensory neuropathy and loss of protective sensation; however, sensory neuropathy does not cause the painful symptoms associated with a nerve entrapment. So, here was a patient with loss of protective sensation and yet he had a painful foot.

An X-ray was negative for fracture, tumor, or joint dislocation. In consideration of both his diabetes and arthritis, I outlined a conservative treatment plan to which he agreed. During that visit, I gave him a low dose steroid injection to both of the painful sites in one foot. Following the injections, he stood up from the treatment chair pain free. He was delighted. He smiled as he kept looking at his foot moving it around, and bending his toes in great wonder that he could feel so good so quickly.

As he walked out the door of the treatment room, he turned, looked me in the eye and said, "Thank you, Dr. Hinkes. I have not been pain free for so long; this is wonderful."

For me, there is no greater reward than receiving a thank you from a grateful patient.

In reviewing JP's case, it became clear to me that he had been misdiagnosed and inappropriately treated. His case was complex, but an adequate history and physical exam combined with appropriate care provided him with dramatic and lasting pain relief.

## Treatment for Pain

We should not treat foot pain with our eyes closed. We should find out *why* a patient has foot pain because a legitimate diagnosis usually assures the correct treatment. Pain medications only mask the problem and give people the idea that they don't have to go the foot doctor. Instead, they stop by Walgreens and pick up a pain reliever and learn to live with foot pain. Many patients with diabetes end up with a tragedy when they ignore pain. Many people suffering foot and leg pain think their aches are due to growing old. Frequently, something far more serious (and often preventable) is taking place.

Pain is a symptom common to many foot conditions, but there are some therapies that a person with diabetes—especially someone who has lost sensation—should never use. For instance, an ice pack or a hot foot soak. Don't apply ice or gel packs that you can either freeze or heat in the microwave to an inflamed area. Instead, see your doctor—preferably a podiatrist. If your skin feels warm to the touch or is swollen, this is an indication that your foot is inflamed and possibly infected.

Let's look at some common methods for treating pain:

- Analgesics are a class of orally-administered pain relievers such as acetaminophen (Tylenol™), which relieve pain without relieving inflammation. I only suggest using pain relievers after a legitimate evaluation has been made rather than as a method of self-treatment.

- Topical analgesics available in lotion, cream, or gel form are applied to the skin where they penetrate to relieve mild foot pain. Some topical preparations containing menthol, eucalyptus oil, or turpentine oil reduce pain by distracting the nerves with a different type of sensation. We also use 5 percent Lidocaine patches called Lidoderm™. Another type of topical analgesic delivers salicylates (the same ingredient as in aspirin) through the skin. A third group counters a chemical known as substance P (Capsaicin), which is a neurotransmitter that transmits pain signals to the brain. Capsaicin is derived from a natural ingredient found in cayenne pepper. For that reason, it may burn or sting when first used. Be sure to use gloves when applying Capsaicin to the body. Getting this product in your eyes would be severely painful.

- Non-steroidal anti-inflammatory drugs (NSAID) include aspirin, ibuprofen (Advil, Motrin), and naproxen (Aleve). Patients with decreased kidney function may choose to avoid these drugs as they can decrease kidney function.

- Morphine-like analgesic drugs contain opioids such as codeine, hydrocodone, or morphine and provide stronger pain relief because they block certain chemical pathways that send pain signals through the central nervous system. These drugs may only be prescribed by your doctor.

- Nerve pain medications are prescribed for pain caused by nerve damage that does not respond well to opioids. Two drugs for treating nerve pain in the feet include the antidepressant amitriptyline (Elavil™), which increases the levels of brain chemicals that calm down pain signals, and the anticonvulsant/seizure medication known as gabapentin (Neurontin™). There are two other drugs that may be of value in treating neuropathic pain. They are Pregabalin (Lyrica™) and Duloxetine Hydrochloride (Cymbalta™), which work by interfering with nerve signaling. We can do a nerve block injection to numb a particular nerve to prevent pain signals from reaching your brain (much as Lidocaine or Xylocaine™ does for your teeth in a dentist's office).

- Corticosteroids are synthetic forms of naturally occurring hormones produced by the adrenal glands. These may be given topically, in pill form, or by injections to decrease inflammation and relieve pain. Topical corticosteroids, applied directly to the skin, are useful only in treating rashes. Pills and injections can be used for treating nerve entrapment and heel pain, however, these drugs must be used wisely. They do incredible things such as provide relief by decreasing inflammation, but they can also cause atrophy of the skin, decreased strength of soft tissues, and they increase blood sugar, and elevate blood pressure.

## Gaps in Healthcare

The reality about healthcare for patients with diabetes is that because of financial issues and time constraints, doctors are hard pressed to spend the time necessary to deal with all of the issues confronting patients. What tends to happen is that the patient will come in and the doctor will say, "Your finger stick test results (a random blood sugar test), show that your blood sugar is 290. That's way too high. I'd like to see your blood sugar around 110, so we're going to bump up your insulin, or add this pill. Make an appointment in eight weeks and we'll take another blood sugar test." Then, the doctor is out the door. This scenario is frequently repeated.

What happened? The doctor did what was medically necessary to treat you, but he failed to find out why your blood sugar levels were high, and to tell you continued elevated blood sugar levels can cause blindness, loss of kidney function, or the loss of a leg due to painless trauma from neuropathy. Doctors should be better educators. Not telling you about these potential outcomes is an example of a gap in care.

In my interview with him, James Powers, MD gave another example as the lack of a foot examination during routine a visit to the doctor. Dr. Powers is an associate professor of medicine at Vanderbilt University and Medical Director of the senior care service. He is also chief of geriatrics at the VA Tennessee Valley Healthcare System Hospital in Nashville. While the stories he shares are terrible, they are more the norm than one might expect.

*Among internists taking care of diabetics, the examination of the foot is not often the first priority. In fact, we should be faulted for forgetting to examine the foot. From my own clinical experience when I was an intern, we had a diabetic patient who had an ingrown toenail removed by a practitioner who did not pay attention to the pulses.*

I saw the patient on a medical service and he was having several toes amputated. He had peripheral vascular disease and he just did not heal. That just imprinted in my mind how important it is to take care of feet. The practitioner operated and tried to repair the injury of the ingrown toenail without taking the patient's underlying disease into consideration. As a result, the operation intended to help the patient ended up causing more destruction. It was just an awful introduction to how quickly a diabetic can lose a limb.

During my time with geriatrics, I've seen patients from many different perspectives and had the chance to care for older veterans. In fact, I saw a WWI veteran who was over 100 years old. He had some dementia but was living alone. He did not realize that his diabetes had caused peripheral neuropathy. His feet felt cold so he lit a fire in his wood stove and put his feet into the open oven. Not touching the metal, of course, but to feel the warmth. It caused irrevocable damage to his feet. The burns and the non-healing ulcers that ensued caused him to end up having bilateral below-the-knee amputations.

Most of the time when we care for chronic illness, we're trying to keep the high points under control. Making sure the blood sugar doesn't get too high or low, making sure the cholesterol is at an appropriate level, blood pressure is checked, metabolic syndrome is checked irrespective of the patient's age. But it's also important to be aware of the rest of the end organs that can be affected by diabetes. Checking the feet is something that all internists should be reminded to do frequently. You can't do it too many times. The minimum standard of checking once a year is certainly very reasonable. We all stand to be reminded to do the right thing at the right time and to the extent that electronic records, our panel management tools, dashboards can be developed to help remind particularly primary care providers to check diabetic feet. I think we'd all stand to benefit from that, as certainly will our patients.

I've been an educator for many years in university settings. In my experience, healthcare professionals know their own fields very well but it takes effort to make them think outside of their traditional spheres of expertise. For instance, it isn't common for surgeons to be worried about the diabetic biochemical profile (medications); for internists to be aware of the ulcers, the neuropathies, and how to treat these conditions, and how to appropriately refer for assistive ambulatory devices. Young physicians in training tend to ignore the areas they don't feel comfortable with. When you quiz them about what can be done for ulcers and foot deformities they don't know. When asked, "Why don't you consider *a referral to podiatry for this patient?" they may reply, "I don't know what they can do."*

*"Have you addressed the ulcer that's developing on the foot?"*

*"Well, no."*

*"Is the ulcer about to get worse?"*

*"Yes, but I don't know what to do for it."*

*Again, in a teaching role, kindly but positively, steering the practitioner to recognize when they need to call another healthcare professional with a different sphere of competency and expertise. We'd like to do all things for all patients, but to think about what someone else can do to help that patient is the next level of learning. It has been a joy and a constant effort in my work with young healthcare professionals to get them to think beyond their own areas of expertise, particularly in the care of diabetic feet.*

Foot specialists often hold the key to unlocking the mystery of foot pain and can return patients to their normal lives when other medical practitioners fail. Oftentimes, podiatrists are the last medical professionals consulted about a foot problem when, in fact, they should have been the first. It is because of this awareness-gap that patients often miss opportunities to receive appropriate diagnosis and proper treatment for their problems in a timely fashion. In some cases, this lost time can be critical and can mean the difference between keeping or losing a foot or leg. This is where a multi-disciplinary team would greatly benefit the patient. Each professional would know what care/education the others on the team are giving the patient. Together, they would be able to provide the right combination of drugs and therapy to help the patient heal quicker.

The development of the educational process has given podiatrists much credibility, and today, they are involved in all varieties of research involving the foot and lower leg. It is true that podiatrists still cut nails and trim corns and calluses, but our expertise and skills are far greater. In many communities podiatrists live in the shadow of orthopedics, so we're kind of like Avis™: we have to try harder.

I'm very proud of my profession because it serves a legitimate medical need. It's always wonderful when someone comes in with pain and leaves saying, "It feels better." I always say to the patient, "Aren't you glad I went to school the day they taught that?"

## Foot Notes: Five Foot Problems That Shouldn't Be Ignored

Many people choose not to see a doctor when they have foot problems; however, there are five foot problems that should never be ignored:[1]

1. Heel pain is usually caused by soft tissue inflammation but can also be the result of a broken bone, a tight Achilles tendon, a pinched nerve, or other problem.

2. Ankle sprains require prompt medical attention. Choosing to skip medical care increases the likelihood of repeated ankle sprains and the development of chronic ankle instability.

3. Big toe joint stiffness and pain usually develop over time as the cartilage in the big toe joint wears down and eventually leads to arthritis. The sooner a doctor diagnoses it, the easier it is to treat.
4. Achilles tendonitis causes pain and tenderness at the back of the foot or heel. This is usually the result of a sudden increase in physical activity. The risk of an Achilles tendon rupture can be reduced by promptly treating the symptoms.
5. Ingrown toenails can pierce the skin, allowing bacteria to enter the body. You should never attempt to perform dangerous "bathroom surgery." A doctor can perform a quick procedure that will stop the pain and permanently cure an ingrown toenail.

You may want to watch one of the very informative videos at http://www.asiasbestdoctors.com/story_1385.html

**Six Questions Every Patient with Diabetes Should Ask His Physician:**

1. Will you please examine my feet?
2. Can you do a monofilament test to determine if I have sensory neuropathy?
3. Can you check my pulses and tell me about my circulation?
4. Do I have any bone, soft tissue, or nail deformities?
5. If I qualify for diabetic shoes (from Medicare), can you help with the paperwork?
6. Can you refer me to a podiatrist for foot care?

# Chapter Four

## The Role of the Caregiver

### Tweeners

He's in a white tee shirt, has a really big belly and is wearing red and blue striped suspenders. Or, perhaps he's wearing overalls with a plaid shirt and his chapeau is an old baseball cap. Maybe he has on a military-type jump suit and looks like a cross between Jack Lalane and my father when he returned home from the South Pacific in WWII.

Female tweeners are not that common in our office. When she does come out, her daughter or granddaughter usually accompanies her. More likely than not, she is a widow. If her spouse is still living, sometimes both he and she are, as Paul Harvey would say "on the road to forever together," and are accompanied by family to the office. She's still properly dressed, and with a little help still manages to get some makeup on. Her straw purse remains her favorite. She is generally in better shape than he is, but not always.

If he lives alone, sometimes his clothes are not clean and neither is he. He doesn't see or hear very well and his feet look like they have not been washed in the past month. He walks slowly with a cane or walker. He shuffles his feet with an occasional stumble that would make most folks fearful that he might fall, but he is not concerned.

He usually lives close enough to his family that they can keep an eye on him, but they don't visit him too frequently because of work and family pressures. He may live alone or with his wife of fifty-plus years, and in some cases the behavior between the two of them makes me wonder how they get through the day. Sometimes he is confused about what day it is, or if he took his medicine that morning. He may not remember what he ate for dinner last night.

In the best of situations, his wife is still with him and makes all the decisions about the daily issues of his life. She makes sure he takes medicine, gets a bath, and has food to eat. In general, she runs the home while he watches TV or reads the newspaper. Many times he refuses to cooperate with her because he is just plain stubborn. In some cases, he has a legitimate medical reason for not cooperating; he may have Alzheimer's disease or a mild form of dementia. Regardless of the reason, this patient is in between being able to understand what is happening around him and being willing to take his medications, control his behaviors or do whatever is necessary to heal a foot wound. He is in a category that few recognize and even fewer want to talk about because it is so tough. He is a "tweener."

I first heard the word tweener as a child listening to the legendary Pittsburgh Pirates announcer, Bob Prince, on the car radio while riding with my father. Dad played pitcher at Peabody High School in Pittsburgh. And, at age 85, Dad still loved baseball. When I would go home to visit him and Mom in Albuquerque, I would usually find him in his favorite lounge chair, feet tipped toward the sky with a baseball game on the tube. It could be the pros, it could be a college game, and I have even seen him watching high school games. He especially enjoyed seeing the Cubs against the Pirates and would tease my Chicago-raised mom with something like, "My Pirates are going to beat your Cubs." I bought him a Pirates Cap for his last birthday. My dad passed away during the writing of this book.

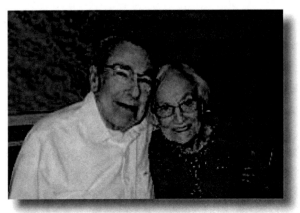

**Mark's parents**

A tweener was a ball that was hit in such a way that it landed between two outfielders. Even though both of them ran at top speed trying to catch the ball, neither was able to get to it before it hit the ground and dropped in for a single base hit. The term seems to appropriately describe those patients who are not completely able to take care of themselves but really don't fit into the category of being unable to self-care. I also use the word for patients who are barely able to understand what we are talking about concerning their foot problems and those who don't have a clue.

Some tweeners are fortunate because their family recognizes when they have become a tweener and makes adjustments for them. They may move closer to or actually move in with their tweener. In many cases, tweeners have money and can relocate to an adult living facility that lets them live alone but with assistance. Some tweeners have neither family nor money, and it is these folks who need to be identified. Our social services safety net should be there to catch them before they fall. Fortunately, there are home healthcare services that can come to the rescue. Unfortunately, these services tend to be for temporary emergency care, and once they depart, the scene reverts back to where it was.

Being the wife or husband of a tweener is not easy. Being the caregiver of a tweener can be a relentless full-time job. I have seen mostly women serving as the caregiver for their husbands. In many instances these caregivers suffer as much or more than their mates but in different ways. They suffer from feelings of guilt; they worry about finances and how they are going to afford medication; they stress over their inability to convince their mate to "behave" properly; they take them to and from doctor appointments and perform home health treatments; they make a frustrated attempt to get their loved one to take their medicine and make healthy food choices. Many caregivers are closely involved with blood sugar control and some even have to prick the tweener's finger to get a blood sample for the glucose monitor.

I have often heard caregivers in my office say, "See? The doctor also says not to use your penknife to cut your nails."

Over the years, I have noted that when a patient has a significant other in their life, they seem to do better than those who live alone.

"Put your shoes on!"

"Did you take your medicine?"

"Have you eaten anything?"

Could it be that the gentle, constant, loving harassment and reinforcement of good prevention behaviors makes the difference?

## KC and Glenda

Mr. KC was a seventy-year-old, type 2 diabetic who came to the clinic on an emergency basis. He was referred by his PCP because of a suspicious skin lesion on the bottom of his left foot. KC was accompanied by his wife, Glenda. I could barely see her face when she sat down in the visitor chair in our treatment room. She was carrying both of their coats, several bags of holiday gifts they had purchased in the hospital gift shop, and a large clear plastic bag filled with bottles of her husband's pills. The hospital policy asks the patient to bring all of their pills with them for their visits. I have seen patients walking around with large bags filled with pill bottles containing as many as twenty or more medications. Some patients even bring their medication in gym bags or back packs.

KC wore thick glasses. The lenses were so dirty I wondered how he could see anything through them. He had a habit of looking over the top of them that I found a bit unnerving. I wondered why he didn't just take them off and clean them, but such is common with a tweener.

"I have a thick piece of skin on the bottom of my foot that bothers me," KC grumbled.

"He picks on it while watching TV," Glenda tattled. "He will get a corner loose and tear off the skin. The last time he did this was a few days ago and now the area is red, swollen, and warm. I told him not to do that, but he never listens to me."

Our examination revealed an area below the big toe on the left foot that showed thickening of skin, and the area where KC had torn the skin off was infected. After debriding and removing the remainder of the thick skin and devitalized tissue, we found an ulcer approximately one centimeter in diameter. A weight-bearing X-ray was taken with a wire marker on the site of the ulcer to determine if there was a bone infection under the ulcer. The marker permits us to see the relationship between the skin lesion and the underlying bony structures and learn whether a bony structure was involved in the skin lesion, ulcer, or infection.

KC was wearing diabetic shoes at the time of his visit, which might suggest that his feet were protected, but this is not always true. The bones in the foot can rub against the shoe, and cause infections and ulcers. In KC's case, the head of the first metatarsal, which is located just behind his big toe, was lower than the level of the other four metatarsal bones. This means that the first metatarsal was hitting the ground before the other bones and was bearing more weight and pressure with each step. Routine evaluations of KC's shoes and insoles might have revealed the faulty insole, and he might not have developed the callus that led to his ulcer if the insole had been changed when it bottomed out. If KC's foot had been evaluated for biomechanical function, he might have been wearing a biomechanical orthotic instead of the Plastizote® insole that came with the shoe.

We treated KC with oral antibiotics, a topical debriding agent, and a special surgical shoe that repositioned his foot to relieve the pressure on the affected area. We replaced his worn-out diabetic shoes with a new pair and provided him with biomechanical orthotics and ongoing foot care to prevent a reoccurrence of the callus. KC was instructed to inspect his shoes, insoles, and feet daily, and to stop picking at his foot. We see KC for ongoing care every six months. By following our suggestions and Glenda's pleading, he has not had any further problems.

## Mr. Biggun's Story

Mr. Biggun came to my office weighing over 300 pounds. He was a former alcoholic who had been told multiple times to eat less and exercise more, but he couldn't pull it together. His issues were more complex than I could help him with, so I referred him to the kinesio-therapist to get him started on an exercise program, and to the nutritionist to help him figure out what he should and shouldn't eat. We even talked about gastric bypass surgery. He said, "My head's not together enough to do that."

Mr. Biggun and many patients with diabetes have psychological issues and could benefit from therapy with a professional. "Why don't you put a picture of yourself on your bathroom mirror—one from a time when you felt better about your weight?" I suggested. He needed to love himself, but he had stopped doing this. "I want you to look into the mirror and say, 'I love you, and I'm going to take care of you. I'm going to do the right thing starting today.'"

He laughed at the thought of doing this, but there was a sadness in his laugh. For a physician to suggest to someone that they have got to lose weight typically frustrates the patient, and can cause him to be overwhelmed by the burden of having to accomplish weight loss along with everything else they must do. Ultimately, the responsibility for losing weight and most preventive practices must come from the patient.

**Foot Notes: Checklist for Caregiver**

Here are a few things you can do to take care of yourself while you care for your tweener.

- Take time off! Even if it is only thirty minutes a day, do something for yourself. Separating yourself from the demanding scene will enable you to rejuvenate your own energy level and recharge your batteries before returning to your duties. You might enjoy a hobby that gives you a chance to be creative. Spend time alone or with a friend. The stimulation of friendship and laughter can go a long way to help relieve stress and lighten your load.

- Ask other members of your family to assist you. Perhaps you could ask a friend or neighbor to sit with your tweener while you get out for a while. A change of scenery can give you a fresh perspective as you walk back into your situation.

- Get some exercise and make sure you maintain a healthy eating regimen. Keeping your own body in good shape will help you manage your stress level. A yoga class is a good choice because it gently stretches and works all the muscles in your body.

- Hire someone to help with the chores. Ask a responsible teenager in your neighborhood to do your grocery shopping from a list you prepare. You might consider paying the teen or someone else to prepare meals ahead of time. Then, you can take the meal out of the freezer and heat it in the microwave. There are services that will deliver prepared meals to your door. A cleaning service could tackle the household work once a week.

- Talk to someone. It could be a friend or you could see a therapist who will let you vent and get the stress off your shoulders. Keeping all your thoughts and feelings to yourself only leads to internal stress for your body and emotions.

# Chapter Five

## Putting Your Best Foot Forward (Biomechanics)

> *Feet: One pair must last a lifetime*
> —American Podiatric Medical Association

The foot is an unusually sturdy, not to mention complex, structure. Each foot has more than forty muscles and tendons, thirty-three complex joints, 107 ligaments, and twenty-six bones (which together adds up to more than one-quarter of the 208 bones in the body). Each foot also has two sesamoid bones below the big toe joint. Knowing this, one would agree with Michelangelo: "The foot is an engineering masterpiece and a work of art."

People watching is one of the great attractions of life. If you watch people on the sidewalks, in a crowded airport terminal, in an office building, or in a shopping mall, you will see one of the best shows on earth happening right before your eyes. These people are doing something miraculous and yet few realize that they are even doing it. What is this mysterious activity? Walking.

Most of us take the ability to walk for granted, and most of us barely give our feet a second thought unless we are having a problem with one of them or perhaps when shopping for a new pair of shoes. However, our ability to walk takes a series of complex actions that involves all of our body systems—nervous, musculoskeletal, and circulatory—controlled by our brain. We don't typically put much thought into how each body part contributes to the process unless we're watching a baby take her first steps, seeing a loved one in a wheelchair or sickbed, or if we're having to learn to walk again because of a stroke or accident.

The circumference of Earth is 24,901.55 miles at the equator.[1] The average person walks approximately 115,000 miles in a lifetime, which equals 4.4 trips around the Earth. Walking gives us the freedom to choose where and when we want to go and how fast we want to get there. Walking allows us to freely conduct the affairs of our daily lives without depending on others. While we go through life without giving much thought as to how we get from point A to point B, this concern is much different for an amputee. Ask any person who has lost a foot or leg and they will tell you the world is a different place when you lose the ability to walk. Patients with a below-the-knee amputation must work three times harder to walk with a prosthesis. Patients with an above-the-knee amputation exert five times the effort to walk as compared to those of us with all of our original parts.

Walking is one of the healthiest exercises you can do. Walking is good for your heart, brains, bowels, and spirit. Though exercise improves most anyone's health, for the patient with diabetes, it is even more essential. Exercise improves insulin resistance, increases the circulation, decreases cardiovascular disease, decreases blood sugar levels, and helps control weight.

Our feet were designed to function on uneven terrain, but the necessity of travel and commerce has led to our walking on hard, flat surfaces, on which they were *not* designed to function. Podiatrists have special understanding of not only the physiological functioning of the foot but also of how the foot functions biomechanically. The foot of the patient with diabetes is subjected to the same physical forces as everyone else's foot; however, because of immunopathy, vascular and neurological disease, the diabetic foot is at a disadvantage when it comes to wound healing. It is the understanding of the interaction between the foot, the shoes, the supporting surface, and the effects of physics that give the podiatrist an advantage over other medical providers when it comes to healing a diabetic foot wound. Without understanding the biomechanical functioning of the foot, even the best wound care is doomed to failure.

It is easy to understand why podiatry is an important part of maintaining good foot health. Let's look at several of the issues that affect the diabetic foot and how a podiatrist helps a person with diabetes sustain their ability to walk.

## Biomechanics

In the last half of the twentieth century, research on the diabetic foot has provided new information concerning its diagnosis, pathology, and treatment. Evidence-based medicine techniques have given us a better understanding of the best and most cost-effective types of foot care in the area of anatomy, physiology, or biomechanics. We understand how these three entities can work harmoniously to achieve the normal function of the foot. We have developed sophisticated tools to diagnose and treat complex and everyday foot problems that have affected the lives of millions since humans started walking upright on two feet.

If you have diabetes, it is critical that you understand how the foot functions, what might cause a foot problem and what opportunities are available today for you to take advantage of to prevent a foot ulcer, or worse—losing part of your foot or leg. As a preventive measure, you should take action to address any problems that affect your foot. You can do this with a foot exam for biomechanical evaluation, footwear, medication, or surgery.

Podiatrists literally wrote the book on walking, the gait cycle, and biomechanics. In the early 1960s, Dr. Merton Root, one of the most influential educators in the podiatric profession, developed his structural theory of biomechanics and established the early pioneering foundations of modern podiatric biomechanics. Dr. Verne Inman wrote a series of articles on the functioning of the human foot from the late 1940s through the 1970s. Dr. D.J. Morton published articles on feet and function from the late 1930s well into the 1950s.

Over the past eighty years, investigators have gone from forming opinions of how the foot functions by visually cataloging arch height and foot width to a sophisticated analysis of the bones, gait and foot function. In the biomechanical exam, we look at the position of the foot bones, joints, and range of motion. Specifically, we look at:

- the ankle joint (the joint formed by the two long bones of the leg, the tibia, and fibula, and the square-shaped foot bone that fits between them called the talus),

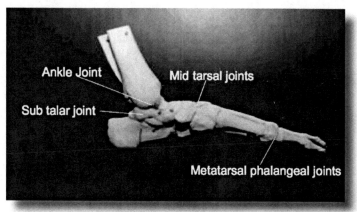

**Foot joints side view**

- the subtalar joint (the joint between the calcaneus and the talus)

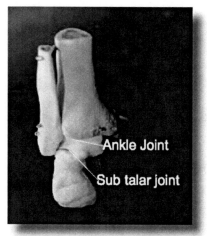

**Ankle & Subtalar Joint**

- mid-tarsal joint (the bones that run across the middle part of the foot)

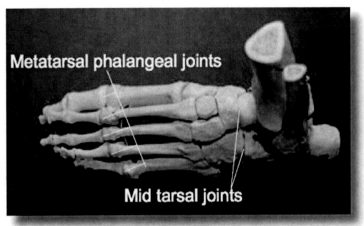

**Metatarsal & Midtarsal Joints**

- great toe joint.

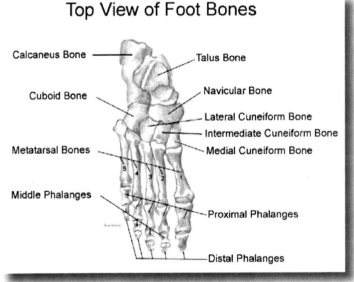

**Foot Model Top**

# Side View of Foot Bones

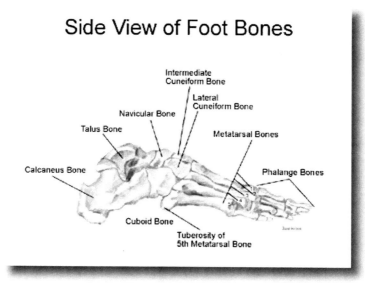

Foot Model Side

Structural or bony deformities such as bunions, tailor's bunions, digital deformities, and soft tissue deformities such as corns and calluses are the markers that might indicate there is a biomechanical or functional problem with the foot. The feet are like the foundation of a building. If the foundation is solid, the walls won't crack and the floors don't creak. Otherwise, there will be problems. The human body reacts in similar ways. I often see patients who suffer with ankle, knee, hip, or low back pain that may be partly caused by faulty foot mechanics and function.

## Balance

Our eyes, ears, and central nervous system are key to maintaining our stability. Our vision tells us where we are in relation to the rest of the world and is a tremendous help in our everyday activities. Our balance is also helped by our inner ear. When we move, our central nervous system receives information from our nerve receptors embedded in muscles and tendons.

Most people are introduced to the concept of balance (and gravity) when they learn how to walk, ride a bicycle, or roller skate. As we age, we tend to lose our ability to balance ourselves and some older adults fear falling. In fact, some senior citizens do not want their family to know they have problems with their balance for fear their family will remove them from their home and relocate them to assisted living facilities.

A study by Chamberlain and colleagues in 2005 identified patients they called "fearful walkers." These patients adopted a slower walking speed and shorter stride length than fearless walkers. Foot problems like corns, calluses, hammertoes, or bunions may result in uneven balance. Another reason for falling is a result of taking too many drugs, since some medications cause dizziness or lightheadedness. Podiatrists are able to identify patients who have higher risk of falling by watching and analyzing their gait.

Dr. Jim Powers, associate professor of medicine at Vanderbilt University in Nashville, and his colleagues have developed a geriatric program and serve many community agencies fostering services for seniors. He says that the older patient rarely comes to his office with only one illness; most elderly patients come with multiple comorbidities. Therefore, your guidelines or standards of care for each individual illness tend to accumulate. You may find that some of the guidelines actually interact negatively with the patient's care. For instance, keeping blood sugar low or blood pressure under control may predispose a patient for more falls.

Many have poly-pharmacy issues with drug interactions. A patient may spend the entire day taking medicines and checking their blood sugar level. That's not an appropriate quality of life when you've got to follow guidelines for three or four or five diseases. It comes down to clinical judgment, but where we have guidance in literature, it's a big support for what we do. For instance, with a patient who's losing weight and falling, it may be appropriate for the blood sugar or blood pressure to run high. Sometimes we have to ignore the need for lowering cholesterol just to make sure the patient has an adequate diet. Otherwise, that patient's risk for falling is increased. If that patient sustains a fracture, we would have to deal with other consequences such as pneumonia, urinary tract infection, or perhaps institutional care.

There are common, and not so common, foot problems that can lead to bone or soft tissue deformities, pain and functional disability. These include bunions and digital deformities, heel or nerve pain, and corns, calluses, and ingrown toenails. In some patients, we see problems of gait and ambulation that manifest as tired feet and legs or difficulty standing for long time periods. Some patients report difficulty walking for medium to long distances, others may have knee, hip, or low back pain, while still others may have problems with balance and falling.

## Gait Cycle Interruptus

Walking is nothing more than a series of controlled falls, and our feet have a starring role. In walking, as your center of gravity moves forward (for men this is generally closer to the shoulders, for women it's generally closer to the hips), if your foot doesn't come out in front of you, you can expect to fall right on your face. Scientists refer to the complex musculo-skeletal events that occur when you walk as the "gait cycle." The gait cycle is divided into three phases: contact, mid-stance, and propulsive phases. When everything goes right, you get from here to there without even thinking about it. When things don't go right, you can develop foot, leg, and even low back problems.

Gait (the manner or pattern in which a person walks) and ambulation (their ability to move) are of particular interest to me and this is an area that most general medical practitioners don't understand. Podiatrists have the training, skills, and knowledge to understand the relationship between gait, ambulation, and foot biomechanics, and how these three affect each other and the patient's foot health.

Understanding gait cycle and biomechanics is critical to understanding foot function and why people develop foot deformities and pain. Biomechanical theory also gives me a tool to understand why faulty foot function causes patients with diabetes to develop ulcers on their feet. It gives me the understanding so I may control foot function to prevent a re-occurrence of that ulcer. Understanding biomechanical function is critical to the foot health of patients with diabetes. Podiatric biomechanics is considered a core subject that is universally taught in podiatric medical education. It takes two years to complete the full course of study and a lifetime to perfect the implementation of this special science.

There are several systems that must function harmoniously and simultaneously in order for us to move in space or walk. These include the anatomy (how it's made), the physiology (how it lives), and the mechanics (how it moves or functions) of the foot. The foot has multiple joints that perform complex functions. The most miraculous is changing a vertical force from the leg into a horizontal force in the foot, thus allowing us to walk. This is achieved because the bones and joints of the foot have a range of motion that can permit them to change their position relative to each other during the gait cycle.

Foot function is influenced by a series of factors that include:

- The size, shape, position, and condition of foot bones and joints they form
- The normal functioning of the vascular, neurological, and musculo-skeletal systems
- The surface we are standing on
- The speed at which we are moving and
- The type of footgear we are wearing

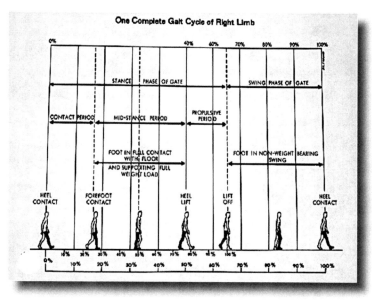

During the gait cycle, the foot should be in a particular position at a particular time in order to function as nature intended. The phases of the gait cycle and the functions of the foot in normal gait include:

- *Phase 1, Contact*: The foot is in the "loose" position as it contacts the ground, and the function of the foot is to be a mobile adaptor to the terrain—whether standing on rocks, sand, gravel, and whether going uphill or downhill. The foot should come out in front of our body as it moves forward to prevent falling.

- *Phase 2, Mid-stance*: The foot should be neither loose nor locked—it should be neutral. The function of the foot is to support the body's weight, and the entire bottom of the foot is involved.

- *Phase 3, Propulsive*: The foot should be in the "locked" position. The body weight has passed over the foot and the function of the foot changes to that of a rigid lever for propulsion moving the body forward. The toes help the body balance, and the great toe, especially, does the work of pushing the body forward to take the next step.

If the feet have faulty biomechanical function, the gait or the way a person walks may vary from the normal gait cycle. A person may have difficulty standing for long periods of time or walking for long distances. A patient with diabetes should see a healthcare provider about preventing bony and soft tissue problems that can lead to amputation.

Why do some people develop foot deformities and have pain while others seem immune to the problem? A large part of the answer lies in the biomechanics of foot function. Staying in the "loose" position in the propulsive phase of gait is one reason why patients develop foot problems. If your foot remains "loose" during propulsion, we say that you walk with a pronated gait. That is, your foot rolls over and flattens on the inside instead of being "locked" in a straight position.

One might think that when the foot rolls over and flattens, that you have a flat foot. That may not be true. Caution: when it comes to understanding the foot and its function, one can't necessarily go by what the foot looks like when it touches the floor, bearing weight. It's what the foot looks like when it's not weight bearing that helps determine if the foot has a high arch or low arch. This very common problem means that the first metatarsal (the long bone behind the big toe) may have a larger than normal range of motion and fails to support the foot, which stays in the "loose" position for too long during the gait cycle. When the foot flattens out, this causes the muscles, tendons, and joints to be overused. As per Newton's third law of relativity, for every action there's an equal and opposite reaction. When the foot rolls over and pushes down on the floor, the floor pushes back with an equal force. That motion causes several common foot problems including joint misalignment, heel spurs, and pinched nerves.

Foot dysfunction may contribute to knee, hip, or low back pain that may not respond to conventional therapy. These problems do respond to restoring normal biomechanical foot function. In the diabetic foot, faulty mechanics can create excessive pressure against a bony surface. This activates the body's natural protective mechanism causing a thickening of skin that we see as corns or calluses. Left untreated, these soft tissue lesions can become a trigger for amputation.

## Balance, Falling, and Peripheral Neuropathy

In *Diabetes Care*, Ann V. Schwartz, PhD, Associate Adjunct Professor, Division of Clinical Trials & Multicenter Studies and her team at the University of California, San Francisco, published an article that revealed, "Diabetes-related complications of reduced peripheral nerve function, reduced vision, and renal function are associated with increased risk of falls. Reduced balance, strength, and gait are likely intermediaries in any association between diabetes-related complications and risk of falls."[2] Improved glycemic control (blood glucose control) prevents progression of nerve and eye problems in patients with diabetes and is likely to prevent falls. This is another benefit of keeping blood glucose levels under control.

## Foot Notes: How Smart Is Your Right Foot?

Try this. It will boggle your mind and you will keep trying over and over again to see if you can outsmart your right foot, Chances are you can't. It's preprogrammed in your brain!

Without anyone watching you (they might think you are goofy) perhaps while sitting at your desk in front of your computer, lift your right foot off the floor and make clockwise circles.

Now, while doing this, draw the number "6" in the air with your right hand. Your foot will change direction, and there's nothing you can do to stop it!

I experimented with the foot circle by keeping my foot connected with the floor. I was able to draw the number 6 with my right hand without my foot changing directions only when I kept my foot in contact with a surface. I have no idea why the brain can process opposite motions when touching a surface, but not when suspended.

Perhaps there is something we can learn from this experiment. This experiment shows one way we can learn how our own nervous system works. We can get a "feel" for the complexities and subtleties of its function and our ability to control it.

The patient with diabetic neuropathy may not experience the sensation of their foot moving or changing direction or position.

# Chapter Six

## Common Foot Problems

> *I can't think when my feet hurt*
> —Abraham Lincoln

More than 70 percent of Americans suffer from painful foot problems at some time in their lives. My grandmother, Grandma Honey, as we called her, would occasionally mention that her feet hurt. I remember her taking off her shoes and rubbing her feet. Her toes did not look like my toes; they were stubby and crooked and she had a knot at her big toe joint. Her big toe tucked under her second toe. On one occasion, she even mentioned to me that she went to the foot doctor. She said, "He put a needle to my foot because I had so much pain."

As a young child, I wondered why grandmother's feet looked so bad and hurt so much. Foot deformities can be a trigger that starts the cascade of events leading to soft tissue infection, ulceration, and bone infection that can result in amputation. Deformities of the foot come in three categories: bone (osseous), soft tissue, and nail.

When we deal with a person's body, we must know what anatomical structures are located in what location in order to understand why something has gone wrong. Without knowing the anatomy of the foot, it is virtually impossible to diagnose one of the over three hundred problems affecting the foot, and even more difficult to fix it.

### Bone (Osseous) Deformities

Common bone problems include bunions (a deformity of the big toe joint), bone spurs, digital deformities like hammertoe, mallet toe, claw toe, and tailor's bunion. By the way, tailor's bunion gets its name because before the use of sewing machines, tailors would sit cross-legged on the floor allowing the outside of the fifth toe to rub against the floor as they stitched. Each of these bone deformities presents an opportunity to develop a corn or a callus (a keratosis).

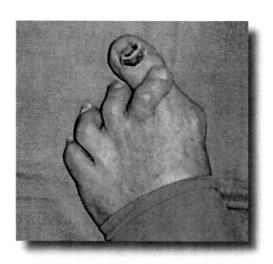

**Mallet Toe: 4th toe
is contracted at the distal joint**

The digital deformities are the result of faulty biomechanical function that leaves the normally straight toes deformed. The deformities are classified by their location. Since there are three bones in each of the toes except the big toe, there are opportunities for deformities at each of the joints.

Hammer toe is a toe with a deformity at the proximal joint. Sometimes a corn forms on the top of the toe.

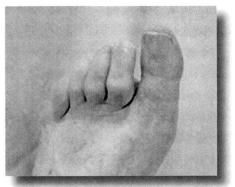

**Hammer Toes**

The mallet toe is a toe with a deformity at the distal joint. You can have a corn on the tip or top of the toe.

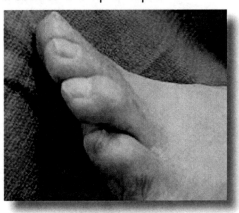

**Mallet Toes**

Claw toe is the worst deformity because both joints are deformed, so it's an equal opportunity problem—you can have a thickened skin anywhere on the toes.

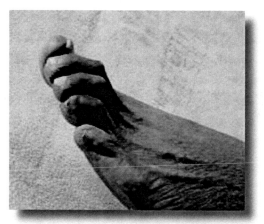

**Claw Toe: 4th toe is contracted at both at the proximal and distal joints.**

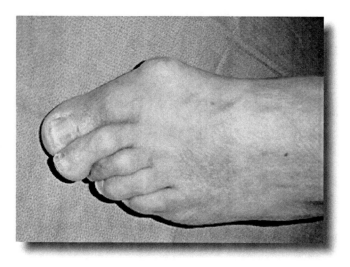

**Bunion**

A bunion is the result of the big toe joint being out of alignment. The first metatarsal bone begins to move toward the opposite foot and the great toe moves in the opposite direction, toward the fifth toe of the same foot. At times the second toe may overlap the great toe. Normally, the great toe joint functions as a freely-moving hinge. It's not supposed to rotate or move crossways; only up and down. Because of the deformity, the head of the first metatarsal can rub against the shoe and cause a blister. These are dangerous in the at-risk and patient with diabetes because an abscess or ulcer can develop, which can become infected and lead to a bone infection (osteomyelitis).

A tailor's bunion is similar to a bunion of the great toe joint, except it occurs at the fifth toe joint. It too is the result of a misalignment of the metatarsal-phalangeal joint in the smallest (fifth) toe.

Patients with diabetes who have bone deformities need to pay special attention to their footgear. They must use shoes that have enough room to accommodate the deformities and won't rub against the foot.

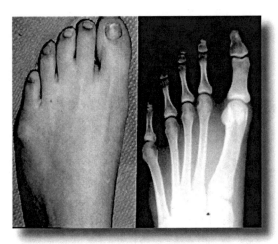

**Tailor's Bunion**

In the foot, most people have two sesamoid bones located within the long flexor tendon that runs under the first metatarsal, the bone just behind the big toe (hallux). While they can greatly benefit the ability to walk, they also can be the source of pain, functional disability, and the secret cause of foot ulcers. Sesamoid bones are part of a sophisticated system of natural pulleys and levers to provide the muscles with mechanical advantage in function. They help the big toe with the power to propel the body forward in the push-off phase of gait.

## The Charcot Foot or Neurogenic Arthropathy

The Charcot foot is a foot deformity that is the result of sensory neuropathy, a malfunction of the sensory nervous system resulting in loss of protective sensation (LOPS) in the foot. It was first described in the nineteenth century by neurologist, Jean-Martin Charcot. Then, it was mostly seen in patients with syphilis. In modern times, is it mostly seen in patients with diabetes.

An offshoot of *sensory neuropathy*, Charcot foot, occurs when the mid-part of the foot literally collapses because the bones give out. It's rarely painful but it causes the foot to become unstable; the mid-foot can become flat as a pancake. These bones can easily fracture, and the joints can dislocate and cause a collapse of the mid-foot. When the mid-foot begins to protrude, it may cause the bottom of the foot to ulcerate. It can take a year or more to heal a Charcot foot using a cast-like device called a cam walker, or a total contact cast. The best solution is to place the patient in a below-the-knee, non-weight-bearing cast and get him off of his feet completely.

The Charcot foot is characterized by increased blood flow, which results in a loss of calcium in the foot bones. It is a progressive, destructive condition usually accompanied by redness, elevated skin temperature and swelling, as well as bounding pulses. It can be difficult to diagnose because it may appear that the patient has a bone infection. Lab testing, X-rays as well as bone and soft tissue scans are helpful to determine if there is joint inflammation, fracture, dislocation, or an infection of the soft tissues or bone.

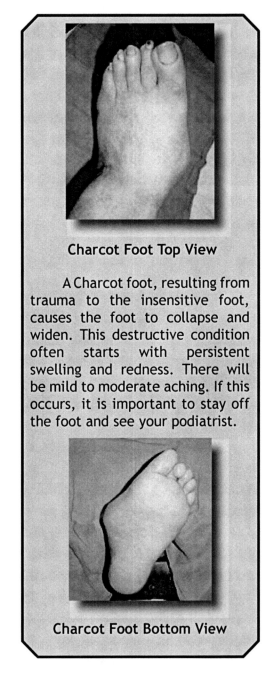

**Charcot Foot Top View**

A Charcot foot, resulting from trauma to the insensitive foot, causes the foot to collapse and widen. This destructive condition often starts with persistent swelling and redness. There will be mild to moderate aching. If this occurs, it is important to stay off the foot and see your podiatrist.

**Charcot Foot Bottom View**

Some patients with the Charcot foot can benefit from reconstructive surgery that can be performed by foot and ankle surgeons who have special training in this condition. The recovery is a very involved ordeal and non-compliant patients who are not willing or able to go through the follow-up care, may be just as well off with a below-knee amputation.

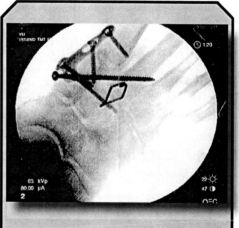

In early cases of the deformity, before the bone and joints collapse, surgical stabilization of the foot can be accomplished by using screws, plates, or wires.

This is not always in the best interest of the patient, but all aspects (physical, mental, emotional well being) of the patient should be considered before any decision is made for reconstructive surgery or amputation.

## Soft Tissue Deformities

Common soft tissue problems include corns, calluses, porokeratosis, (plugged up sweat gland ducts), and scar tissue. People with abnormal function of the foot or faulty biomechanics typically have foot problems involving gait and ambulation including: difficulty walking, problems with balance and inflammatory soft tissue problems (the "itis" family) falling, and injuries due to overuse or micro-trauma. The "itis" family includes bursitis, capsulitis, tendonitis, myositis, fasciitis, and neuritis.

### Corns and Calluses (Keratosis)

Keratosis is the technical name for soft tissue lesions of the foot. Keratosis are formed as a natural protective mechanism when an abnormal pressure is noted against a bony structure. Whether corns or calluses, keratosis can be trimmed by your podiatrist for foot comfort. A pad can be used to protect the area and these soft tissue deformities can be surgically corrected on a permanent basis. In the case where one piece of bone rubs against a piece of bone in the adjacent toe, the answer is an in-office or out-patient procedure. We make a small incision, file the bone down, put in one stitch, and the patient goes home. Many times patients only need minimal pain medication.

Heloma durum, or a hard corn, is typically located on the top or distal tip of toe.

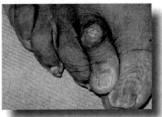

Hard Corn on
2nd Toe

A soft corn is called a heloma molle. It is called a soft corn because it is located between the toes and is kept soft by the moisture between the toes.

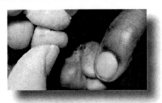

Soft Corn
between Toes

Calluses are located under the metatarsal heads and are often mistaken for a wart.

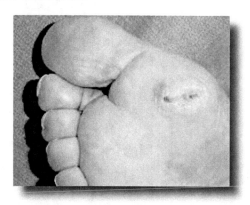

Callus with Hemorrhage.

## Porokeratosis

Porokeratosis is a common skin lesion that is usually found on the non-weight bearing surfaces the bottom of the foot. It appears as a small seed-like skin lesion. It appears like a miniature callus. Patients describe the feeling of a porokeratosis as "like standing on a stone." It is often misdiagnosed as a wart.

## Warts

There are so many physicians who think that no matter what it is, if it's on the bottom of the foot, it's a wart. This is not necessarily true. A wart (or verruca) is caused by the human papaloma virus family. Warts take their oxygen and nourishment from the body and excrete their metabolic waste products into the body.

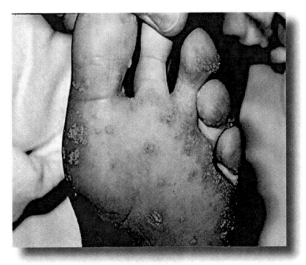

Warts

To identify warts, note how the normal skin lines are spread around the skin lesion. Pin-point bleeding occurs when a wart is debrided. There are little black spots that show where the wart has set up housekeeping and taken residence and sent a capillary (a little blood vessel) and plugged into the system. When we shave a wart, we slice through the capillary, and it starts to bleed, and a little black dot is left there. Multiple warts may indicate the patient has a compromised immune system or HIV.

Man has devised many torturous ways to treat warts. They can be frozen, burned electronically or with acid, or surgically removed. The problem is that they're so virulent that if we leave one cell, another whole lesion comes back and usually with a vengeance. The best way to treat them is by using a laser because the laser beam destroys all the wart cells and turns them to smoke.

## Neuroma, Foot Tumors, and Cysts

While the previous discussion has focused on superficial skin problems, no discussion of the diabetic foot would be complete without mentioning tumors of the skin and the deep structures. A tumor of nerve tissue, or a neuroma, is a common problem seen in women more than men. If I have ten patients scheduled, three of them will probably have nerve pain that might be caused by a neuritis or neuroma. Similar to a nerve entrapment, neuromas occur where the nerve passes between the foot bones and gets pinched. Think of a nerve as an electrical cord. There's the copper wire in the middle, which is the nerve, and the plastic covering, which is the nerve sheath. When there is pressure against the nerve (such as when the bones are pinching), the nerve sheath begins to swell to protect itself, and can become extremely painful. It can be difficult to know the source of a patient's foot pain, especially in a situation where there are local and systemic problems that affect the foot. For example, a patient may have diabetic peripheral neuropathy that causes numbness and pain, and he might have an unstable foot-type combined with faulty biomechanical function resulting in a local nerve entrapment, which can mimic neuropathy, or the nerve can be entrapped behind the ankle causing "tarsal tunnel syndrome." He may also have problems in his back like a pinched nerve or an arthritic bone spur that may cause radiating pain into the foot. This is called radicular pain or radiculopathy. How do we know which problem is the source of the pain? By understanding how both local and systemic factors can affect the foot and using all the tools available to test the patient for each possible diagnosis.

Tumors of the foot do occur, but luckily the majority of them are benign. The most common non-cancerous tumors of the foot are lipoma, fibroma, and neuroma. Cancerous tumors found on the foot include: kaposi sarcoma and malignant melanoma. Primary cancer malignancies of the foot are rare.

Cysts are fluid-filled soft tissue masses that usually originate from a joint capsule or tendon sheath. They usually contain a viscous fluid, are palpable, and easily treated.

Another area where soft tissue problems occur is on the bottom of the foot and the fat pads—they are amazing! Fat pads are made in chambers and are located under both the front of the foot and the heel. That's why the feet have such terrific shock absorption. There can be tumors of the fat pad (lipoma), derangements of the fat pad, or a person can lose the fat pad. This usually happens under the forefoot leaving the metatarsal heads unprotected and prone to ulcers. This is most commonly seen in patients with rheumatoid arthritis.

## Nail Deformities

Not a day goes by without someone asking me a question about toenails. More than any other foot problem, toenails are associated with podiatry. Perhaps it is because for millions of patients, only the podiatrist has the right tools, training, and special expertise necessary for proper foot care—especially nail care.

Perhaps the most common of all foot problems involves the toenails, and there are several types of problems that can affect the nails. The nails may be invaded by dermatophytes, mold, yeast, fungus, or bacteria. Ingrown toenails and thickened and deformed nails are also very common.

## Totally Dystrophic Nail Syndrome

The totally dystrophic nail syndrome occurs when there's been some damage (perhaps blunt force trauma) to the growth center of the nail called the matrix.It produces a deformed nail that you would swear had fungus on it, but the culture or PAS (Periodic Acid Schiff) test does not confirm the diagnosis. The PAS test is used to analyze anatomic pathology. If this nail problem is treated as a fungus infection without taking a specimen and sending it to the lab, the patient usually sees little, if any, clearing of the nail after treatment. The patient comes back in three months and says, "Doc, my toenail is as bad as it was when you gave me the medicine." The doctor says, "Oh, we must have had a medication failure." No we don't; we have a doctor failure. The doctor didn't do the right thing when he failed to send a specimen to confirm the diagnosis before prescribing the medication.

## The Ingrown Toenail

Also called onychia or paronychia, an ingrown toenail happens when a piece of nail gets imbedded in the soft tissue adjacent to the nail. To understand this problem and how to fix it, a short anatomy lesson is appropriate.

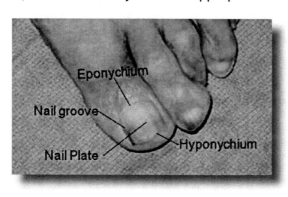

Toe Nail Diagram

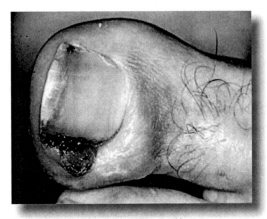

### Ingrown Toenail

At the base of the nail, under the skin near the eponychium, there is a specialized tissue called the matrix from which the nail grows. Think of the matrix as an envelope. The cells are on top and underneath, and the nail comes out from in between the two surfaces of the matrix. If you get an ingrown toenail, it's probably caused by one of three reasons. The first two are caused by improper nail trimming. When you trimmed the nail, you may have left a little piece near the edge or trimmed the nail too far back along the nail border. As the nail grows out it eventually becomes imbedded in the soft tissue next to the nail. The third reason is hereditary. A normal nail should have a nice, flat arc to it. Some people have very curved nail borders, and as a result, they're always fighting ingrown toenail problems.

Skin islands are portions of the nail bed that grow along with the nail. This small portion of soft tissue becomes surrounded by a deformed nail that is centrally elevated and deeply curved on both sides. This nail deformity can be seen on any of the toenails. It may be caused by a bone spur under the nail or by wearing narrow toe box shoes that deform the nails due to lack of appropriate space in the shoe and crowding of the toes. Patients may not recognize this small portion of soft tissue and when they trim their nails they actually cut the end of their toe along with the nail. Unnoticed and unfelt in the patient with diabetes and neuropathy, this self-inflicted wound can trigger a soft tissue infection.

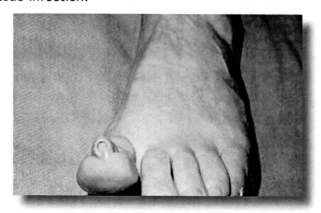

**Ingrown Toenail with Skin Island**

Typically, primary care providers like to treat this problem with antibiotics. They are paid to diagnose your health but they usually don't do procedures. It inevitably ends up with the doctor ripping a prescription off her pad and saying, "Take this antibiotic and have a great day." Primary care providers will look at an ingrown toenail not realizing that there's a piece of nail stuck in the skin. You can take antibiotics from now until they stop making them. The ingrown toenail is not going to go away because it's a mechanical problem that must be locally treated. The nail is growing into the skin. In order to make this problem go away on a permanent basis, we must use a tried and tested method to remove the nail spicule from the skin and prevent it from reoccurring:

- The toe is put to sleep with a local anesthesia block that can be done literally without any pain (fear of needles is a major cause of patients fearing foot care. If they only knew we can do this without hurting them.)

- A tourniquet is applied to the toe to prevent bleeding

- A sharp chisel-like scalpel or an English anvil nail splitter is used to cut out the piece of ingrown nail back to the matrix tissues. You have to permanently remove the offending portion of the nail in order to prevent reoccurrence. Taking a part of the nail or even the entire nail, will not prevent future problems. It may give temporary relief, but after the nail grows back, the nail is likely to grow back into the skin again. I have seen far too many patients who have had the entire nail removed, some more than once, only to be disappointed when the nail grows back and becomes ingrown and infected again.

- After the small portion of the nail is removed and the site is prepared, I put two applications of acid such as phenol (88 percent carbolic acid) to destroy the matrix cells that generate the small portion of the nail that was ingrown and removed. Some doctors use sodium hydroxide; however, phenol is a tested procedure that has been acceptable for patients with diabetes for about forty years. Then, I flush the site with alcohol and dress the wound.

A surgical shoe is important for the patient to wear after the procedure as we don't want to place a freshly operated foot into a closed and perhaps not clean shoe. This procedure kills the cells that generate the portion of nail that becomes ingrown. So, we're permanently getting rid of the problem. Actually, we're trading one problem for another—an ingrown toenail for a chemical burn. Now we have to heal the patient's chemical burn. There is "homework" in taking care of the operative sites but it is minimal. Still patients love me for fixing this problem. The good news is that this procedure is acceptable for patients with diabetes as long as they have adequate circulation and are willing to do the post op care.

**Nail Infections**

No discussion of foot infections would be complete without mentioning fungus infections of the nails, a common problem found in patients with diabetes. Since many have lost protective sensation and cannot feel pain, have poor vision, or don't inspect their feet, they may not be aware of this problem until there is pus or blood on their socks, and by then it is usually too late. Once there is an infection, it may be difficult to resolve without prolonged therapy with intravenous or oral antibiotics and surgery to remove any infected bone.

A fungal infection can cause the nail to thicken. A deformed and thickened toenail can lacerate the adjacent toe and cause an ulcer on the injured toe. Toenail deformities can cause an abscess to develop under the toenail when it rubs against the shoe. If this goes undetected, it can result in a bone infection. So, we need to pay attention to these types of infections.

Unfortunately, there continues to be a lack of understanding about this malady in the general medical community. Many medical practitioners fail to realize that a mycotic nail infection *is* an infection, which can be spread to others and that patients afflicted with this problem suffer both physical pain and have psychosocial issues because of the condition of their nails. This is why patients with diabetes with neuropathy and a toenail deformity should have professional foot care that includes debridement and trimming of the nail to prevent abscesses and lacerations.

Toenails are not usually affected by bacteria, but it can happen. Patients who have black-colored nails usually have a secondary infection contaminated with a bacteria known as aspergillis niger.

Dermatophytes, known as mold, yeast, and fungus, seem to thrive on skin and nails. A nail infected with a dermatophyte is called onychomycosis. The term onychomycosis is used to describe the combination of onycho=nail and mycosis=fungus or fungal toenail infection.

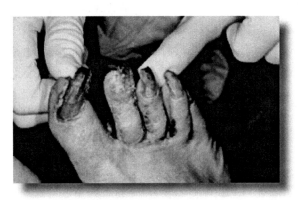

**Onychomycosis**

The great majority of thickened and diseased toenails are usually caused by an organism named T. Rubum or Tonsorinis Rubrim. The second most prevalent critter that can cause a fungal nail infection is named T-Mentagrophytes. Both of these dermatophytes can cause fungal skin infections that can be recognized by their typical redness, swelling, and itching. Understanding which fungal organism caused the fungus infection of the nail allows us to understand what we need to do to get rid of it. A nail specimen should be sent for laboratory testing to confirm that the nail is infected; and a blood test to check liver function should be done if oral anti-fungal medication will be used for treatment. Topical antifungal creams are not approved by the FDA for treatment of fungal infections of toenails and their use will not cure fungal toenails. Tests for fungal infections include dermatophyte test medium, fungal culture, and PAS (Periodic Acid Shift). The PAS is the same procedure used when a biopsy is done on tissue. For the nail deformity, we take a piece of nail, send it to the lab for a pathology exam where the specimen is frozen, sliced, put on a slide, and stained to look at it on the cellular level to identify the organism causing the nail infection. Additionally, the patient with diabetes and onychomycosis should have a professional foot exam, be evaluated for their circulation, have the monofilament test, and be checked for foot deformities.

Onychomycosis infections may be classified into five distinct categories:

1. Distal lateral sub ungual onychomycosis, which is the most common type of nail pathology;
2. Superficial white onychomycosis, which is a white layer of mycotic tissue that is easily removed with a nail file or emery board;

3. Proximal white onychomycosis, which is a white discoloration of the nail at the eponychium (the area of the nail that has the small white semi circular area). This problem is associated with HIV;
4. Chronic muccocutaneous onychomycosis, which is a topical infection with a bug named Candida;
5. Totally dystrophic nail syndrome, which is a nail deformity that appears to be a fungal infection but is really caused by trauma to the growth plate (matrix) of the nail.

Most medical practitioners have traditionally ignored toenail infections as they lacked training in this area combined with the fact that there was not an effective method to treat it. Prior to the release of oral antifungal medications, patients with onychomycosis had little choice for treatment except for permanent removal of the nail and "root" called the matrix tissue. Patients have reported that they used tea tree oil or Vicks Vapo Rub™ on their nails, but there is no scientific evidence to show these treatments actually work.

Penlac™ is a unique, topically applied medication that is now available to treat onychomycosis. It has a very limited scope of use and a relatively low success rate in comparison to the oral medications in treating this problem. It is a nail lacquer that is applied to the nail daily with a small brush like nail polish, and requires significant patient involvement in terms of cleaning and filing the nail. It can take up to a year for the nails to respond before returning to their normal pink smooth and shiny appearance. It requires follow-up visits to a physician or podiatrist for nail debridement. While in limited cases it has shown the ability to produce a clean nail, I prefer to use oral medications with my patients and will reserve the use of Penlac™ for those who cannot take the oral anti-fungal medications.

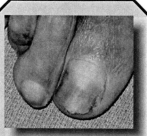

This is a typical response from a patient that is taking oral Lamisil® for treatment of onychomycosis. Note that the new growth of the nail is clean while the old portion is still affected with fungus. As the nail grows, the fungal portion will be trimmed off leaving a clean toenail.

In the late 1990s, oral Terbinifine (Lamisil™) and Itraconazole (Sporanox™) became available. Each drug has specific strengths and weaknesses and the decision to use one of these drugs should not be taken lightly. When oral anti-fungal medications became popular for treating toe nail infections a lot of resources and time were devoted to marketing them. The market is still huge (upwards of $6 billion) and worldwide. It is estimated that over 60 percent of the world's population has a dermatophyte infection on their toenails.

Each of these medications are powerful and when used properly are very safe and effective in treating nail infection. However, lab testing for positive identification of fungal element on the nail is the best practice before starting therapy with these medications. There has been much publicity and fear created by competitive adverting that these medications can cause serious harm. Over the past decade I have written many prescriptions for these mediations and my experience is that when used properly, these medications are safe and effective.

Over and above the physical pain that a patient might have with thick, deformed toenails, patients with nail problems may also experience psychosocial pain. Many patients with diabetes have thick discolored and painful nails. Comfortable shoes are often hard to find and some patients cannot wear closed-toe shoes due to pain. This is extremely risky for patients with diabetes, as using open-toed shoes leaves their feet vulnerable to painless trauma. Since they don't want their feet to be seen, they may avoid wearing open toes shoes or having their feet exposed in public.

## Seeking the Right Professional Care for Foot Problems

While most general practice physicians tend to overlook the feet and the nails, patients are left with an unsolved problem. They are carrying a living infection that can spread to other parts of their bodies and others who come into contact with them and their surroundings.

There are many physicians who do not understand the foot's anatomy, physiology, or function. Regardless of your foot problem, when you make an appointment for care, ask yourself, "Will my physician know what my foot problem is, and can he or she treat it?" While some problems are uncommon and rarely seen in the foot, such as a primary malignancy or cancer, others are very common.

Many people have never heard of a podiatrist, so they do not know about the education, training, and services that are offered. On top of that, many people feel that a deformed or painful foot is "normal" and fail to seek care at all. Nothing could be further from the truth.

Regardless of the foot problem that brings a patient to my office, there usually is some treatment that can be done to resolve it and relieve their foot pain—even if only on a temporary basis. The two most motivating forces that bring patients into the office are pain and fear. I believe there should be a third and more positive reason why patients come to visit a podiatrist: for preventive foot care and education.

## A Day in the Life of a DPM

A podiatrist's day is varied. Some days, I am trimming nails, debriding corns and calluses, fixing an ingrown toenail, injecting a patient for a painful nerve entrapment or heel spur, making foot impressions for custom insoles, or setting fractures. Other days, I am in the operating room replacing old arthritic joints with new artificial joints in the toes, fixing a bunion, removing a tumor, or tending to the athlete's needs in sports medicine. Every day, I deal with the feet of diabetic and at-risk patients, treating ulcers, infections, and the effects of diabetic neuropathy and peripheral vascular disease. Every day is a bit different and I enjoy the variety of people I meet and the opportunity to serve them.

The most enjoyable part of my day is the interaction I have with my patients as I listen to their history and concerns about their feet. It gives me the opportunity to help them solve a foot health mystery by asking a few pointed questions. Patients usually tell me what they think their foot problem is. Sometimes they know what it is, and sometimes they don't, but this starting point gives me information I can use to help them. Your history can provide "hidden information" that I am looking for—key elements that will help me make the diagnosis and plan the treatment.

If you are diabetic, we need specific information concerning both your general and foot health history. For instance, have your blood sugar levels been under control? Do your feet feel numb or cold to you? Do you lose your balance? Is there a history of an open wound in your skin or an ulcer? Have you had any previous infections, any previous foot surgery, or a previous amputation? This information is critical in determining what evaluation and management category to assign you to and allows me to organize a plan for your foot care. I am always interested in how my patients spend their time. If they work, I want to know what they do and what their leisure activities include. Do they stand, walk, or work on hard surfaces for long periods of time? Has anyone in their family had foot problems, and if so, what were the problems? Often patients are poor historians and are unable to provide much information concerning their foot health history.

Cultural and social differences affect how people relate to and care for their feet, though my experience has been that many people have a limited education and vocabulary when it comes to foot problems. Several times a week, a patient sits on my treatment chair and identifies a problem on his foot as something that is nowhere near what the real problem is. For example, patients tell me all the time that their bunions hurt when it turns out that their real problem is a callus or a hammertoe. Many patients think their foot problem has to do with something they can see. They don't realize that there could

be an internal problem that is an additional or secondary source of their foot pain. A perfect example of this is the patient with a callus who is sure that this is the reason for the foot pain. A thorough exam reveals that, indeed, they do have a callus and pressing on it causes pain. But they *also* have pain near the callus that is the source of their major foot pain: a neuritis caused by a pinched nerve in their foot.

Recognizing a foot deformity is just the first step in preventing an amputation. There are complex sets of variables that must be considered in order to heal a wound or successfully treat a foot problem. These can include anatomy, physiology, biomechanics of foot function, vascular and neurological status, and footwear. Also critical to the overall prevention scheme are the specifics of the general health, behaviors, and the social support situation of the patient.

An organized approach to foot health works wonders in preventing amputations. When we organize our efforts to a set of universal standards, patients benefit. When we provide a framework to identify the triggers that can lead to an amputation and provide individualized preventive care everyone benefits: patients, their families, and those financially responsible. By understanding the three specialized classes of foot deformities based on our anatomy: bone, soft tissue, and nail, we can devise a strategy to provide preventive care. To understand how people's feet develop bone, joint, and soft tissue deformities, you must have some knowledge of the science of podiatric biomechanics.

An oft-repeated truism of medicine is "You have to have the right diagnosis in order to provide the right treatment" (unless you are extremely lucky). Sounds simple, but it is frequently

a tremendous challenge to accomplish this especially when it comes to a patient with foot problems. When medical providers do go wrong, they may start with the wrong diagnosis, or they may be unaware that there may be multiple diagnoses involved in a patient's foot problems and that each one needs to be identified and treated. Delaying identification of the correct diagnosis could leave the patient with chronic pain or a lingering open wound that is vulnerable to infection. We know there are systemic diseases whose origins are not in the feet but that can affect the feet. Diabetes is an example of this. The key concept is to recognize that a problem not directly associated with your feet may have its origin in another area of your body and can affect your feet. If you are a patient with diabetes, your foot problem may be caused by a factor in or not in your foot.

Patients with diabetes respond differently to foot problems and they have different risk factors than a patient without diabetes. We need to gather pertinent supporting information that will lead me to the correct diagnosis and help me provide the right care.

## Neuropathy vs. Neuritis

Patients with diabetes might tell their primary care doctors that they have burning or shooting pain, or tingling sensations in their feet, which are classic symptoms of a neurological problem. The first diagnosis the doctor might consider is "diabetic sensory neuropathy" because these are some of the common symptoms caused by neuropathy. But wait; could there be another reason for the pain? In order to find out if there is a neuritis in the foot, there is an easy test to check the foot. Just

take your fingers and press between the toes where they attach to the foot and watch the patient's face, not her foot, for a response to pain. A good history will help to identify the source of the pain too. The question to ask is whether it's burning on the whole foot or just the front of the foot. If the pain affects the whole foot it may be due to neuropathy. If it's the front of the foot, then ask if it's episodic in nature or constant pain. Neuropathy would be constant pain, and nerve entrapment would be episodic. By taking a good history, asking the right questions, and performing a quick foot exam, we can usually figure out the source of the patient's pain. Remember that there can be even more reasons why a patient may have pain in their foot and all of them should be investigated. If the pain is due to a local nerve entrapment I can treat it with a cortisone shot, and see if that helps alleviate their pain. Patients need to know that if we give them a cortisone shot, their blood glucose may become elevated. In this case, the easy way to reduce the blood glucose levels is for the patient to take a walk. We can make orthotics, or have them go to physical therapy, too. If those conservative treatments fail, we can do surgery to remove the affected portion of the nerve.

## This is a Test, Only a Test

Tests that I might order to help diagnose and treat a foot problem in a patient with diabetes might include:
- ABI or Duplex Doppler exam
- Bone Scan/Soft Tissue Scan
- Complete Blood Count (CBC)
- C-Reactive Protein

- Gram Stain and Bacterial Culture and Sensitivity (if there is an infection)
- HLAB27 (to diagnose arthritis)
- Hemoglobin A1c
- Kidney and Liver Function Tests
- Nerve Conduction Study
- MRI
- Random Blood Sugar
- Sedimentation Rate
- X-Ray

These tests rule out certain diagnoses or a list of possible reasons for a patient's foot pain or problems and should be evaluated. Heel pain is a diagnostic challenge and I see this problem in many patients with diabetes. There are probably thirty different reasons for heel pain. There are nerve entrapments, torn tissue, heel spurs, foreign bodies, tumors, and fractures. "Conservative treatments for heel pain include injections, physical therapy, changing footgear, taking anti-inflammatory medicines, biomechanical adjustments (such as orthotics and stretching), shoe modification, and using ice and heat if the physician believes the patient is able to tolerate these temperature extremes. There is also a surgical option to cut a portion of the plantar fascia and/or remove the heel spur."

**Foot Notes: Questions Your Podiatrist May Ask You**

A doctor of podiatric medicine (DPM) is the specialist responsible for the medical and surgical care of diseases, and deformities of the foot and ankle. Podiatrists also provide preventive foot care for patients with diabetes and other patients who are at risk for amputation and who should not self-treat.

Here are a few questions your podiatrist may ask you and tests he or she may offer:

- Do you use alcohol or tobacco?
- Do you have a history of nephropathy or disease of the kidney?
- Do you have impaired vision, retinopathy, or damage to the retina of the eye.
- Are you overweight or obese?
- Is there any loss of protective sensation (LOPS)?
- Is there a foot deformity causing a focus of high pressure?
- Is there a previous history of foot ulceration or amputation?
- Test for vascular disease using ABI.
- Test for sensation in feet and legs with the monofilament testing device.
- Visual foot deformity, limited joint mobility, high plantar pressures.

# Chapter Seven

## You've Lost that loving Feeling

A loss of feeling anywhere in the body is not good, unless you're at the dentist's office and you have just received a dose of Novocain™ local anesthesia in preparation for dental work. Pain is our body's burglar alarm and alerts us to intruders such as injuries. It is primordial, and as unpleasant as it may be, humans would not have survived without it. Without the ability to feel pain, our bodies are vulnerable to a variety of injuries, or traumas. As a matter of fact, after pulse, respiration, blood pressure, and temperature, pain is considered to be the fifth vital sign. It is crucial that a medical history documents information on all vital statistics including pain and its location, type, intensity, and any factors that trigger or reduce the pain. Without the ability to feel pain, you are vulnerable to being injured without realizing it.

Neuropathy is a degenerative disease or disorder that affects the nervous system and one of the results of neuropathy is an inability to feel physical sensation. In the foot, this is called a loss of protective sensation. As a result, peripheral sensory neuropathy is generally the greatest risk factor and often the root cause for foot ulcers in patients with diabetes. Just because you do not feel pain in your feet, it doesn't mean you should ignore a foot injury. I've had patients say, "Yeah, I have a hole in my foot, but it doesn't hurt, so it must not be a bad thing." A hole in the foot is not harmless, even if it is painless. As a recent ad campaign from a national pharmaceutical company puts it, "A hole in your foot *is* a medical emergency."[1]

The ability to feel pain is controlled by our sensory nerves. They give us information about our environment, and that includes a sense of where our joints are positioned and input from mechanical and thermal receptors that can generate impulses that we recognize as pain.

Patients who come in with complaints of pain in their feet may actually be suffering from pathology that originates in their back. Because many folks never get an appropriate diagnosis, the care they receive may fail to alleviate their pain. Patients with diabetes and plenty of other folks have pains that can be mistaken for neuropathy, and the range of causes for foot pain may surprise you. An arthritic spur radiating from one of the bones in the spinal column pressing against a nerve generates a condition that is called a radiculopathy. This can result in radicular pain, weakness, numbness, or difficulty controlling specific muscles and can cause foot pain! That pain may be felt in only one leg or foot and not in the other. Another "false reading" from nerve sensation might come because of a narrowing of the area where the nerves leave the spinal cord, called spinal stenosis. This, too, can cause foot pain.

## Case Study

Ray was having tingling in his feet. His doctor said it was neuropathy due to diabetes. Then, he started having tingling in his legs, along with lower back pain. Ray's doctor did nothing about it and Ray ended up in a wheelchair.

When he came to me, he had a bleeding fissure on the heel of his foot that was about an inch deep. I shaved it off, treated it and taught him how to take care of his feet. His doctor had told him they were probably going to cut his feet off, but I talked to him about it and assured him we're going to try everything else before resulting to such drastic measures. His doctor misdiagnosed him. We did an MRI and found a tumor as big as a tennis ball in Ray's spine. He had the tumor removed and Ray is gratefully able to walk again without pain.

Data from the GOAL A1c Study (sponsored by Adventis) revealed that the diagnosis of neuropathy was missed in 63 percent of patients examined by generalists *and* specialists.[2]

Peripheral neuropathy is the most dangerous and least understood of all the complications of diabetes.

If you cannot feel sensation in your feet, you are vulnerable to painless trauma and are at the highest risk level for amputation.

## What is Peripheral Neuropathy?

Diabetic peripheral neuropathy specifically refers to changes to the nervous system. There are three subcategories of problems with the nervous system: autonomic neuropathy, motor neuropathy, and sensory neuropathy. We will look at each of these in this chapter.

Do you know what it's like when you hit your funny bone and your arm feels paralyzed for a few seconds? That happens because you've temporarily traumatized the nerve in your elbow. What if your feet and legs feel like that all the time? That's how some patients with peripheral neuropathy (PN) describe the sensation in their feet.

Others describe PN as feeling like they're walking on nails or glass, or like a lightning bolt is shooting through their feet. Many patients with diabetes have these feelings in their feet and legs non-stop. Other patients with PN do not feel these things. In fact, they don't feel anything in their feet. They tell me they feel like they are standing on a balled up sock or on wood, and ironically some patients can't feel the floor at all while standing—like when your foot falls asleep. Because they can't feel their feet on the floor, these patients may have balance problems or fall. We don't realize how the feeling in our feet communicates to us exactly where we are positioned in the 3-D world until we lose that feeling.

In PN, the nerves have lost their ability to transmit neurological impulses normally. There are four theories for why someone gets PN:

1. Chronically elevated blood glucose levels

2. Free electrons attack the nerve as a result of metabolism

3. Microvascular disease—a shrinking of the blood vessels that deprive the nerves of the oxygen and nutrients necessary for them to function normally

4. Chemotherapy

KEEP THE LEGS YOU STAND ON — Dr. Mark Hinkes

In clinical practice, every patient is unique with different complaints and symptoms. This is especially true with peripheral neuropathy. Your physician's job is to figure out whether you have peripheral neuropathy, or another problem like a nerve entrapment, and how to provide relief. Sometimes the solution is obvious, and sometimes it is not. One of the first predictors of neuropathy in the patient with diabetes is the loss of deep tendon reflexes, which are the patellar (knee) and Achilles (ankle) reflexes. You've probably had this test during checkups—your doctor taps your knee and ankle tendons with the neurological hammer and your reflexes cause your leg or ankle to jump.

Other signs of peripheral neuropathy include *parasthesias*, the sensation of a little lightning bolt shooting through the foot; *hyperesthesia*, where the foot is extremely sensitive to touch and in some patients is so intense that just getting under the bedcovers can cause extreme pain; and *hypoesthesia* when there is a decreased sensitivity to light touch and vibratory sensation, which may be demonstrated by the patient's inability to feel the fibers of a brush or a vibrating tuning fork applied to the foot or ankle.

In addition to the aforementioned reasons for peripheral sensory neuropathy, other ways to get the disease include alcoholism, a herniated disc in the back, heavy metal intoxication (like lead poisoning), vitamin deficiency (especially the B vitamins), cancer, anemia, leprosy, pernicious anemia (a life threatening blood disorder relating to vitamin B 12), uremia (blood poisoning), porphyria (a group of rare, inherited blood disorders) and collagen vascular diseases.

To come to the correct diagnosis, your doctor will take your medical history, then test for range of motion, muscle power, biomechanics, skin, vascular and neurological health, and will probably palpate (examination by touch) your foot. Some patients with diabetes have nerve entrapment in their forefoot. Be sure your doctor checks for this in the physical examination. Diabetic neuropathy can go undetected and therefore an affected area is not taken care of the way that it needs to be.

## Testing for Proper Diagnosis

Sudomotor perspiration dysfunction develops early in PN. A new test can assess this dysfunction. The IPN (Indicator Plaster Neuropad) is a simple high-sensitivity device that can be used for diagnosing neuropathy. The IPN can be performed either in the office or by the patient at home and takes about ten minutes. The fact that this test can be performed at home by the patient is phenomenal and it allows the patient to participate actively in the prevention and detection of diabetic foot complications. Currently, it is suggested that patients utilize the Indicator Plaster Neuropad once a year. This examination results in either a light pink color when the nerve conduction is normal or a blue color when nerve damage is present.

Peter Dyck in the Rochester Diabetic Neuropathy Study from Mayo Clinic found that 5 to 10 percent of those with diabetes and neuropathy had a cause *other* than diabetes for their nerve disease. A full work up is important.

## History of the Monofilament Wire

In the nineteenth century, the H.L. Teuber medical group in Germany used horsehair to test for neuropathy on patients with gunshot wounds. Later, German physiologist Max Von Frey used varying diameters of horsehair to discover the physiological effects of the loss of sensation.

In the 1950s with the invention of nylon wire, Josephine Semmes and Sidney Weinstein took Von Frey's idea and developed the monofilament aesthesiometer. They were working with patients affected by gunshot wounds, to identify changes in sensory nerve function. Inspired by the reduction of lower limb amputations in the leper population, doctors tried the test on the feet of their patients with diabetes.

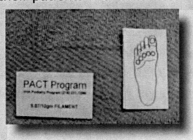

Semmes-Weinstein Monofilament Testing Device

## Monofilament Testing Device (MTD)

The gold standard for detecting loss of protective sensation (LOPS) associated with PN is the Semms-Weinstein monofilament testing device (MTD). It tests your ability to feel a sensation on the bottom of your foot. If you feel it, we say protective sensation is intact; if you do not feel it we say you have lost protective sensation. The MTD is a reliable, fast, non-invasive, and painless test for identifying patients with peripheral sensory neuropathy. A study by the U.S. Department of Veterans Affairs showed that as sensory screening with the 5.07 MTD rose from 35 percent in 1995 to 89 percent in 1998, lower extremity amputations decreased 20 percent. The MTD itself costs about twenty-six cents, and it's the most powerful tool in my toolbox.

One concern in administering a proper monofilament test involves doctor-patient communication which occurs during the testing process. I always show the wire to the patient and touch their arm with it first before going to their foot, so they will know what they are supposed to feel. Patients need to understand the test and how to respond to it appropriately for the test to be valid. I always ask the patient to say "Yes" if he feels it when I touch his foot. For example, you might change your answer due to your perception and give the answer that you think the doctor is expecting. You may say you feel the wire when you *see* the tester's arm move toward your foot before the wire even touches your foot. It is important to keep your eyes shut during the exam. After reading this chapter and book, you should be well-armed with what to expect in an examination and have the ability to give the doctor clear responses.

There are also three elements regarding your doctor's use of the wire:

1. *How to hold and use the wire.* For sensory recognition purposes, your doctor may ask, "Do you feel this?" He or she may use a forced choice method by asking, "Did you feel when I touched your foot the first or second time?" For location identification method, he or she may ask, "Where on which foot did you feel it?" If one method fails, the doctor should try at least one of the other two methods. Inconsistency in these factors can result in inaccurate results. If this happens, the doctor should stop testing and make sure that the patient understands the testing procedure and then repeat the test.

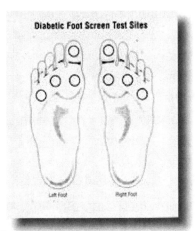

**Where to Touch the Patient's Foot**

2. *Where to touch the wire on the patient's foot.* There is some controversy about where the wire should touch the foot, how many locations to touch, and what constitutes a diagnosis of sensory neuropathy. Some authorities recommend testing the foot in three strategic locations based on the percentage chance of developing an ulcer on the bottom of the foot (visual). Others recommend additional locations be tested, so the criteria for determining whether the patient has sensory neuropathy varies.

3. *When to discard the wire so it will not give false positives.* A recent study indicated that not all 10-gram monofilament testing devices are created equally. Booth and Young showed the difference in manufacturers in increasing flexibility with increased use make the monofilament tests inaccurate and therefore less reliable in assessing neuropathy.

The study's authors suggested that the typical monofilament will survive usage on approximately ten patients before needing a recovery time of 24 hours.

## Vibration Perception Threshold Instrument

Dr. Lawrence Lavery, a podiatrist and co-chairman of the research committee for the American College of Foot and Ankle Surgeons, says he likes to use the vibration perception threshold instrument to evaluate patients. He can perform the test on a patient and their family to demonstrate it for all to feel. Oftentimes, the patient will not feel it, so this is a powerful demonstration of the loss of vibratory sensation that the whole family can learn about. Some relatives can feel as little as five volts of vibration in their hands but the patient may need ninety volts in his foot before he can feel anything. Doctors in the United Kingdom have been using the vibration instrument as a research tool for twenty-five years. Dr. Lavery recognized the value of Dr. Andrew Boulton's work in this field and has been using it in Texas where he practices. Dr. Lavery has had the instrument for nearly twenty years after receiving research money from the University of Texas, San Antonio. "It is a nice complementary tool because probably one-third of people have normal vibration sensation but abnormal monofilament exam," says Lavery. "About one-third have abnormal vibration and normal monofilament and one-third have both abnormal. One tests vibration, one tests pressure."

## Biothesiometer

Evaluation of the patient's ability to sense vibration is critical to understanding each patient's neurological status. Often times the loss of vibratory sensation is the first neurological symptom noted in diabetic peripheral neuropathy. Until now this sensation was tested using a tuning fork and there was much room for error in the testing process. A new technology is now available to more accurately evaluate vibratory sensation, the electronic tuning fork or biothesiometer. This new technology measures vibratory perception threshold. Like the monofilament test is used to detect protective sensation on the foot, the biothesiometer is used to determine the patient's ability to sense vibration on the foot. This test is able to quantify or give us a number to evaluate a patient's ability to feel vibration. Loss of vibratory sense frequently happens to patients with diabetes.

## Autonomic Neuropathy

Autonomic neuropathy is caused by a malfunction of the nerves that innervate the sweat or oil glands in the skin. When this happens, the patient loses the ability to perspire or create the normal oils that protect and keep the skin moist. The result is dry skin that peels or develops deep fissures that can be painful.

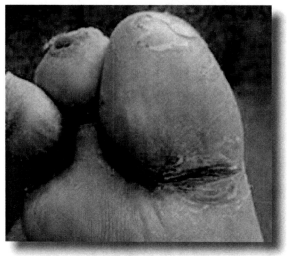

Fissures

These cracks are on the surface of the skin but they may appear to be deep (these actually have a thickening of the skin on either side of the crack that makes them look deeper than they are). They are commonly found on the bottom of your foot where the toes bend or on the back of the heels. The danger associated with fissures is they offer a portal of entry for bacteria, yeast, mold or fungus that can lead to an infection. And, once a patient with diabetes has an infection, it is much more difficult to treat because of a decreased ability to heal from the infection due to PAD and immunopathy. I have seen patients with autonomic neuropathy whose skin is so dry, that when we roll up their pants legs to examine them, there is a miniature "snow storm" of dead, dry skin. Patients suffering from autonomic neuropathy should use a moisturizing cream or lotion daily to keep the skin moist.

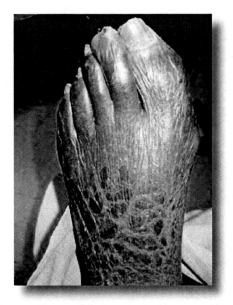

Severe Case of Autonomic Neuropathy.

## Case Study

We often see patients who travel great distances, even from other states, because our facility is the closest one to them. Traveling two to three hours by car each way, a visit to the clinic becomes an all-day event for these patients. TC was a 44-year-old African-American diabetic male who drove several hours to be seen in the clinic.

TC controlled his blood sugars by oral medications, diet, and exercise. The remarkable finding from his physical exam was that his feet were completely numb. He was not able to feel the 5.07 monofilament device on any part of either foot, yet he was able to feel pain from a skin condition. He had painful, cracked skin on the bottom of both feet.

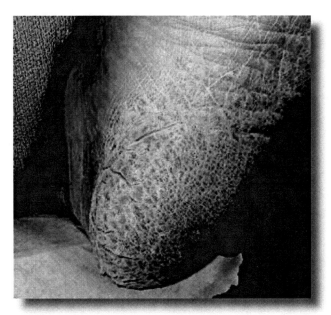

KPPH Misdiagnosed as Autonomic Neuropathy

The onset of TC's problem started many years previous, but he had been unable to find a doctor who could provide him with a correct diagnosis and appropriate treatment to heal the fissures and relieve his pain. TC could hardly walk because it hurt so much. Typically, patients with this problem have fissures along the heel or in areas where the skin "bends" such as the flexion crease under a toe or the heel where there is excessive pressure. TC had fissures in different locations on both feet. There was one fissure on the heel that was larger than the others; it was particularly red, swollen, and painful.

Further examination of TC's hands revealed a similar thickening of the skin, but without the fissures. We diagnosed him as having a variant of KPPH—keratosis palmaris plantaris heredicita—a genetic skin condition caused by an autosomal recessive gene. KPPH causes the skin to grow faster in areas where there is pressure against it. This genetic problem contributes to the creation of the fissures.

When evaluating dry skin lotions check the label for the amount of alcohol in the product. Those products that are more runny and thin contain more alcohol and should be avoided. Alcohol tends to dry the skin so stay away from these products and look for products that are less runny and a bit thicker; these will contain less alcohol.

Instead of subjecting TC to a series of uncomfortable mechanical debridements with a scalpel, I decided to treat the fissures with a regime that has worked successfully for many of my patients for many years—a topical exfoliating ointment I call Dr. Hinkes' Fissure Compound. This ointment consists of salicylic acid, urea, and white petroleum jelly. TC was instructed to apply the ointment to the fissures at night, cover with plastic wrap, put a white sock on and go to bed. The action of my Fissure Compound was to chemically debride the thick skin adjacent to the fissure. In the morning, TC was instructed to use a surgical scrub brush and soap to remove the dead tissue, and then apply a urea-based moisturizing lotion. Over the next several months, TC dutifully followed the procedure with great success. We did some local debridements that were not painful because of the home treatment. We were able to eradicate all of the fissures except for the large deep one on the heel.

KEEP THE LEGS YOU STAND ON — Dr. Mark Hinkes

Medicine is an art based in science and that is why you might hear a physician refer to what they do as "practice." This is a legitimate term because medical care is very much an art, but also based on experience and wisdom. It is very common to adjust our treatment regime depending on the positive or negative results of a previous treatment. Since we had evaluated TC's vascular and neurological status, we needed to complete our evaluation by evaluating TC's biomechanics.

In treating foot wounds, not only is it necessary to consider the vascular and neurological status, but also to look at how the patient's feet function (see Chapter 5 for more information on gait cycle and podiatric biomechanics). Understanding a patient's foot function can provide important information to solving the puzzle of why the patient developed an ulcer or a fissure, and worse, why they re-ulcerate or re-fissure.

When we evaluated TC's biomechanics, it became clear that he had some unusual foot function that was placing an extra amount of stress on the heel and contributing to the large, deep, painful fissure. To solve this problem, we fabricated biomechanical orthotics to change his weight-bearing pattern, provide him with the most efficient mechanical function, and relieve pressure from the heel fissure. After using the orthotics, TC was healing well. However, on a return visit, he complained that he had a small, reddened area adjacent to the fissure. Further inspection revealed a possible granuloma to the site. We took a bacterial culture and two skin samples from the site on the outside chance we had an undiagnosed dermatological problem. One sample was sent to the pathologist, the other for culture and sensitivity (C&S) test. The C&S is a powerful test. Not only does it tell us which bacteria are in a wound, it even tells which antibiotics would take the smallest doses to do the most damage to the bacteria. This information becomes very important in the process of selecting antibiotics because we need to consider the patient's specific set of medical circumstances.

The culture revealed a possible Methacillin-resistant *staphylococcus* aureus (MRSA) Infection (for more information, see Chapter 11 on infection). His biopsies were negative for any additional dermatological problem. So we wrote a prescription for the appropriate oral antibiotic feeling sure this would end the problem.

TC returned in a week reporting he had taken the antibiotics and done the local treatment for the MRSA infection that was healing well. He casually mentioned he thought he might have an infection of the other foot since there was some drainage on his sock. TC assured me he had not walked barefooted or without shoes. There was a small area of devitalized tissue on the bottom of TC's foot near the middle. With a #15 blade, I started to debride the area. As the debridement progressed, I saw a dark grayish material that felt hard against the scalpel and heard a familiar sound. I had struck a metal object! I took a hemostat (medical tweezers), grasped the object and gently pulled on it. Thinking it was a small foreign body on the surface, I expected it to come out easily, but to my astonishment, I kept pulling, and pulling, and pulling. To my total astonishment TC had a three-inch nail embedded in his foot, yet he had been able to walk with no pain for several days. TC was given a tetanus shot and antibiotics. We ordered an X-ray to make sure nothing else was in his foot. Miraculously, TC healed without getting an infection from the nail.

Surely, there can be no better illustration of the danger of diabetic neuropathy that makes a patient vulnerable to painless trauma.

## Motor Neuropathy

Why should I keep my blood glucose levels normal? One reason is that chronically elevated blood glucose levels damage the nervous system. Subtle changes in nerve function may lead to muscle loss. Motor neuropathy occurs when the nerves that supply the foot muscles controlling fine movements of the toes are damaged. This causes the toes to shift into an abnormal position. The result is a variety of digital deformities known as hammer toe, mallet toe, and claw toe. The bony prominences in the toes caused by these deformities can become triggers for mechanical injuries. New pressure points and changes in gait occur.

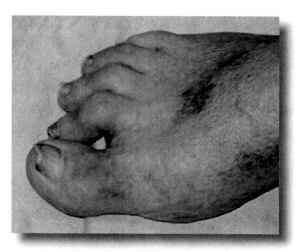

**Hammer Toe Due to Motor Neuropathy.**

Using MRI technology, scientists have been able to see the smallest muscles in the foot, thirteen in all: six lumbricales and seven interossei muscles. In patients with diabetic motor neuropathy, the muscles were seen to be smaller in size when compared to patients without neuropathy. Findings also suggest that changes in the muscles occur early and often before other recognizable changes to the foot associated with neuropathy are noted.

## Sensory Neuropathy

Sensory neuropathy is the most dangerous of the three types of neuropathies because patients affected by sensory neuropathy can be injured without knowing it. They have lost the ability to feel pain, or what is called a loss of protective sensation and are vulnerable to painless trauma.

Painless trauma can be caused in three ways: one is by *chemical injuries* due to patients using over-the-counter products containing salicylic acid, which destroys tissue painlessly on their feet. Salicylic acid can be found in medicated corn pads and in topical wart, ingrown toenail, and callus removers. I tell my patients that acid has no brains; it eats everything it touches—both the affected tissues and healthy skin, so it is best to avoid these products due to the risk of a chemical burn creating an ulcer.

The second type of painless trauma is due to *mechanical injuries.* These injuries can be the result of minor trauma, which includes injuries caused by stepping on a sharp object like a nail, or the foot rubbing against improperly fitted footwear, or a foreign object like a stone inside the shoe causing a blister. Or they can be caused by deformities of the bones, soft tissue, or nails interacting with footgear, which would include a bunion or hammer toe rubbing against an improperly fitted shoe. If you have one of these bony foot deformities and it is rubbing against your shoe, your body will try to protect the area by creating thick keratotic skin lesions known as corns and calluses. And absence of the normal plantar fat pad under the metatarsal heads is a bad sign. Those areas are vulnerable to repetitive micro-trauma, and when a patient has neuropathy, it's very easy to develop a callus, which can lead to an ulcer. If left untreated, pressure against the calluses can lead to abscesses, soft tissue infections, ulcers, bone infections, and ultimately amputations. Your podiatrist can help by periodically debriding these thick skin lesions and may be able to provide you with an insert or recommend a change of shoes that will alleviate the problem. One patient developed a foot ulcer due to a portion of his sock overlapping itself causing excessive pressure. In an effort to provide their patients a measure of pain relief, some podiatrists are injecting medical-grade silicone into the area to replace the protective cushioning effect of the plantar fat pad. While this procedure appears to be beneficial, the FDA has not yet approved the use of silicone for this purpose.

Mechanical injury can also involve toenails that are thickened by fungal infection. They are sometimes overlooked even in the most comprehensive exam. If the thickened or deformed nail rubs against the shoe, it can cause an abscess under the nail. If the deformed toenail is rubbing against another toe, it can lacerate the adjacent toe. In a patient with poor circulation, this type of injury can also start the sequence of events that leads to amputation.

The third type of painless trauma is *thermal trauma*

resulting from over-exposure to heat or cold, but mostly burns caused by an artificial heat source. Many patients with diabetes have cold feet due to vascular disease. They might try a number of ways to warm their feet and in the process burn their feet, thus creating a thermal trauma. Thermal trauma can be caused many ways, but includes the use of a heating pad, a hot water bottle, standing too close to an open fire or a radiator, putting cold feet on a hot brick for warmth, or soaking feet in water that is hot enough to make tea. Every holiday season a patient who has received a foot bath or spa-like item as a gift comes to the office with second degree burns up to his ankles because he couldn't feel the scalding-hot water.

I remember a patient who came to the office with a burn on his big toe. When I questioned him about this he replied, "We was makin' cracklin's." Many southerners know that cracklin's, or pork rinds, are made by boiling pigskin in hot oil. Apparently this patient had been warming his feet by an open fire and his shoe caught on fire resulting in the burn on his foot. He never even felt it.

Another patient we treated in our office had already lost a portion of his foot and was well aware of the issues of amputation prevention. He used a heating pad to treat a muscle pull on his thigh. He fell asleep, rolled over and his heating pad ended up on his big toe. This patient lost his toe because of a thermal injury combined with poor circulation that resulted in a non-healing wound.

## Alcoholic Neuropathy

Alcoholic neuropathy occurs through the abuse of alcohol.

## KEEP THE LEGS YOU STAND ON — Dr. Mark Hinkes

On a Friday at about 11:30 in the morning, I was slammed with new patients at the foot clinic, and was falling into the "Valley of Fatigue." My thoughts were more on lunch than being a healer; nevertheless, I still had five or six patients to see.

My next patient was Mr. XY, a jovial, gray-haired man who came in wearing khaki shorts and a polo shirt. He had bathed and looked fresh. He came in because not only had he lost feeling in his feet, but also in his legs almost up to his knees.

In my usual manner, as I was taught by my internal medicine professor, Dr. Murray Hurwitz, I said, "How can I help you?" Implying to the patient that I was indeed going to help him.

"I just found out about my diabetes," he quickly pointed out, proud that for most of his life he was "normal" like the rest of us. "Doc, it's the damndest thing. I can't feel the floor with my feet. Sometimes I have to grab onto something to keep from falling, and sometimes I fall anyway. See?" He showed me several black and blue spots on his arms and legs that were obviously the result of previous falls.

He had been diagnosed as a type 2 diabetic. Several physicians had told him that he had diabetic neuropathy, but the degree of numbness puzzled me. This was unusual in patients with diabetes who have neuropathies.

After some further questioning he shared with me, "I gotta tell you, Doc, I'm not proud of this, but there was a time when I was doin' some drinkin'—nearly a case of beer and a fifth of whiskey every day for about seven years."

I was honestly shocked that someone who had drank so much had not already died of cirrhosis of the liver. After a thorough work-up, Mr. XY was diagnosed as having alcoholic neuropathy. In testing him, it was true he was totally numb up to about his knees. I was able to take a 25-gauge needle and touch him in multiple locations and he felt nothing.

## Treatments for Peripheral Neuropathy

The most common medical treatment for painful neuropathy is a medication named Neurontin™ (gabapentin). This medication has plusses and minuses and not all patients do well with it. It has no effect on painless neuropathy and some patients are prescribed it in error.

Sometimes vitamin therapy using B complex works well in combination with Alpha-Lipoic Acid and can help reduce the symptoms of neuropathy. When combined with Vitamins C and E, Alpha-Lipoic Acid removes free-electrons that might be attacking the nerves and can help you get some pain relief. ALA it is sold in the U.S. as a food supplement, though in Europe, it requires a prescription.

The most common treatments of neuropathy have included narcotics; non-steroidal anti-inflammatory drugs called NSAIDS, and tricyclic antidepressants such as amitriptyline (Elavil™). The presence of diabetic peripheral neuropathy (DPN) is estimated to be 20 to 24 percent among patients with diabetes. It is also estimated that 10 to 20 percent of patients with DPN have pain severe enough to require treatment.[2]

In 2004, the FDA approved a drug named Cymbalta™. Its original focus was to treat depression but it also works well for diabetic nerve pain. The newest drug for treatment of neuropathy is Lyrica™ (pregabalin) touted as the new generation of medications designed to treat diabetic neuropathic pain. Another drug named Ranirestat™ is in clinical trials. This drug differs from other drugs as it is the first to address the underlying cause of diabetic sensorimotor polyneuropathy (DSP), also known as diabetic neuropathy, These drugs have real promise for the pain caused by neuropathy that is not relieved by other drugs.

An important part of the treatment for peripheral neuropathy is not always discussed—psychological counseling and emotional support for those who feel overwhelmed by this illness. A patient with a foot ulcer may hear their doctor tell them to stay off their foot. The patient may wonder why they have to stay off their foot if it doesn't hurt them? Some patients who want to get off their feet just don't have the support system or can't afford to do this when their employers don't offer time off. You may find yourself thinking: "If I don't stay home and get off my foot, I might lose my leg, but if I don't go to work, I'll lose my job, my house, my car, and I won't be able to feed my family." A mental healthcare worker should be a part of your inter-disciplinary team in the treatment process of this psycho-social dilemma.

## Is It Neuropathy or Nerve Entrapment?

Problems can arise with nerves when trauma causes the nerve sheath to grow larger to protect itself. The nerve then outgrows its original space causing an entrapment syndrome and creating a very painful mass inside the foot. This may occur either due to a blunt trauma (for instance, a foot slamming the floor during an automobile accident), or in a repetitive micro-trauma from abnormal foot function (for instance, a person with a biomechanically unstable foot type who works, runs or jumps without corrective footwear or insoles). Pain can be very deceptive, and figuring out which nerve is causing a sensation can be tricky. This makes for a frustrating situation for both patients and doctors.

**Basic Rule of Anatomy #1:**
Body parts are functional. All the materials—the bones, muscles, hair, and eyes—everything that comprises our bodies is in the size and shape it is because of its function.

**Basic Rule of Anatomy #2:**
The body does what it must to protect itself.

## Hide-and-Seek: Locating the Offending Nerve

Nerve pain is common in patients with diabetes. If we establish that your pain is from a nerve entrapment and not peripheral neuropathy, we need to know which nerve and the location of the real problem. Even though the site of pain from a local nerve entrapment is often located between the second and third metatarsals and between the third and fourth metatarsals in the forefoot, we must determine if there is also a nerve entrapment behind the ankle or even in the low back that can affect the foot. A nerve entrapped behind the ankle is called tarsal tunnel syndrome (the ankle's version of the wrist's carpel tunnel syndrome). A nerve problem in the low back that can affect the foot is called lumbar radiculopathy.

To diagnose tarsal tunnel syndrome clinically, using a neurological hammer, the doctor taps along the area of the nerve, typically behind the ankle, looking for a response called a Tinnel's sign that would be considered a parasthesia—the little lightning bolt described earlier that starts at the ankle and can either radiate toward the toes or up the leg. A positive Tinnel's sign indicates that the pain may indeed be coming from a nerve entrapment behind the ankle.

To be certain about the origin of the pain, you can be referred to a neurologist to have electromyography (EMG) and a nerve conduction study. Although these tests can be uncomfortable, they are worth the effort to identify the location of the affected nerve(s) and provide a better chance to help. It is your doctor's job to figure out whether you have peripheral neuropathy or nerve entrapment and to use the best treatment.

## Treatment for Nerve Entrapment

There are a variety of conservative treatments available for nerve entrapment. Your doctor might recommend a series of cortisone injections, physical therapy, stretching exercises, an orthotic placed in the shoe to control abnormal biomechanical function and lift and separate the bones so they don't pinch the nerve, or a simple change of shoes to a wider toe box often provides significant relief.

If you are a patient with diabetes with a local nerve entrapment and your blood sugar levels are in the normal range, we will consider treating it with an injection, called a "trigger-point" injection, of a short-acting, non-crystalline steroid called dexamethasone (Decadron™) in combination with a local anesthetic. The injection is given through the top of the foot to minimize any discomfort, and if done properly, it can be painless.

We caution patients that the injection does not guarantee that they will be instantly cured, but rather, it can provide a variety of results: (1) minimal pain relief lasting several hours, (2) relief for a couple of days, or (3) long-term relief with one injection. Some patients may benefit from several injections without risk. The other benefit to these injections is that if the pain returns, it usually is at a lesser intensity. This treatment does have the potential to dramatically raise blood sugar levels, so you must know how to regulate and decrease your blood sugar levels if this happens. One of the easiest ways to do this is by walking in order to burn off the extra blood sugar. Since the foot usually feels better after the injection, the walk should be pleasant.

If, after using conservative care treatments, you still have pain, then we're left with two choices. The first is a series of sclerosing alcohol solution injections into the area where the nerve is located—much like the cortisone shot. Sclerosing therapy chemically destroys the nerve, so this remedy is painful.

The second choice is surgery: open up the foot, identify the nerve, section it, and remove it. When a nerve is removed from the foot, the area will be a bit numb after the procedure. My experience shows, whenever a patient has this operation the post-operative pain is so much less than the pain that was present before surgery, that they are very happy, even though it's sore and hurts a little bit. Nerve pain is horrific.

The very foundation of amputation prevention is education. Patients need education for understanding their disease and how to deal with it successfully. You now have an advantage over peripheral neuropathy as you have learned what it is, how it affects your body, and what steps to take to prevent or halt its progress. When patients know about their disease they will be more inclined to be our partners, and that translates into a winning combination of better patient quality of life and cost savings.

If the doctor asks the right questions, you should be able to provide the information to identify the cause of your pain.

1. Is the pain constant or episodic? Neuropathy causes constant pain; a local nerve entrapment causes episodic pain, at least in the early stages, and can happen while you are seated or lying in bed.
2. What does the pain feels like? You might say, "It's a burning, tingling, sharp, or electric shock-type of pain," or that you have numbness.
3. How strong is the pain on a scale of 0-10 (0 represents no pain and 10 is the worst pain you have ever experienced).
4. What is the location of the pain? Is it on the entire bottom of the foot or toward the front of the foot under the weight bearing part behind the toes?
5. Does the pain radiate into the toes or back up the foot toward the legs? At times there are multiple or overlapping diagnoses, and the ability to identify each is critical.

Knowing the difference between the symptoms of peripheral sensory neuropathy and nerve entrapment can lead to prompt treatment and pain relief. Your doctor can only provide the correct treatment if he or she has the correct diagnosis.

## Foot Notes: Tips for Temperature Testing

Use a bath thermometer to test the water temperature before stepping into a bath or shower. There is a product on the market called ScaldSafe™ available for less than five dollars on the Internet: http://www.kidzmed.com/p-16-scaldsafe-bath-thermometer.aspx. It is a floating disc that you can drop into the bath or hold under running water to test the temperature for safety. The disc color will change indicating whether the water is too hot, or the perfect 93.2 degrees Fahrenheit.

And, speaking of thermometers, there is a device called TempTouch® made by Diabetica Solutions, Inc. (www.diabeticasolutions.com) that can test the temperature of the skin and provide the patient with an "early warning" of inflammation and potential ulceration. The device can be used daily at home as a self-management tool by the patient. In the clinic, it gives the doctor an idea of whether or not there is inflammation that occurs before an ulcer actually breaks the surface of the skin. If inflammation is detected, patients are able to off-load the foot to avoid serious problems. TempTouch® only costs about $100 but a prescription is required for the instrument. A reading of more than four degrees difference in temperatures of one foot (or leg) to the other in like position can indicate inflammation is present and ulceration is imminent. Please read our interview with Ruben Zamorano for more information about this product.

# Chapter Eight

Circulation: Round and Round It Goes, Hopefully!

> *Red Gold (blood) is necessary to heal an ulcer*
> —David Allie, MD

Human tissue requires oxygen and nutrients to survive. Adequate circulation is essential for a foot wound to heal. Without it, tissue dies. Problems of the circulation are the number one concern after sensory neuropathy. The circulatory system in the leg is considered a "closed" system. This means there is no way to get more blood flow into it, until you get some out of it. No fresh, oxygenated blood that carries, nutrients, and medications can get to a foot wound until some blood containing metabolic waste products is moved back toward the heart.

People with adequate circulation, including patients with diabetes, should be able to heal wounds from minor traumas—like a blister from improperly fitted shoes or a cut caused by improperly trimming calluses or toenails at home. Patients with impaired circulation have a more difficult time healing a foot wound, and may find that it will not heal.

## Understanding the Circulatory System

There are three systems working under the name of the vascular system: the arterial, venous, and lymphatic, and each must function properly for wound healing to take place. Vascular disease affects the function of every system of our bodies. If a vascular problem is suspected in the foot or leg, we have painless, non-invasive technologies that can measure the blood flow both into and out of the leg from the thigh to the toes. We can even figure out if there is a blood clot or decrease in blood flow, which artery is affected and how bad the problem may be. Armed with this information, appropriate care decisions can be made. Programs that emphasize prompt vascular evaluation and management are successful in preventing amputations.

Malfunction of the circulatory system that fails to provide adequate blood supply leaves damaged tissue at risk for infection, ulceration, and amputation. One of the first visible signs that something is wrong with a patient's circulation might be seen in the legs. The patient may have:

- Cool or cold skin, especially in the feet
- Delayed capillary return
- Diminished hair growth on the legs and feet
- Non-detectable blood flow in the foot arteries
- Color changes in the foot to a more pinkish, purplish, or bluish hue
- A history of leg cramps with exercise
- Pain in the feet or legs while at rest
- A history of cigarette smoking
- Signs and symptoms of peripheral arterial disease (PAD).

## The Arterial System

The circulatory or vascular system can be divided into two broad categories: the *arterial system* that carries blood from the heart to the organs and the extremities via the pumping of the heart, and the *venous system* that returns the blood from the organs and extremities back to the heart. There is a third circulatory system not involved with the circulation of the blood that is rarely mentioned but is important for wound healing. It is called the lymphatic system. This system works to remove debris such as dead cells and other waste products. It, too, must be functioning properly if it is to aid the healing process.

Arterial circulation can be further divided into two categories: large vessels and small vessels. The large vessels are found in the core of the body and extend out to the extremities while the small vessels are within the organs and at the end of the vascular tree in the extremities.

## Macroangiopathy

Macroangiopathy is a term often associated with arterial large vessel disease and is characterized by stenosis (narrowing of the artery) or occlusion (blockage) in a major artery in the leg. The most likely place for this to happen is behind the knee where the femoral artery divides into three segments going away from the heart toward the foot at an anatomical location called Hunter's Canal. The solution to this blockage is usually a surgical procedure called a femoral-popliteal (fem-pop) artery bypass. This operation connects the good portion of the arteries back together and bypasses the clogged portion of the artery to re-establish circulation to the rest of the leg. A vein is usually harvested from the patient's leg, turned inside out, and connected to either side of the blocked artery to bypass the blockage. It is becoming more and more common to see long scars on the legs of patients with diabetes who have had veins harvested for bypass and open heart surgery.

## Microangiopathy

Microangiopathy is a disease of the arterial systems that affects the kidneys, eyes and extremities. In the patient with diabetes, chronically elevated blood sugar levels are known to cause a decrease in blood flow in the body's smallest vessels. The narrowing or complete closure of the small vessels in the body is considered the hallmark of diabetes.

There is a debate as to whether there actually is small vessel disease. What was thought to be a disease characterized by loss of circulation to the smallest vessels is now suspected as being the effects of a lack of circulation in the large vessels. In other words, these vessels are not the cause but the victim of the lack of circulation. Nonetheless, this loss of small vessel circulation will show itself in two ways: (1) the circulation to the toes will be cut off, which may cause gangrene (total loss of circulation causing tissue death) to develop in the toe and, as a result, the patient may lose a portion of or the entire toe, or (2) the skin of the feet and legs will become dry and scaly with the tendency to crack. Fortunately, this problem is easily treated with constant visual inspection of the limb and the use of a moisturizing lotion to keep the skin well hydrated.

Disease of the small or smaller vessel presents clinical situations that may be infinitely more difficult to heal because it is difficult to bypass those very small vessels. There have been studies using lasers, especially the Excimer cold laser that uses ultraviolet light to open some of these vessels. Most sutures are too thick to repair tiny arteries. Even the smallest diameter sutures used by the ophthalmologists in eye surgery are too thick.

Problems that can occur with small or large arterial circulation include stenosis: when the artery narrows resulting in a decreased volume of blood being circulated, and occlusion: when the blood flow is totally cut off in the affected vessels. Often it is not clear whether a patient's problem is due to small or large arterial vascular disease until testing has been done to discover the true nature of the problem and which vessels are involved.

## The Colors of Vascular Disease

In clinic, we see all varieties of problems and many patients have symptoms and foot problems consistent with vascular disease. Frequently, I see localized changes to the color of their skin on their legs and feet. These colors can tell us a lot about circulation.

- White or grey indicates acute vascular occlusion.
- A red and warm foot is a sign of early injury.
- A red and cool foot (dependant rubor) is a sign or peripheral vascular disease and *not* infection.
- Purple indicates loss of adequate blood supply. The most common cause of the purple toe is from plaque being dislodged from large vessels and getting stuck in the smaller vessels.
- Black means the tissue is dying and gangrene is present.

If you develop a foot wound, you should also be highly suspicious of developing circulatory problems in other parts in your body that will also need attention. As podiatrists, we're happy you come to get your feet evaluated, but you should also have your other organ systems checked. This can be done by your primary care provider but may require a specialist such as a cardiologist, ophthalmologist, or optometrist, dentist, and if necessary, a kidney specialist who can evaluate those other systems to be sure that they are functioning properly.

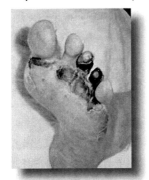

Gangrene

## Case Study

Mr. W came to the office accompanied by his wife. He had been diabetic for over twelve years and controlled his blood sugar levels by insulin injections. He managed his end-stage renal disease with peritoneal dialysis at home. The years of chronically elevated blood sugar levels also contributed to Mr. W's vascular disease and resulted in his becoming legally blind. He had developed an infection between the third and fourth toes on his left foot about twelve days earlier, and his wife was very concerned when his foot got red and warm to the touch.

Mr. W was seen by his PCP and placed on oral antibiotics, but was not given a surgical shoe to place his foot in a better environment for healing and help offload the pressure that was in part responsible for creating the wound. Nor was he given a follow-up appointment within a reasonable amount of time, which is typically about ten days. His wife told me that since Mr. W had taken the antibiotic pills, the infection had decreased, but she said, "I still thought he needed to be seen by a doctor who knows about feet."

When we took Mr. W's shoes and socks off, I was concerned, too. His left foot was cherry red almost up to his ankle. His foot was locally hot to the touch, and both the third and fourth toes were blackened and ulcerated on the conjoined sides. The infected skin on the bottom the foot looked like it was rolling over on itself, there was pus coming from under the bottom of his foot, and there was a foul odor from between the toes. Mr. W had developed gangrene, and his infection was worse than before his last office visit twelve days earlier.

Mr. W was admitted to the hospital and treated with intravenous antibiotics that stabilized the infection but that treatment did not help his black, gangrenous toes. Due to the number of other medical conditions that complicated his health, the vascular surgeons decided to try a bypass instead of taking off the toes with hopes that they could they could reverse the infection and bring more blood flow to the foot and save the toes. Mr. W successfully underwent the bypass surgery and our hopes were high that his foot infection would be cleared and his toes saved. However, within thirty-six hours, it became evident that the procedure had failed as the adjacent toes blackened and he developed fever. Clearly his life was at risk. It was decided that he would need a guillotine above-the-knee amputation procedure to save his life. Mr. W survived the procedure and was returned to the intensive care unit where he passed away soon after.

## Peripheral Arterial Disease (PAD) aka Peripheral Vascular Disease (PVD)

Peripheral vascular disease (PVD) has been the name used as a catch all phrase for a multitude of circulatory problems that can affect the feet. With more understanding of the pathological processes both the arterial and venous systems undergo, better descriptors have been used. Now PAD is used to identify patients who specifically lack arterial blood flow to the extremities and organs like the heart, brain, or kidneys. This disease affects about eight to twelve million Americans, and most are over the age of fifty. Older, obese adults (more women than men) are especially prone to asymptomatic PAD.

PAD refers to problems with arterial blood flow or circulation from the heart to the organs and extremities. It is one symptom of a bigger problem: generalized vascular disease that can affect the heart, brain, and the functioning of all vital organ systems in the body. Patients with diabetes often have poor circulation. The arteries in their legs may become narrow and hardened (atherosclerosis), and are frequently blocked when cholesterol and scar tissue build up plaque inside the arteries. This "hardening of the arteries" is the same disease that can cause heart attack and stroke.

PAD is a systemic disease. Clogging in one area of the body indicates clogging is occurring in other parts of the body as well. This is why almost all patients who have PAD also have problems with other organs. To prevent amputation when a patient has severe ischemia (pain caused by the lack of circulation) or gangrene, balloon angioplasty and stenting may be done to restore blood flow in the lower extremities. The procedure is done through a minimal incision in the groin area rather than the traditional procedures where the limb has to be surgically opened to replace the defective artery. If there is a re-clogging of the artery after having angioplasty or stenting, the surgeon can re-treat the limb.

PAD can be an independent disease in its own right. However, it is also one of the consequences of uncontrolled blood sugar levels. Many patients with diabetes do not know they have peripheral arterial disease since one type (asymptomatic) doesn't have symptoms such as aching in the legs, pain in the leg muscles, and possibly non-healing ulcers. Even the type with symptoms (symptomatic), comes on silently in the early stages.

Frequencies and incidences of PAD are increasing as the population gets older. Diabetes and vascular disease are systemic problems. Whatever condition you have in your leg arteries, you also have in your heart and brain. As Dr. Robert Frykberg recommends, we need to be "...getting physicians, doctors, nurses, clinicians, and health providers to start looking for [PAD] problems early on. Often the first time these patients are diagnosed is when they present with an ischemic lesion or a gangrene." Detecting PAD early can save your life.

## Risk Factors for PAD

PAD can affect patients with or without diabetes (though less often) and result in the loss of a limb. Without question, the combination of peripheral arterial disease in patients with diabetes with peripheral neuropathy can generate deadly consequences.

Those at the highest risk for developing PAD include former and current smokers, those who are obese, people with diabetes, kidney disease, high blood pressure, high cholesterol, history of cardiovascular disease, or a family history of the disease.

## Common Warning Signs of PAD

Often, you will not know you have PAD because the symptoms are subtle and few. If symptoms are present, they likely include fatigue or pain in the feet and legs from walking, foot or toe pain that often disturbs sleep, and wounds or ulcers of the feet that are slow to heal. Common symptoms of PAD are:

- Discomfort, cramping or heaviness in the toes, feet or legs
- Poorly healing or non-healing wounds on the toes, feet or legs
- Walking impairment
- Pain at rest that is localized to the lower leg or foot
- Abdominal pain that is provoked by eating
- Familial history of a first-degree relative with an abdominal or aortic aneurysm

The PAD Coalition is a helpful resource where you may find more information. See their Web site at http://www.padcoalition.org/.

## Venous Circulation

Venous circulation refers to the pathway the blood takes as it travels back toward the heart from the limbs or organs. The limbs have two pathways that return blood back to the heart: the deep path and the superficial path.

As its name indicates, the deep system is deep in the body usually embedded between the muscles. The superficial system is the one most people are familiar with, because we can see the blue-colored veins just under our skin. More than one patient has come to my office complaining of "very close" veins. They mean to say varicose, but I know what they are talking about and it does seem to describe the appearance of the veins since they are very close to the skin's surface and more visible than the deeper veins.

The veins appear to be blue because the blood in them does not contain any oxygen. Just like there are two and sometimes three backup systems in airplanes, the body has backup systems as well. The blood coming back to the heart may return via one of two systems, the deep system or the superficial system. So, if one system goes out, the other system picks up for it. If you are one of those people who develop venous disease where the veins become incompetent, you'll appreciate knowing that your body has this capability.

Think of the vein like a garden hose where every so often there's a three-leafed valve, and these valves open towards the heart. When you walk, the muscles contract and compress the vein. This action squeezes the vein and pushes the blood up to the next little compartment where the valves open up, and then they close capturing a small amount of blood bringing it closer to the heart. In people who stand a lot, or who don't move a lot, these valves may become incompetent. What happens is the muscle contracts, and a small amount of blood shoots up to the next compartment, but it falls back down to the compartment from which it was just released. The amount of blood now in the vein is too large for the capacity of the vein and it causes the vein to dilate, and that's what causes a varicose vein, which is an indication of a particular type of vascular disease called venous insufficiency. Fluid tends to leak out of the veins into the tissues and we see swelling of the legs that is called edema.

## Venous Insufficiency

The complication of these incompetent valves in the veins leads to venous disease or venous insufficiency. The danger of venous insufficiency is that patients can develop edema and venous stasis dermatitis (VSD), which usually causes the skin to become dry, inflamed, and itchy. Some patients will scratch their legs thereby complicating an already bad situation and causing the area to ulcerate causing venous ulcers. The bad news is that these drippy weeping lesions can become large and extremely difficult to heal. I've seen patients start with small, localized venous ulcer on their legs and end up with a gigantic ulcer that seems to encompass the entire lower leg and stay that way indefinitely.

Some patients develop an ulcer in a specific location on the inside of the ankle where a perforating vein is located that connects the superficial and the deep systems. Sometimes that perforating vein becomes incompetent and we see back flow from the deep system to the superficial system. The pressure from the deep system, being greater than the superficial system can handle, causes an ulcer to develop. These wounds are among the most difficult to heal.

There are many physicians who may not be acquainted with the anatomy in that area of the leg, and patients treated by these physicians may have a tough time healing because they are fighting the pressure gradient. The solution is to have a vascular surgeon tie off that little vein between the deep and the superficial system so the ulcer can heal. Unfortunately, most of the folks with advanced cases of VSD use motorized carts instead of walking, so they sit most of the time not using nature's built-in pump to return fluid back towards the heart, which adds to the complexity of the problem.

When we diagnose a patient who has VSD, if they have adequate arterial blood flow, we can use compression stockings as soon as possible to prevent further VSD, chronic edema to the leg and possible ulceration. The most common treatment for venous ulcer is to apply an absorbent dressing followed by a compression dressing called an Unna boot. Many patients benefit from compression boots that are large balloon-like devices that fit over the legs and use external compression to mimic the function of the muscles and literally force the fluid from the feet and legs toward the heart. The Normatec PCD (Pneumatic Compression Device) technology (www.normatecusa.com) uses twenty-first century technology developed by Laura Jacobs, MD, PhD. It uses the idea of peristaltic compression, the same mechanism that your intestines use to move food through your digestive tract to remove fluid from the legs. This boot compresses the fluid from the foot toward the heart in small amounts without letting the fluid fall back. Two to thirty minutes treatment is all it takes and can be done in the privacy of the patient's home.

Anytime a patient gets an ulcer on his foot, we need to determine the reason for the ulcer. It could be arterial, venous, or neurotropic, caused by peripheral neuropathy. Regardless of the reason, we know that there's a vascular component to it. We can try healing that ulcer by getting the patient off his foot and into a surgical shoe or using a cam walker; taking a tissue sample for a culture; checking the neurological and vascular status; and giving the appropriate topical as well as oral antibiotic if there is an infection. If the ulcer doesn't heal, we have to re-think the cause of the ulcer. In most cases, the problem is the patient does not have enough arterial circulation, and healthcare providers don't realize the situation. This may happen with doctors who don't treat this type of problem frequently or who are not familiar with the alternative of treatment for such a wound. I have encountered several patients reporting his previous doctor saying "Well, let's just put a little cream on that hole on your foot. It's not infected, so we'll just take a look at it next month." That's the wrong thing to do.

## Case Study

Peter was a 58-year-old male with type 2 diabetes who was accompanied by his wife to the clinic for a diabetic foot evaluation. He had a family history of diabetes and was deeply concerned about his foot health. Peter told me that he had been diabetic for almost twelve years and recently it had been difficult for him to keep his blood sugars under control. He thought he was taking good control of his diet by not eating too many sweets, but he did mention he liked pasta and spaghetti and ate it several times a week. Because of the recent serious elevation in blood sugar levels, his PCP had recently changed his medication from pills and started him on insulin injections.

As Peter walked into the treatment area I noted something peculiar about his gait. He held his hands up as if to balance himself like a child who is just learning to walk. Peter reported he did not see well and had episodes of falling. His wife interjected, "He falls a lot and we are afraid he will break his hip. We just don't know why he is falling or what to do about it."

In further discussions, we learned that problems with his eyes were becoming progressively worse over time but not necessarily attributed to his diabetes. He had been seen by his optometrist, was wearing glasses, and reported his vision was fine because he could still read the newspaper. But, that had not altered the pattern of his falling. Since the family was not sure of the type of doctor to see about the falling problem, Peter had not received any treatment. On first review, it seemed that his problem might be better served by an ophthalmologist, neurologist, and orthopedist. But I reserved my decision until I completed his exam.

His exam showed diminished pedal pulses, delayed capillary return, dry skin, decreased elasticity in the skin, and cold skin temperature—all signs of peripheral vascular disease. But, further complicating the picture was the fact that he was unable to feel the monofilament testing device or a vibrating tuning fork when applied to several bony prominences on his ankles and feet. This confirmed to me that he had sensory neuropathy.

The picture was becoming clearer and I was beginning to understand why he was falling. "Can you feel the floor with your feet," I finally asked him.

"No," was his response.

"Have you told your primary care provider about this?" I asked.

"No."

Looking him straight in the eye, I asked him, "Why not?"

He replied, "Because my doctor never asked me about it. He almost never looks at my feet."

I reviewed his chart and was astonished to see that his most recent Hemoglobin A1c test result was 13.2! The upper limit of normal of this test is less than 7. Below is a chart of values to know about the Hemoglobin A1c test.

Normal: Less than 7
Excellent: 7-7.5
Good: 7.5-8.5
Fair: 8.5-9.5
Poor: Greater than 9.5

When I asked Peter if he knew about this test and his results he again said, "No." A result of 13.2 in a hemoglobin A1c test translates into an average blood sugar level of over 330! We would expect normally controlled blood sugar levels to be close to 110 and an A1c value less than 7. Clearly Peter had an unacceptable test result and his doctor had done nothing to educate him about the seriousness of this condition. We discussed the test results with Peter. We also mentioned the ABCs of diabetes: A is for the A1c test, which should be less than 7; B is for blood pressure should be below 130/80; and C is for cholesterol (LDL) which should be below 100.

This ongoing and chronically elevated blood sugar problem led Peter to develop sensory neuropathy. The numbness that prevented him from feeling the floor with his feet caused him to be unable to sense where his body was in space and resulted in his falling. That was why he walked with his hands in the air for better balance. The pieces of the puzzle all fit together.

In order for Peter to try to get sensation back in his feet and to prevent future falls, it was imperative for him to get his blood sugar levels back into the normal range. We ordered him a cane for mild support and balance, and consultations with a nutritionist to refresh his knowledge on foods and how they affect his blood sugars. We sent him to a kinesiologist to start an exercise program to help burn blood sugars, and to the orthotics and prosthetics department for diabetic shoes. We made sure he had adequate diabetes education.

Peter stayed adherent to his treatment plan and over the coming months reported better blood sugar control, exercising more, and a better ability to feel the floor. He still occasionally stumbles, but the cane saves him from falling.

## Edema, It's the Pits!

Another sign of disease in the venous circulatory system is edema—fluid in the tissues of the legs. This is caused from either a systemic disease that affects the heart, liver, and kidneys, or by varicose veins or a blood clot in the legs. With these conditions, not enough blood is pumped back to the heart. This causes a difference between the pressure inside the vein and the pressure outside the vein. This retained excess fluid occurs when the body retains too much salt. Excess salt attracts water into the spaces within the soft tissues in the leg. Diuretics or "water pills" like Lasix™ can help reduce the extra fluid in the legs by accelerating the function of the kidneys.

Edema may be categorized as non-pitting or pitting. To identify pitting edema, press your finger to the skin of the tibia bone along the front of your leg. If there is an indentation after removing your finger, you have pitting edema. The danger associated with pitting edema is the development of venous stasis dermatitis (VSD), which can have serious effects that may lead to amputation. Some patients who suffer with VSD have legs that look like partially cooked pieces of meat with bronze to rusty orange skin color. These are called hemosidirin deposits.

In non-pitting edema there is no indentation of the skin when you press your finger to your leg. It still causes accumulation of fluid in the interstitial spaces of the tissues just like pitting edema, but diuretic medications or "water pills" don't work to reduce the fluid. Non-pitting edema is not related to venous disease, but may be caused by an inflammatory disease of the lymphatic system. The lymphatic system is known as the sewer pipes of the body because it carries away dead cells and other debris to be removed by the kidneys or liver.

Pitting edema causes the skin to become discolored, dry, and itchy. Scratching the itch can cause the area to ulcerate. Fluid may drain from those wounds. If you have pitting edema but have not developed an ulcer, you should be greatly helped by moisturizing lotions and compression stockings. The lotion keeps the skin supple and prevents dry and itchy skin. Compression stockings keep adequate pressure on the leg so fluid won't collect. Be sure to put the stockings on *before* you get out of bed and before your legs start to swell.

## Ischemia

Ischemia is the condition where there is not enough blood flow to adequately maintain the tissues. With ischemia there is insufficient oxygen and nutrients delivered to the tissue and there is a buildup of metabolic waste products. Ultimately ischemia can lead to tissue death. It can be caused by a stenosis or occlusion of an artery and often complicates and delays the healing of wounds in the feet and legs such as ulcers and infections, and may necessitate a revascularization procedure or amputation.

> Press a finger against the toe until the skin color blanches. Remove the finger, and count how long it takes for the toe to return to normal color. More than three seconds is abnormal and indicates problems with the microcirculation to the toe.

## Diagnostic Testing

The International Working Group on the Diabetic Foot recommends evaluation of the following three areas when it comes to your foot and assessing your personal risk for amputation.

1. Pulses/circulation
2. Protective sensation evaluation
3. Identification of bone, soft tissue, and nail deformities.

### Ankle-Brachial Index (ABI)

When one of my patients has a delay in wound healing, the first consideration is always the patient's circulation. I must suspect that their circulation may not be adequate enough to bring sufficient fresh oxygenated blood, nutrients, and antibiotics to heal the wound. In that case, the first test I order is an Ankle Brachial Index (ABI) with segmental pressures. The ABI test is the safest and most reliable test to measure the circulation in the leg. It is a non-invasive measurement of the blood flow in the leg that involves inflating a series of blood pressure cuffs and measuring blood flow in the leg, foot, and toes, and comparing those measurements to the blood flow in the arm.

Ankle Brachial Index (ABI) Test and Pulse Volume Recordings (PVR) help the vascular specialist determine whether you have vascular disease due to diabetes and PAD. Therefore, if you have a wound or ulcer in your foot that won't heal and wonder whether or not a vascular surgical procedure can help resolve your problem, you'll want to understand how your doctor interprets the ABI results.

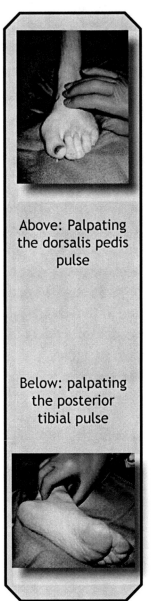

Above: Palpating the dorsalis pedis pulse

Below: palpating the posterior tibial pulse

232

The results are calculated both in numbers and a descriptor of the quality of the exam or "waveform." The normal resting ankle-brachial index value is 1. This is when the blood pressure at the ankle is the same as the pressure in the arm indicating there is no significant narrowing or blockage of blood flow. A resting ABI value of "greater than" or "less than" 1 is usually an indicator of abnormal circulation. However, some patients will have an ABI value of greater than 1 because of calcified (loss of elasticity) arteries, which is a very common finding in patients with diabetes. A resting ankle-brachial index of less than 1 is also abnormal:

- Less than 0.95: there is significant narrowing of one or more blood vessels

- Less than 0.8: pain in the foot, leg, or buttock may occur with exercise such as walking.

- Less than 0.4: symptoms may occur when the patient is at rest.

- Less than 0.25: the chances of losing a limb due to a failure to heal are very high.

The waveform indicates the quality of the circulation. It's similar to an EKG exam that shows the quality of the heart function. The waveform displays the results of the exam in a graphic display as opposed to a numerical value and helps us evaluate the circulation. Changes in the waveform indicate changes in the circulation. Comparing pressures with waveforms helps to avoid errors in the interpretation of the exam. The waveform can be triphasic (the best), biphasic (acceptable), or monophasic (not good) and depends on the functioning of your heart. In some cases where the circulation of the digit is very poor or there is almost no blood flow into the digit, the ABI may be less than 1, and there may not be a waveform at all.

The results of an ABI are calculated by dividing the results of the blood pressure reading of the ankle by the blood pressure reading of the arm (brachial). The test will identify whether there is a problem with the circulation and, most importantly, reveal the location in the foot or leg where the circulation is decreased or absent. Why is the ABI such an important test? It can save someone from returning over and over for surgeries to remove devitalized tissue due to non-healing wounds. For the amputation surgery to be successful the first time, the exact location of where the blood supply ends must be determined. For patients with diabetes, or other at-risk patients, that means the location where the body has sufficient circulation to heal the wound. I have seen cases where patients did not have the ABI test before the decision was made to amputate a toe, foot, or leg at a particular location. In some of these cases, the patient had to return to the operating room for amputations farther up the leg with hopes that the site would eventually heal.

Imagine that you have an infection so severe in your toe that your first operation is to have your toe removed. Several days later it becomes apparent that the surgery site is not going to heal, so you go back to the operating room a second time, for a procedure called a below-the-knee amputation (BKA). If this site fails to heal, you go back a third time for a procedure called an above-the-knee amputation (AKA). Imagine having three trips to the operating room, three general anesthesia inductions, and three parts of your body taken away from you all within as little as two weeks. The stress on the body, mind, and spirit is enormous, and in some cases, patients fail to survive the procedures. Of course, surgery is not the first method of care for dealing with inadequate circulation, but when non-surgical therapies such as medication fail to bring enough fresh oxygenated blood to the affected leg, it is up to the vascular surgeon to decide whether the affected vessels can be repaired and, if so, what is the best method to use.

## Case Study

James was a patient who had a tiny ulcer on his fifth toe for more than two years. It would "cover over" but it would not heal. He visited a surgeon who recommended the best way to heal the ulcer was from the inside out. James' wife was instructed to probe the wound two times daily with the wooden end of a Q-tip. This maneuver not only failed to heal the wound, but when James had an X-ray of his infected toe it showed a serious bone infection. Since the wound was two years old, it was determined the best treatment was to remove the toe. However, he had no palpable pulses in his feet. He had delayed capillary return, and his feet were cold to the touch. I sent James for an ABI exam to evaluate his circulation.

The results of the ABI were shocking to both James and his wife revealing that there was not enough circulation in his foot for me to successfully remove the toe and for him to heal from the procedure. Amputating James's toe might invite a disaster because he had developed a serious case of peripheral arterial disease from his diabetes. I referred James to a vascular surgeon who placed him on medication that failed to bring enough blood to his toe. Eventually, he had a bypass procedure in his leg that was successful. Shortly after he healed from the procedure, I was able to remove the toe and thankfully the operative site healed.

## Peripheral MRA

When I identify a patient whom I believe has PAD, there are several diagnostic tests available to identify the location and extent of a vascular lesion. Imaging of the arterial system is necessary in determining if limping or impaired gait is occurring as a result of reduced blood supply to the leg muscles. It can also help us discover why a person has pain while resting, or why foot ulcers are not healing. This information helps the vascular surgeon decide what type of treatment may be best for you. Open general surgery, minimal incision balloon angioplasty, or amputation—the choices are based on the type and location of the lesion, and any issues concerning your general health.

MRA stands for magnetic resonance angiogram. Like MRI scanning used to evaluate the deep soft tissue structures in your body, the peripheral MRA serves as a diagnostic tool to evaluate the vascular system or blood vessels. The noninvasive test is fast and easy and does not involve catheters, radiation, contrast materials (which can be toxic to the kidneys), or the risks of angiograms. With this technique, the whole vascular system from abdominal aorta to the foot can be seen in less than two minutes. This will undoubtedly change how we diagnose and treat patient with peripheral vascular disease.

The MRA was initially studied in the late 1980s and continued into the 1990s. Today, an MRA can detect blood flow in the foot with an 81 percent accuracy rate and can be performed to locate the level of the vascular disease so the vascular surgeon can perform the proper intervention at the right location. Peripheral MRA uses a magnetic field and pulses of radio wave energy to provide pictures of blood vessels in the body. It can provide information not available by X-ray, ultrasound, or CT scan.

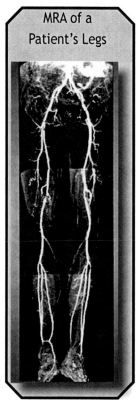

MRA of a Patient's Legs

Often there are red flags or signs of vascular problems before the patient's leg is affected, but you have to know what to look for. Patients may have had heart attacks or strokes, and they or their doctors may not have made the connection between these various vascular problems and their diabetes. Patients who know they have circulatory symptoms in their legs may never realize that other systems are simultaneously being affected by vascular disease until it is too late. They may develop serious complications like a stroke, blood clots, or heart attack. The legs may be the first external sign, but by the time that damage is visible, there must be internal damage that is equally threatening.

Reasons many people get to an advanced stage of circulatory problems might include: (1) lack of education about diabetes and what it does to their bodies, and (2) denial about the disease. They do not understand that chronically elevated blood sugar levels cause generalized vascular disease that affects the eyes, kidneys, heart, brain, and the function of all vital organ systems in the body, as well as the lower limbs. The effect of diabetes against the circulatory system is cumulative. So the decisions we make today concerning blood sugar control and practicing preventive behaviors have long-term consequences.

There is the risk that at some point a patient with diabetes will have an incident with his feet. It might be a blister, an ingrown toenail, or ulcer that would seem simple enough to treat and heal—but if you have diabetes, it may not be. If a patient has failed to do his part by keeping blood sugar levels in the normal range and preserving the normal function of the body, my treatments may not work. If they do work, it may take longer than normal.

## Foot Notes: Treatment for Arterial Disease and Aids to Circulation

In addition to behavioral changes, there are medicines such as Pletal™ and Plavix™ that can be of some value for patients with peripheral vascular disease. Pletal™ is used to treat the symptoms of intermittent claudication (pain in the legs). Pletal™ helps people walk a longer distance before leg pain occurs. Plavix™ is used to prevent platelets, the building blocks of blood clots, from clustering together and forming a blood clot. Plavix™ is also used to prevent and treat heart attack, stroke, and acute coronary syndrome. An 81-milligram aspirin will help prevent blood clotting.

Unless you understand the vital role of the circulatory system, especially the arterial system, and how to protect it, chronically elevated blood sugar levels can eventually destroy the circulation that provides your body with the very essence of life: fresh oxygenated blood. The easiest and most cost-effective methods to increase a patient's circulation are under the control of the patient:

- Take your meds.

- Stop smoking.

- Keep blood sugar levels within the normal range. This is the most important step—all other efforts are secondary to this. Failure to do this will cause complications in the circulatory and neurological systems that can lead to an amputation.

- Tell your doctor if you notice any color changes to skin or if a wound seems to be slow in healing.

- Eat the right foods and in reasonable portions.

- Start or increase an exercise program. Walking is the best exercise for your feet. Swimming is a good exercise, but cold water should be avoided. Special protective swim sneakers are available for foot protection.

- Do not wear garters or constricting girdles that may cut off circulation.

- When sitting, use a rocking chair or footstool. When traveling and sitting for long time periods, use range of motion exercises every hour to aid circulation.

## Vascular Survey

- Do I have vascular risks that will delay healing of a foot wound?

- Do I smoke?

- Do I have peripheral neuropathy? If so, what type of neuropathy is affecting me, autonomic, sensory or motor?

- Have I had a foot exam this year?

- Do I have problems with my vision?

- Do I have problems with my teeth?

- Do I have problems concerning my urinary system?

- Do I know about silent or painless trauma and why it is dangerous?

- Do I know what a "triggering event" is and how to prevent/protect myself from these often disastrous events?

- What must I know and do to prevent a triggering event (painless trauma to the foot caused by loss of protective sensation in the foot) causing me to have pain or feel numb at the same time?

# Chapter Nine

## The Foot Ulcer, Causes and Cures

> *Skin ulcers and wounds are the most expensive dermatological problems followed second by acne.*
> ~ Peter Cavanagh, Cleveland Clinic, Cleveland, Ohio

At any given time, approximately 5 percent of the diabetic population will have a foot ulcer, and almost half of them are infected by the time a patient seeks medical attention.[1] A foot ulcer can develop and escalate quickly into a significant problem and if an infection occurs, it may require hospitalization, intravenous antibiotics and perhaps vascular surgery to avoid an amputation.

> *The foot is the crossroad of several pathological processes. Because each of these components can contribute to foot ulcers, a multi-disciplinary approach is needed.*
> —Dr. Nicolass Schaper[1]

A 2007 study by Peters, Armstrong, and Lavery showed that 71.6 percent of ulcers healed; 12.3 percent did not heal; and 16 percent had lower extremity amputations.[3] Healing the foot ulcer is much like solving a puzzle because ulcers are complex wounds, and usually there are multiple contributing factors. If each of these factors has not been identified and treated correctly, the ulcer usually fails to heal. A healed ulcer might return, or worse, the patient might lose a limb. Therefore, understanding the reason the patient has developed the ulcer helps us decide how to treat it. Numerous factors contribute to the development of the diabetic foot wound. The most common factors for re-ulceration include:

- Being male
- Being older than sixty
- Having Type 2 diabetes
- Duration of diabetes longer than ten years
- Alcohol abuse
- Tobacco abuse
- Nephropathy (kidney disease)
- Retinopathy (eye disease of retina)
- Neuropathy (nervous system disease)
- Peripheral Vascular Disease
- History of amputation
- Elevated A1c (higher than 9%)
- Elevated pressure on foot
- Rigid toe deformity or Charcot foot
- Extra sesamoid bone in the big toe

No matter what type of injury a patient has, PAD delays or prevents wound healing. In the best-case scenario, the circulatory problem can be repaired and the wound will heal. In the worst-case scenario, the circulatory problem cannot be repaired, the wound will not heal, and the patient will pay the ultimate price: the loss of a leg.

## Dry Skin

Dry skin is a condition that should be taken seriously by patients with diabetes. An examination by a physician will assure the skin condition will be appropriately diagnosed and treated. Unfortunately, most people do not know the difference between dry skin and infected or diseased skin.

While there are various medical reasons for dry skin, at the top of the list we should consider autonomic neuropathy. This malfunction of the nervous system is considered to be a variant of diabetic peripheral neuropathy where the nerves that innervate the glands that secrete oil and sweat fail to function. The results are dry flaky skin that seems to affect the entire leg can be very itchy and therefore dangerous. Repeatedly scratching this dry skin can lead to an ulcer on the leg. Without realizing that some skin infections can also be fungal (such a tine a infection or athlete's foot), or bacterial many people do not seek medical treatment. Thinking they have dry skin, they try to treat it themselves. They may apply over-the-counter moisturizing lotion, petroleum jelly, or baby oil. I have spoken with patients who have done this exact treatment for years but the affected patch never seemed to go away. More than likely they are trying to cure a pathological mold, fungal, or yeast infection known as tinea pedis or athlete's foot. The bad news is that this type of infection can be spread to other parts of the body or to other people. I normally give patients a surgical scrub brush to use with antibacterial soap and instructions to vigorously scrub their feet to get all the dead skin off, rinse and dry them well, and apply a topical anti-fungal powder or cream.

Another reason for dry, itching skin is venous insufficiency where the veins fail to function correctly and fluid collects in the legs. This problem leads to venous stasis dermatitis, where the skin of the legs can become discolored and itchy. Scratching this type of dry skin can cause a venous ulcer. In advanced cases, a rust to orange-brown discoloration can be seen in the skin. This change in the pigmentation of the skin is the result of hemosidirin or iron from the pigment in the red cells depositing in the skin. An ulcer should be seen as a wildly waving red flag that gets your attention, particularly if you have diabetes.

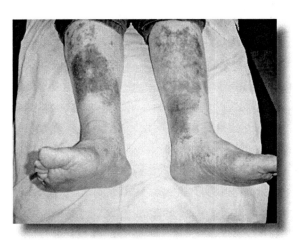

**Hemosidirin Deposits in Legs**

If it turns out that your problem is indeed dry skin, one treatment I use is an emollient lotion containing urea. Urea has the unique ability to moisturize dry skin by drawing moisture into the cell structure in the top layer of the skin. It is available in several strengths and is one of the best products for this condition. If you can't reach your feet, maybe you can recruit a family member or friend to help you apply lotion. Hydrating the skin is one behavior that actually helps to prevent ulcers and amputations.

## Biomechanical Problems

There are multiple causes for development of diabetic foot ulcers related to biomechanical problems. These include bone, soft tissue, and nail deformities associated with faulty biomechanics, mechanical instability, connective tissue disease, muscle atrophy, fat pad loss, and calluses. Other reasons a person with diabetes might develop a foot ulcer is having a previous ulceration or amputation. Elevated blood glucose levels lead to the damage of connective tissue. This results in limited joint mobility, high peak pressures during gait, and loss of the normal heel and forefoot cushioning that can lead to the formation of ulcers. Ankle equinus, which causes a person to have a limited amount of heel contact, moves more pressure to the front of the foot. In an attempt to correct this kind of a problem, an Achilles-tendon lengthening surgical procedure can be done. This procedure reduces the amount of pressure across the mid-foot during walking. This procedure significantly reduces forefoot pressure as well and therefore reduces the risk for ulceration. The shortening of the calf muscle (gastroc-soleus equinus) causes an inability to move the toes upward, which is essential in the gait cycle of normal gait.

Bone deformities in the toes and feet can rub against your shoe and cause abnormal pressure. Ill-fitting footwear can also contribute to ulcer formation. When there is abnormal pressure against an underlying bony structure, your body tries to protect itself by forming a thickened skin or a natural protective pad commonly called a corn (located on the toes) or a callus (located on the bottom of the foot under the metatarsal bones). Patients with diabetes and sensory neuropathy may not feel the pressure caused by the thickened skin pushing against the bone. If that thick skin is not removed, you may develop an abscess under the corn or callus. The abscess can lead to an infection of the soft tissues called cellulitis. If the cellulitis is not treated promptly, it can cause a bone infection called osteomyelitis.

## Neuropathy

The next factor affecting the start of an ulcer is peripheral sensory neuropathy. PAD and PVD complicate ulcer healing but are not responsible for the creation of ulcers. Patients with diabetes having this condition or the loss of protective sensation in their feet from a variety of other reasons, such as cancer, medications, back problems and exposure to heavy metals may not feel pain when they injure themselves. Cuts, scratches, or lacerations that might go unnoticed in most patients can cause a catastrophe for the patient with diabetes or the at-risk patient. These wounds should sound big alarms because when things go wrong for patients with diabetes, they can go very wrong seemingly in the blink of an eye.

A variant of sensory neuropathy is the Charcot foot deformity. This problem is caused from increased blood flow with loss of bone (mineral) density and a propensity for micro fractures and destruction of the joints across the mid foot. With the bones in abnormal positions combined with faulty biomechanical function, ulcers are commonly seen on the bottom of the mid foot.

**Trauma**

A foot ulcer in the foot that has no feeling is usually the result of painless or silent trauma of mechanical, thermal, or chemical origin—we're not talking about events like major car accidents. In the foot of a patient with diabetes, a trauma can be something as minor as too much pressure against the heel from the bed sheets that are tucked in too tight and do not permit the feet enough room to move under the covers.

Trauma can also occur when you bump your foot against the doorframe on your way to the bathroom at night, when you walk barefooted on the sizzling hot blacktop to get the mail, or when you use a medicated corn pad with salicylic acid that causes a chemical burn to your skin. These are all examples of silent, painless traumas, unfelt, unnoticed, yet dangerous to the diabetic patient.

A foot wound provides a point of entry for bacteria and causes the risk of a soft tissue infection, which can turn into an ulcer or the most-feared complication a diabetic patient can face—a bone infection (osteomyelitis). In either case, you will spend significant time and money to treat these infections, including possible time in the hospital. In fact, foot infections account for the largest number of diabetes-related hospital admissions and are the most common non-traumatic cause of amputations. If left untreated, these infections can threaten life and limb. Proper healing of a foot ulcer and intervention to reduce the rate of recurrence can reduce the risk of a second ulcer, infection and the risk of lower-extremity amputation.

Eighty-five percent of all lower extremity amputations are preceded by a foot infection or ulcer in patients with diabetes. Preventing these ulcers is one of the main goals in preventing lower limb amputations. Professor Andrew J.M. Boulton, MD, FRCP, is in the department of medicine at the University of Manchester, Manchester, UK, and the Division of Endocrinology, Metabolism and Diabetes, University of Miami. Professor Boulton says, "People at the greatest risk of ulceration can easily be identified by careful clinical examination of the feet, education, and frequent follow-up is indicated in these patients." Yet, most medical doctors do not ask to see a patient's feet during a routine examination.[4]

## X Marks the Spot Where Can Ulcers Be Found

Gait platforms and in-shoe measuring devices are used to analyze pressure against the foot during gait and show where the highest forces are on the bottom of the foot. The areas of the foot that receive the highest forces are the most likely to ulcerate, so this technology provides the key to building proper orthotics or placing padding to offload the site of highest pressure to protect your feet.

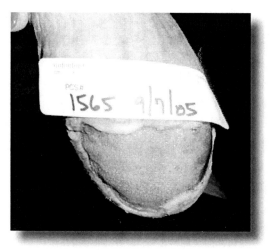

**Debrided Heel Ulcer**

In a recent article in *Diabetes Care*, Dr. David Armstrong shared his research findings when comparing the location of ulceration and the probability of reulceration. Ulcers on the top of the toes are due more to footgear or ill-fitted shoes. Changing shoes to a deeper and wider toe box can prevent re-ulceration. Ulcers on the bottom of the foot are due more to pressure issues. Reducing pressure or offloading the site of the ulcer with accommodative pads or biomechanical orthotics has worked well for preventing recurrent ulcers.

The incidence of diabetic ulcers on the bottom of the foot is quite high. Twenty-five percent of all diabetic ulcers occur under the first toe, 19 percent occur under the first metatarsal, and 15 percent occur under the fifth metatarsal. By protecting these specific locations, we have the opportunity to prevent almost two-thirds of the ulcers on the diabetic foot.

Anatomically, the back of the heel has a small surface space to absorb a large amount of pressure. Ulcers generated by pressure or friction where the bed sheets rub against the foot are usually seen in patients who are bedridden for long time periods. This often occurs after a stroke or while the patient is recovering in bed from an amputation. Because of their location and the fragility of the tissues in that location, heel ulcers often require substantial treatment. Ironically, an ulcer on the back of the heel or on ankle bone is almost 100 percent preventable. Some hospitals and extended care facilities seem oblivious to this ongoing problem.

## Testing for Infection

Testing must be done for patients with infection. We take a social history of smoking or alcohol use, nutritional status, and the degree to which the patient monitors blood glucose levels. We start with an ABI test to see if there is a blockage of blood flow to the foot. We may do an MRA that produces a 3-D image of the vascular system. We test the patient's blood glucose levels and hemoglobin A1c, and get a complete blood count, sedimentation rate, a C-reactive protein test—both indicators of inflammation, and a creatinine level, which is an indicator of kidney function. Other lab tests include liver and kidney function tests, check for vascular profusions, sensory acuity, and joint mobility. X-rays should be taken and if there is any question as to whether the bone is infected or if only the soft tissues are infected we can do a white cell (indium) scan. If we feel that the patient has a bone infection, we can do a technetium, or gallium scan. When a bone is infected, a bone culture is taken in conjunction with a biopsy.

## Types of Treatment for Ulcers

Getting a foot ulcer to heal is an art based in science. It takes great patience, can be costly, and takes the best science to help our patients recover. In treating a foot ulcer we need to maintain a moist wound environment, offload areas of pressure, protect against further infection, maintain control of blood glucose level, establish the level of arterial supply, initiate appropriate wound care including removal of necrotic or non-viable tissue as needed.

## Debridement

The primary goal for the care of foot ulcers is to achieve closure as quickly as possible. But before we can close the wound, we have to clean it.

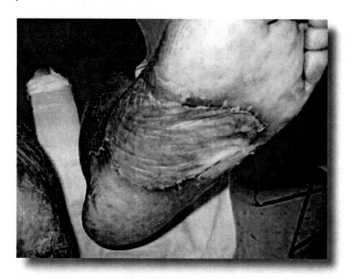

**Healing Blister**

Debridement, or the removal of necrotic (dead) tissue, is imperative in the treatment of ulcerative wounds and to protect against bacteria. There are various types of debridement including autolytic (which occurs naturally on its own), mechanical, enzymatic, sharp/surgical, and biosurgical.

- *Mechanical debridement* is usually accomplished with a dry dressing or whirlpool.

- *Enzymatic debridement* involves the topical application of a debriding enzyme to the wound.

- Papain urea agents are not particular to the type of tissue to which they adhere. These enzymes go after all proteins that have the amino acid known as cysteine to digest and strip away the fibers on the wound that hold dead tissue in place. Accuzyme™ and Panafil™ ointments use Papain urea. The U.S. Government recalled Papain in September 2008. All wound care products containing Papain were stopped being manufactured.

- Collagenase enzymes are used for removing dead tissue from wounds. Collagenase enzymes only eat denatured collagen without negatively affecting the other proteins in the wounded area. It also contributes to the formation of healthy granulation tissue. Santyl™ ointment contains collagenase.

- *Sharp or surgical debridement* remains the preferred method for debriding wounds in patients with diabetic foot ulcers. Removal of dead tissue on a regular basis (decreasing bioburden) can expedite the rate at which a diabetic foot wound heals and recently has been shown to increase the probability of obtaining full wound closure.

- *Biosurgical debridement* includes hydrosurgery systems that use specialized water jet-powered surgical tools designed to cut and remove unwanted tissue from ulcers or wounds without driving microbial contamination into the wound. The VersaJet™ system appears to cause less bleeding than traditional knife debridements and promotes more rapid wound healing.

- *Ultrasonic debridement* is a new and virtually pain-free way to prepare the wound bed. This method allows the clinician to control the rate of fluid flow, therefore increasing the level of precision. It has an antimicrobial effect sub-dermally. These devices offer rapid results, safety, and efficacy while providing exceptional formation of healing tissue with minimal or no bleeding. This technology is being used within in-patient and out-patient clinics throughout the country. This relatively gentle wound bed preparation tool offers hope to patients whose wounds have stalled in the healing process. This new equipment makes a great alternative to the scalpel for debriding diabetic foot wounds.

- *Polyacrylate debriding systems* provide quick, simple, safe, and pain-free debridement in a trouble-free, user-friendly dressing that provides 24-hour simultaneous rinsing and debriding. The dressing is activated by Ringer's solution, the most perfect physiologic fluid. The dressing only needs to be changed once per day; therefore it is an ideal choice in acute care. Management of this type of dressing can be taught to the family for home care at discharge. Another plus is that this system is the only dressing that does not require wound cleansing, further reducing costs of saline or wound cleansers. It provides constant cleansing of the wound bed, removing devitalized material and biofilm[5]. Bacterial and fungal absorption properties of a hydrogel dressing with a super absorbent polymer core[6] debriding wounds at a mean rate of 38.11 percent per week.[7]

## Negative Pressure Wound Therapy

A wound with bacteria and devitalized tissue is a challenge to heal because it is not clean. Negative pressure wound therapy makes cleaning the wound possible, so it accelerates wound healing. One treatment that helps is the Wound VAC™ (Vacuum-Assisted Closure) or negative pressure therapy (NPWT). We use negative pressure every day when we use a straw to drink, and this twenty-first century wound care device uses the same principle to help heal large, deep, and draining wounds such as heel ulcers. It literally sucks out the debris and excess fluid through a suction hose that runs to a machine. The Blue Sky Versatile Vacuum System™ is another device that uses similar technology with different dressing configurations also for patients who may benefit from a suction device to promote wound healing.

The name brand, Wound VAC™ (developed at Wake Forest University School of Medicine) has been in use since the mid-1990s for treatment of burns, traumatic wounds, pressure ulcers, and surgical wounds. In 2006, the use was expanded to include the treatment of diabetic ulcers. NPWT promotes wound healing as it draws the wound edges together, provides a moist healing wound environment, promotes blood flow, removes wound debris and infectious materials, reduces swelling, and promotes granulation tissue formation. NPWT is also known as topical negative pressure, sub-atmospheric pressure, sub-atmospheric pressure dressing, vacuum sealing technique, and sealed surface suction. Regardless what you call it, sub-atmospheric pressure helps increase local blood flow and granulation tissue formation, decrease bacterial load, and promote wound closure.

## Offloading/Pressure Redistribution Strategies

An estimated 90 percent of foot ulcers develop due to abnormal pressure on the foot. Reduction of pressure, external forces, and preventing painless injury to the foot are the key factors in preventing diabetic foot ulcers. Because pressure redistribution reduces shock and shear forces, cushions the foot, redistributes plantar pressure, and realigns mechanically imbalanced structures to permit a wound to heal, offloading is one of the critical issues involved in successfully healing a diabetic foot ulcer.

Patient compliance is critical for successful wound healing. Therefore, the solution is usually tailored to the patient's lifestyle needs. Healing takes place with immobilization and total avoidance of weight bearing. Walking with crutches is often not practical due to poor cardiovascular status or upper-body strength. Bed rest, limited walking, and the use of a removable walking cast, a walker or wheelchair are the most effective methods to offload the ulcerated foot. Padding of the wound and orthotics can be used within a surgical shoe during the healing phase.

The goal of offloading is to permit the patient to stay mobile while preventing excessive pressure to the wound. Custom-molded prescription biomechanical orthotics have been a favorite of mine because this type of treatment offloads the wound and controls the faulty foot function, which usually contributed to the origin of the wound.

The solutions for offloading range from simple to truly innovative twenty-first century care. Even the world's poorest patients with diabetes, those in India, have found success in offloading pressure from foot ulcers in an unusual way. Developed by Kshitij Shankhdhar, a simple roll of one-inch foam sheeting rolled like a jellyroll is placed on the bottom of the foot under the metatarsal heads to offload the injured site. Instead of jelly between the foam layers, he uses glue. This custom-fitted, easily-applied brace can be worn with a sandal. The estimated cost per patient is one dollar.

The other end of the spectrum to offload a wound is the computerized gyroscopically-controlled motorized wheelchair (GCMC). The GCMC can literally walk up steps while the patient sits in the chair. The estimated cost per patient can be $30,000 or higher depending what customized parts are added to the chair.

*Roller Aid* is an assistive device made of tubular aluminum that has wheels on the bottom, hand brakes, and a small place to sit when the user gets tired and needs to rest. Priced at about seventy dollars, this comfortable, portable and maneuverable four-wheeled vehicle offers stability and energy efficiency as it provides its user the ability to move around without crutches or walkers.

In between these options are a range of gismos and gadgets, some custom-made and others mass-produced. These include pads, insoles, biomechanical orthotics, shoes, crutches, braces, boots, walkers, self powered wheelchairs, and scooters.

*Total Contact Cast* (TCC) also known as a full-contact cast is fabricated using a piece of particleboard or plywood placed across the bottom of the foot with a cast that covers everything so that when the patient stands, all the weight is dispersed equally over the wood surface. The TCC can be used for patients with sensory neuropathy and peripheral arterial disease, but it should not be used in patients with an active infection in an ulcer to the back of the heel or the back part of their foot. The TCC requires cast changes and the need for staff trained in the application of the cast and wound care inspection. This six-week treatment is for people who can't get off of their feet due to work or family demands.

An *Instant Total Contact Cast System* has been developed by Med Efficiency of Colorado. This innovative cast comes with a special boot that is easier, lighter, and more stable than the traditional TCC. Although TCC is still considered the gold standard for offloading, for the at-risk foot or the Charcot foot, it is not commonly used in a majority of the wound centers because it is so expensive, time consuming and difficult to apply.

*A Cam Walker* is a walking boot brace that provides degrees of immobilization. One great benefit is that it is easy to remove. Patients can do self-examinations and apply any needed medications, and can bathe and dress easily while wearing it. A cam walker does not hinder physical therapy or diagnostic imaging tests.

*Walking boots* are another alternative treatment for offloading and protecting foot ulcers. The boots are reasonably priced, are easily removed for wound assessment, and require no specialized training for use. A walking boot can be "converted" to become a hybridized TCC by wrapping a bit of casting material around the boot making it irremovable.

Because patients with neuropathy cannot safely ambulate without shoes or orthotics, they must be educated about the importance of wearing their offloading device at all times, even during trips to the bathroom at night.

The patient's decision to wear a prescribed device depends on several factors including appearance, wearing time, comfort, and cost. No one wants to appear oddly different. Even when patients understand the possibility of a serious risk such as amputation, a device's appearance may determine their adherence to the therapy. Adherence to therapy is often related to the comfort level of the prescribed device. If there are problems, adjustments by a podiatrist or pedorthist can improve the comfort. The last factor is cost. Insurance does not always cover the cost of the prescribed devices and, due to that fact, some patients do not have the financial ability to pay for them or use them.

The Centers for Medicare and Medicaid Services have determined that two to four weeks is the appropriate time point for re-evaluating a treatment plan for pressure ulcers should they fail to show evidence of a progression towards healing. At this point, clinicians may want to use therapies that enhance wound healing such as growth factors, matrix enhancement, or biosynthesis wound materials. There have been numerous studies concerning electrical stimulation to show its effectiveness in wound care, but it is still not widely used.

Full chamber total body hyperbaric oxygen has proven efficacy in the treatment of lower extremity wounds from a number of causes. However, topical hyperbaric oxygen has not. We will review these in Chapter 17.

There is no one who has a more vested interest in your health than you. While physicians always practice with best intent for the patient, it is virtually impossible to be up on the current information of every aspect of medical care. Advances in medical care are occurring at a pace that challenges any medical practitioner to keep up. Some practitioners have little training and understanding of the structure and the function of the foot. Wound care of the ulcerated or infected foot is complex, expensive, and time consuming, but in many cases it works and a wound can be healed. If you feel uncomfortable about the progress of a foot ulcer that fails to heal, it's time to put on your "advocacy hat" and look for another provider, or get a second opinion.

## Case Study on Following Instructions

Mr. BG came to my office and complained of a rash between all of his toes. The rash was present for over eight months and no provider had been able to resolve it. When I examined his feet, the skin between the toes was red and raw. It was clear to me that he had this infection for quite a while. After taking my usual history and performing a physical exam, I harvested a piece of tissue for a culture and sensitivity test. I prescribed a broad-spectrum antibiotic and planned to change it to a narrower spectrum antibiotic when I got the culture results back. Recognizing that hygiene was an issue, I prescribed an antibacterial soap and topical antibiotic cream to be applied between the toes two times every day.

When Mr. BG returned for his follow-up visit he reported that he had done the local treatment and had taken the antibiotics. The lab reports on his infection revealed that he had three different Gram-negative bacteria (see Chapter 11 for information on classification of bacteria by Gram stain.) When I looked between his toes, I was surprised to see that his infection had worsened. Upon questioning, he told me he decided not to use the topical antibiotic I prescribed for his toes. He used "horse balm" instead. He reasoned that a barn was not a clean place and that if the balm worked for the horses, it would surely work for him.

Dementia? Diabetes? Tweener? Nevertheless, non-compliant. What made him change his behavior and substitute horse balm for the medication we ordered for him is still a mystery to me.

## Stop Smoking: No Ifs, Ands, or Butts

Another way to assist a wound in healing is to stop smoking. Nicotine constricts the blood vessels decreasing the amount of fresh, oxygenated blood and the amount of antibiotics that could be delivered to the wound.

KEEP THE LEGS YOU STAND ON — Dr. Mark Hinkes

Mr. D was a sixty-year-old type 2 diabetic who presented with a red, swollen, locally warm, and non-painful ulcer on the bottom of his first toe. The onset of the ulcer was two years previous, but his physicians had been unsuccessful in treating the problem. Mr. D had injured his toe walking on a concrete sidewalk while wearing sandals. Shoes are meant to cover, support, and protect the feet of patients with diabetes. Because sandals fail to meet these criteria, we recommend patients with diabetes not use sandals.

Our exam of Mr. D's foot showed an ulcer with a halo of devitalized tissue on the perimeter and gummy tissue near the base. Fortunately, the ulcer did not penetrate to the bone. Mr. D had barely palpable pedal pulses, and, as we suspected, he was unable to feel the monofilament testing device. If this patient had gone to a non-podiatric provider, he might have been given an antibiotic and sent home without any thought about the issues of shoes, debridement, or X-ray. In contrast, we started with an X-ray to determine whether he had a bone infection. A tissue sample was taken for Gram stain and bacterial culture to identify the causative organism(s) and assure that we would prescribe the appropriate antibiotic. We debrided the ulcer, applied a sterile dressing, and sent him for a surgical shoe. A closed-type shoe that most people wear on a daily basis provides a warm, moist, and dark environment and acts as an incubator for the infection. Using a surgical shoe that is less constricting leaves room for both the foot and dressings and promotes healing by preventing a dark, warm, and moist environment and provides an environment more conducive to healing. Additionally, a surgical shoe usually gives the patient a bit of comfort as well.

Mr. D smoked about a pack of cigarettes a day and I felt that smoking cessation would contribute positively to healing his wound. Here is why:

- Twenty minutes after you stop smoking, your blood pressure drops to that before you had your last cigarette, and the temperature of the hands and feet increases to normal.
- After eight hours, your levels of carbon monoxide return to normal. After twenty-four hours, your chances of a heart attack decrease. After two weeks to three months, your circulation improves. Your lung function increases up to 30 percent.
- After one to nine months, symptoms such as coughing, sinus congestion, fatigue, and shortness of breath decrease. Your lung function begins to return to normal. Your lungs have the ability to clean mucous and reduce infection.
- After one year, your chance of having a heart attack is cut in half. After five to fifteen years, your chance of having a stroke is reduced to that of a non-smoker.
- After ten years, your risk of dying from lung cancer is about half that of a continuing smoker. Risks of cancer to the mouth, throat, esophagus, bladder, kidney, and pancreas decrease. After fifteen years, your risk of coronary heart disease is that of a non-smoker.

I recommended that Mr. D stop smoking as soon as he was able. To my surprise, he agreed to attend the smoking cessation clinic. Shortly after, and much to his credit, Mr. D stopped smoking. I believe if more patients would follow Mr. D's example, we would have less wounds and fewer amputations.

Another aspect of our wound healing strategy for Mr. D was to offload the pressure by using a walker that permitted him to be totally non-weight bearing on the affected foot. As the infection receded and the ulcer demonstrated healing, we prepared casts of his foot for custom-made prescription biomechanical orthotics. We also provided him with a wheelchair and diabetic shoes that would accommodate his foot with the orthotics. As Mr. D's ulcer continued to heal, we provided him the necessary prosthetic items to not only heal the wound, but to keep it healed.

Mr. D did well in his part toward healing the ulcer; however, we reached a point where we could not get the ulcer to heal any further. At this point, I considered alternatives and decided that a recombant DNA product made from yeast, Regranex™ would be the best choice of therapy. Mr. D applied the Regranex™ as directed and in a matter of weeks, the wound had filled in and was totally healed.

Speaking of Regranex™, the June 11, 2008 *National PBM Bulletin* issued an announcement showing the death rate from cancer to be higher in patients prescribed three or more tubes of becaplermin (Regranex™). The FDA has recommended a boxed warning be included with the product. So at this point, this medicine should be used only after reviewing the safety recommendations and recognizing the risks, and only then if the expected benefits should outweigh the risks of treatment. We need to be cautious about prescribing new drugs or therapies in general. It is inevitable that a certain number of drugs and therapies will reveal themselves to have both beneficial and harmful long-term effects that perhaps could not have been predicted. Practicing medicine is akin to playing a constant chess game with Mother Nature.

## Bypass Surgery

Good blood flow to an affected area is required to heal a wound. Therefore, vascular surgery may be required before an ulcer will heal.

It was late October in Nashville and it was cool outside when Mr. TR came to our clinic in a wheelchair. He was wearing Bermuda shorts. His wife rolled his wheelchair right up close to the green surgical power table and locked the brakes so the chair would not move. She and my assistant, Deborah, each secured one of his arms and maneuvered him onto my treatment chair. As he leaned back in the chair in a soft and weak voice he said, "I had a heart attack since I last saw you, and I'm sorry I missed my last appointment." He looked pretty ill.

The reason for the shorts was obvious. Both of his legs had scars from harvesting veins that were used to repair his heart. It was as if someone took a red crayon and drew a graceful oscillating line on both of his legs, from his groin to his ankle. Each of the wounds was inflamed and there was a risk of a postoperative infection. On closer examination, I noticed that he had open wounds on both legs without even a gauze pad dressing to cover them. The family was very concerned about the wounds, but had been assured by the young resident doctor treating him that the incision sites looked acceptable. To me, they looked terrible. Needless to say, we went into action. We started the appropriate wound care, and antibiotics and the patient did well and healed.

Here is another story about successful bypass surgery. Melvin was a very unusual patient. With a background in advertising and marketing, he would enter the room with a big smile, a warm personal greeting, and offer a handshake that would engulf my entire hand. And because Mel always had a joke or quip to start our conversations, it was always a treat when he came to the office.

Mel came to see me because of an ulcer to the bottom of his right foot. He was clear about his objective. "Doc," he said, "fix me up so I can go to Florida this winter." Mel's ulcer measured about one by two inches, covered three metatarsal heads, and went deep into the foot. His foot had ulcerated several times previously, but his doctors always managed to heal the ulcer. However, as the years went by, it became more difficult and took more time to get the ulcer healed.

With my patient declaring that he must get to Florida before the first frost of the fall, I went to work to heal his ulcer. I worked for many months with Mel to heal the ulcer. There were some occasions where I thought we had it healed and Mel would disappear for a while. When he did return, it was like starting over again. All the hard work I had done vanished while Mel was out walking on his foot. But with appropriate patient education, antibiotics, and better patient compliance, Mel somehow managed to stay ahead of the ulcer.

He would return with the ulcer a smaller size, but a lot of dead tissue that need to be debrided. He would always kid me while I worked on him. "Am I the first patient you have ever tried to fix up, or are you using a clean blade? I wish you had someone else to practice on."

We methodically worked with Mel to get his blood sugars

under control. He was eventually willing to wear the diabetic shoes we got for him, even though he said they "tarnished his image." We prepared a biomechanical orthotic to remove the pressure from the ulcerated area and we sent him to the nutritionist to help him with his diet. It was a battle all the way.

Mel made his travel plans and secured a waterfront hotel on Ft. Lauderdale Beach. He even bought new white pants for his trip. But, Mel did not get to Florida that year. Despite my admonishments and deep concern, his foot had become so infected that he had two choices left: lose the leg, or attempt a revascularization procedure that the vascular surgeons did not want to do. They felt Mel was not the best candidate for the procedure.

Mel disappeared for quite a while, and then unexpectedly showed up on my clinic schedule. I was pleased to see him but dreading what might be awaiting me. He arrived in the treatment room, smiled, and said, "I have a surprise for you, Doc."

He took off his shoes and socks and there it was—a perfect foot in every way, with no evidence that there had ever been an ulcer. It was like looking at a baby's foot. Mel had the by-pass surgery. The procedure was successful and his foot had healed.

## The Cool Laser Endovascular Surgery

The year was 1978 and I had been in private practice for two years. LK had been diabetic for twelve years and was one of the smartest patients I have met. He read everything he could about diabetes and I had much respect for him because of the manner in which he approached his health issues. LK listened to all of his doctors and followed their directions regarding his diabetes.

He came to my office with an ulcer on the bottom of his left foot. This was especially surprising to LK who felt that his vigilance toward his diabetes should have prevented him from developing the ulcer, but unfortunately the combination of a bony deformity of his foot and microvascular disease had brought him to the point where he had a terrible infection and the ulcer would not heal.

If you were a diabetic patient with PVD in 1978 and had an infected ulcer that would not heal, your choices were very limited. You could either have a large vessel bypass or have your leg amputated. That was it. There were no manmade grafts, no stents, and no lasers that could clear out the small vessels and permit enough fresh oxygenated blood to get to the foot to heal the ulcer.

LK was an impatient patient and a bit high strung. He was not ready to just give up and lose his leg. We talked about his treatment options. None of the physicians he had previously visited offered an alternative to amputation. But he was totally sure that if he could find a doctor who would use a laser on his arteries he could have them "unclogged" and he would be fine. But this was 1978 and lasers were the fantasy of the future. Nevertheless LK moved on. He went to California and met with researchers who were working with lasers to see if there was one that could resolve his problem. After meeting with several of the leading researchers in the field, he was saddened to realize that his timing was just not right.

The laser that he was seeking was the cool excimer laser,

invented in 1971 by Nikolay Gennadiyevich Basov, a Russian physicist and educator. This laser was especially useful for humans because it used gasses that created ultraviolet energy that did not heat up the surrounding air or tissues. One of the most familiar applications of the cool laser is the LASIK eye surgery. At the time, this technology had not been applied to vascular surgery and sadly LK ended up losing his leg.

Had LK come to my office today, I could have referred him to one of over 300 hospitals in the United States that offer cool laser revascularization for correction of peripheral arterial disease. The cool laser works by vaporizing arterial blockages including plaque, calcium, and thrombus (blood clots), thus restoring blood flow, which promotes healing. Spectranetics develops, manufactures, and markets the CVX-300® excimer laser. It is the only system approved in the United States, Europe, Japan, and Canada for use in multiple, minimally-invasive cardiovascular procedures. Another minimally invasive device, known as the CLiRpath® cool excimer laser and catheter procedure, removes arterial blockages in leg and foot arteries that cannot be reached by standard methods. The CLiRpath® procedure often enables patients to leave the hospital the day after the treatment.

## Prevention of Ulcer Reoccurrence

Patients with a history of ulcers are at high risk for ulcer recurrence. Re-ulceration can be prevented but in order to do so, attention and effort must be invested to identify each patient's specific risk factors and to provide individualized preventive care for each problem. Once healed, meticulous care must be provided to prevent a wound from re-occurring. This can be done by regular risk assessment, tight glycemic control, diet, exercise, and a biomechanical assessment. Efforts may also include custom-molded orthotics and specialized supportive footwear.

The triggers to a foot ulcer are: neuropathy, or loss of protective nerve sensations in the feet that result in silent or painless trauma that goes unrecognized; and foot deformities interacting with footgear and leading to a keratosis or infection. Chances of keeping the foot and leg are improved with preventive measures to avoid the triggers that can cause a foot ulcer.

### Ruben Zamorano and TempTouch®

Twelve years ago, Ruben Zamorano's sister-in-law, Janie, went shopping with her daughter and granddaughter one holiday season. As a consequence of wearing flip-flops on that shopping excursion, Janie developed an ulcer on one side of her foot and a blister on the other side. She had been diagnosed with gestational diabetes twenty-nine years before when she was expecting her daughter.

Ruben followed Janie's progress over the next eighteen months: from the first visit with her primary care doctor and a referral to the podiatrist, to having an orthopedic surgeon amputate first her toe, then her foot, and then a total below-the-knee amputation. Eighteen months later, Janie passed away.

Additionally, Ruben's sister-in-law had lost her mom from cardiovascular disease. She had gotten a little ulcer caused by a skin scratch from a kitten one of the grandkids had given her.

KEEP THE LEGS YOU STAND ON — Dr. Mark Hinkes

The ulcer became as large as a 50 cent piece. It took eleven months to finally close that ulcer. These incidences made a big impression on Ruben.

Being a serial entrepreneur, Ruben was approached by a friend of Dr. Lawrence Lavery, who asked him to organize and administer the company that is now Diabetica Solutions. They received National Institutes of Health (NIH) Small Business Innovation Research (SBIR) grants and have gone through FDA approval for two of these on a 510(k) basis: VPT Meter and TempTouch®. They later obtained ISO (International Organization for Standardization) and CE (European standards) approval for the TempTouch®.

Diabetes was a family-related issue that Ruben dealt with on an academic and business basis. It became a personal interest six years ago when his PCP said, "Ruben, your blood glucose levels are extremely high." He did a fasting glucose level study to confirm type 2 diabetes. The doctor immediately sent him to the nurses at a local hospital where he went through his first diabetes education class. A couple of years ago, his wife was diagnosed as a patient with diabetes.

Because Diabetica Solutions has other products, Ruben sees a lot of the patients who want shoes and insoles. One of his products, Glidesole® uses shear technology that passed phase one and phase two testing with NIH grants. "It's really great to know that the technologies I work on may serve to give a good income and also help people keep their toes or feet where God first put them; I really enjoy that aspect of it," Ruben told me. "There is nothing more rewarding than to know that what we think and dream about actually comes to life and affects someone else's life. Through our company, Diabetica Solutions, we give people a better quality life. There's no real dollar value anybody could put on that."

For ten years, Diabetica Solutions' products have been focused in the area of the diabetic lower extremity. Their products are being accepted by clinicians and the company is also providing them to patients, focus groups and patient advocacy groups around the country. Before, people had few tools to help them know when there's a (foot) problem. Diabetica Solutions has a precise diagnostic tool whereby they can take action with their clinician, endocrinologist, a primary care doctor, internal medicine or family practice physician, podiatrist, or nurse practitioner.

Other products on the market are so expensive most people can't afford them. Diabetica Solutions came to the market with products easily within the reach of most people's budget and allowed them to self diagnose a foot problem at home. Between their twelve-week visits to the physician, (because Medicare requires sixty-one days between visits), diabetic foot ulcers can become totally out of control. It's obviously not going to wait for 61 days to present. Diabetica Solutions gives the patient tools to know when a foot ulcer is about to happen.

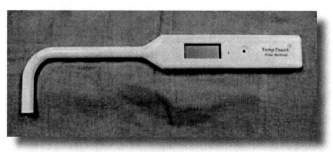

TempTouch®

Some people can't see or reach their feet. That's why the TempTouch® temperature tool is sixteen and a half inches long and ergonomically designed so that even a portly person can sit down in a chair and reach the bottom of his foot to test temperatures on a daily basis. It is designed in such a way that a family member or friend can help a person use it. The product was tested not only with the patients, but with the help of clinicians and especially the nurses, because the majority of patient education is not done by clinicians. Clinicians may not have time, but the nurses have training to tell patients about this tool that is reliable and easy to use. No longer do patients have to wonder if their foot is beginning to ulcerate or if their foot is beginning to present a problem if it is a little pink or red. Patients who are neuropathic can't feel, so Diabetica Solutions gave the device a battery that would last for a long time, made the reading numbers a half-inch tall, and installed an auditory beep to let the patient know when they touch the bottom of their foot.

Patients who have had a previous ulcer can use this thermometer to check their foot temperature once a day. If they note a four-degree difference between one region of the foot compared to the other foot, they can call the nurse who would give them instructions on what to do. This intervention combined with good medical care, proper footwear, and good diabetic education, could drop the ulceration rate almost fourfold. The device is also used for revealing a potential Charcot foot before it starts to break down.

TempTouch® comes with three training tools: a DVD, a user's manual that provides technical background about the device, and a big, bold-print logbook for the patient to keep track of their temperature readings. Anyone should be able to understand the operation of the device. It looks simple, but the device actually goes through a quadratic equation of 160 readings in order to come up with the number you see on the screen. When the device is turned on, it self-calibrates and reads the ambient temperature of the room (must be between 65 and 105 degrees F) as well as the temperature of the hand holding it. It then compares those temperatures as it reaches the foot being tested. TempTouch® is available online at www.temptouch.com or www.diabeticasolutions.com.

Diabetica Solutions has had some success in terms of insurance reimbursement by private insurance carriers, but is still awaiting Medicare reimbursement decision to cover the TempTouch® as a diagnostic product. The device can also display its reading in centigrade for convenient use in the European community.

This device can help patients prevent the cost of treating a foot ulcer or amputation whether it's an above-the-knee or below-the-knee amputation. Since Medicare does not pay for prevention, in order to get them to accept this device, Diabetica Solutions had to refrain from using the word "prevention." Instead, they use "self-diagnosis" or "diagnostic instrument" or "diagnostic tool" to promote the product.

The $100 device can catch a problem area on the foot that could develop into an ulcer ten to twenty days before the surface of the skin breaks down. I'm very impressed with the thermometer and am using it in the clinic. I've had a couple of people with Charcot foot and I've had a couple of people with ulcers and I'm amazed with the temperature measurements I am getting. I'm seeing ten to twelve degrees difference between the patient's two feet. I think it's a wonderful technology that has a bright future for prevention of amputations in patients with diabetes.

The National Institutes of Health had bought some of Diabetica Solutions' TempTouch® devices for use on the Sacaton, Arizona Pima Indian Reservation, where Dr. Wes Yamada works as a podiatrist. When Ruben went to visit Wes, a colleague named Dr. Larry Lavery asked Ruben to come to the reservation and talk to him about the device. Ruben recalls the event:

*The reservation in mid-December looked very desolate. As I drove into the hospital parking lot, there were old manually operated beds sitting outdoors that needed wheels, levers, and other parts or repairs. Sitting cheek to jowl with the clinic was this brand spanking new dialysis center funded by a private dialysis group.*

*Wes' clinic had a humongous number of patients waiting to be seen. I knew he would be staying long after I left in order to take care of all those folks. Every one of the patients there was either missing a toe or a leg.*

*I proposed then, that if there was anything I could do to keep people from losing the toes and feet God gave us, I would do my darndest to help.*

*I've seen the devastation of the diabetic foot problems in all kinds of populations all across this country. I was brought up as a pastor's son. Our family moved from Mexico to Texas in 1953 when I was six years old. Communities back then were segregated; we had a black community, a Mexican community, and an Anglo-white community each having its own schools. The clinics were few and far between. Together with many others, we tried to equalize the situation and bring changes as a consequence of our training and education.*

*I proposed that this company I was working with would do something to help people not only in the United States, but also around the world. Diabetes mellitus is rampant in the United Arab Emirates; it's happening to high-income Spaniards; people in Finland have a tremendously high rate of diabetes and amputations. The UK, Japan—it's a worldwide phenomenon. My parents trained me to share technology and knowledge and help my fellow man in other countries. That's exactly what I propose to do.*

## Foot Surgery to Heal Ulcers

International lecturer, Dr. Bob Frykberg, a noted author and chief of VA podiatry in Phoenix, Arizona, supports the conclusion that diabetes is not a contraindication for prophylactic foot surgery. It is especially worth considering for those patients whose footwear needs cannot be accommodated by extra depth footwear or orthosis. Foot surgery that may benefit patients with diabetes with an ulcer may be divided into three categories.

1. Prophylactic surgery is the correction of a foot problem *before* it can cause an infection or ulcer.

2. Reconstructive surgery may be considered when treating a non-healing or recurrent ulcer that is caused by a bone spur that cannot be treated in a conservative manner with a pad or brace.

3. Curative or ablative surgery includes opening of a deep abscess, debridement of infected or dead tissue and partial or total foot amputation.

## Foot Notes: It's All in Prevention!

With all the bad news about foot ulcers, it is good to know that there are things that can be done to avoid them. Ideally, it is better to prevent an ulcer than to heal it. Preventive foot care can reduce the risk of amputation by 49 to 85 percent. Here are several steps a patient can take to prevent foot ulcers:

- Control blood sugar levels
- Distribute weight equally on each foot when walking or standing
- Do not smoke
- Eat a healthy diet and exercise regularly
- Improve your personal hygiene
- Moisturize feet if they are dry by using a cream or lotion containing urea
- Not cutting your toenails too short
- Use foot powder or cornstarch if feet are sweaty
- Visit your podiatrist annually (or more frequently if necessary) for proper care of toenails, corns, and calluses
- Wash, rinse, and thoroughly dry (particularly between the toes), and inspect feet daily
- Wear clean socks each day making sure they are not too tight (no elastic bands) and do not have irritating spots such as an area that has been darned
- Wear properly-fitted shoes at all times—around the house or yard, or swim sneakers when you go swimming in a pool or at the beach

Prevention is cost effective because it stops the problem before it starts and costs virtually nothing, except for a bit of patient time to inspect feet and practice preventive foot care. It is the key to better health and to controlling healthcare costs.

While prevention is the most effective way to minimize the risks of foot problems, certain segments of the population may not be up to the task of self-care. Examples of those patients include those who have crippling arthritis, those with low vision or who are legally blind and cannot see or reach their feet, or those with mental conditions that make them unable to self care. These people need the help of their family, friends or social service agencies that will ensure that they get the services they need from specialists who can provide preventive care.

### First Aid Treatment for Diabetic Foot Injury

Prompt treatment should be given for cuts or scratches. First, wash the area with warm water and mild soap. Then, use a mild antiseptic such as Bactine™. Next, cover the area with a dry, sterile dressing. Avoid adhesive tape, moleskin, or other occlusive dressing that may pull off skin when removed. If a lesion occurs on the foot, rest with the foot elevated. Call your doctor if the area involved does not improve within 24 hours.

### Avoid Athlete's Foot

- Avoid excessive perspiration. Bathe feet and change socks as frequently as necessary to maintain dryness.
- If feet sweat excessively, gently rub them with alcohol.
- To keep feet dry, use talcum or foot powder.
- Never use patented athlete's foot remedies without consulting your doctor.

# Chapter Ten

## Wound Care and Dressing Types

In treating an ulcer or other type of infection, dressings are the next consideration, both as the type of dressing and how often the dressing is changed. The primary function of a wound dressing is to promote a moist healing environment, which is necessary for wound healing. Dressings can range from plain gauze to sophisticated bioengineered tissue. Regardless of which dressing is used to treat the wound, we try never to use a dressing that uses adhesive to secure it to a diabetic foot. We use non-adhesive type dressings that stick to themselves to secure wound dressings. While these dressings cost a bit more, the benefit in skin protection outweighs the risk of a wound complication.

Since the cave man first cut himself, probably fashioning farming tools or creating sharp hunting instruments, humans have been looking for better materials and methods for dressing wounds. The sleeve was most likely to be the very first wound dressing. Realizing that we could do better, that idea was followed by several hundred years of tinkering with various chemicals, materials, and adhesives to create today's specialized wound dressings.

## Types of Wound Care Dressings

We will hear from a wound care expert in this chapter, but for now, here is a quick review of dressings and how they may be used:

*Alginates* are non-woven sheets or ropes of natural fibers derived from brown seaweed. A moist gel forms when wound fluid contacts the dressing, an advantage of this dressing.

*Antimicrobial* dressings contain agents such as poloyhexethylene biguanides, silver, or iodine to combat bioburden and superficial infection.

*Collagen dressings* come in gels, pastes, powders, pads, but are not injectable. They are derived from purified animal collagen to accelerate wound repair after debridement. These dressings can be expensive (ten 4-inch squares run about $500) and difficult to apply.

*Collagens* are produced by fibroblasts and are the most abundant protein in the body. External tissue engineered products, like Dermagraft™, contain human fibroblasts from neonatal foreskins. They are seeded onto a bioabsorbable mesh and frozen until they are used on a wound to replace the skin.

*Composites* combine two different types of dressings in one to address different needs such as absorption and wound barrier.

*Contact layers* are made of woven or net mesh that are best used to protect a wound from sticking to a dressing.

*Acticoat™* from Smith and Nephew consists of two layers of a silver-coated, tightly-knit mesh that enclose a single layer of a non-woven rayon and polyester fabric. Acticoat™ provides a rapid and sustained release of silver ions to the wound bed for three to seven days.

*Foams* are non-adherent, absorbent dressings that provide for moist wound healing, thermo-regulation, and protection.

*Honey dressings and gels*, as well as tubes of manuka honey, have been gaining in popularity overseas as their medical the dramatic recovery of patients with longtime wounds successfully treated with honey dressings. Dr. Robert Frykberg, Chief of Podiatry at the VA Medical Center in Phoenix, said the Medihoney™ product has worked successfully on about half the patients with diabetic foot ulcers who have used it. He said the Medihoney™ dressing can prevent the dangerous drug-resistant staph infection known as MRSA from infecting open wounds.[1]

*APMA News* reported a patient who incurred $390,000 in foot care for ulcers (including four surgeries) over a fourteen-month period. The patient had three toes removed, refused below-the-knee surgery, and decided to return home where he was told he would die without the amputation. At home, he applied a thick layer of store-bought honey once daily and covered the wound with a four-by-four-inch gauze and wrapped it securely. All other medication was stopped. New tissue appeared within two weeks; in six to twelve months the ulcers healed. Two years later the ulcers have not recurred.[2]

*Hydrocolloids* are the most used dressing for wound management.

*Hydrogel* dressings are water-soluble polymers that come in gauze form, on sheets, in strands, or closed-wound dressings. They have special properties that permit them to bring moisture to the wound for relief or to help with wound debridement.

*Transparent film* or see-through dressings permit visualization of the wound. They are coated on one side with an adhesive but they are water-proof while permitting oxygen to pass through. Use of this dressing has shown lower wound infection rates as compared to traditional gauze dressings.

*Silvadine* is a silver-based cream that is frequently used on burns and wounds to prevent bacterial and fungal infections. Silver dressings have an antibiotic effect. Silver seems to be more universally effective than antibiotics. It is a broad-spectrum agent effective against a number of Gram-positive and Gram-negative bacteria including MRSA and Vancomycin-Resistant Enterococcus (VRE), two very feared bacteria. Silver has been used for centuries in a variety of ways to help treat infections. Silver dressings are "patient friendly" as they do not promote bacterial resistance and show little risk to the organ systems. Metallic silver is relatively inert, but the presence of liquid releases the silver ion responsible for its biological activity. There are considerable differences between commercially available silver-containing dressings in terms of their overall structure, and the concentration and formulation of the silver compound responsible for their antimicrobial activity.

*Arglaes*™ made by Unomedical/Medline comprises a mixture of an alginate powder and an inorganic polymer containing ionic silver. When moist, the alginate absorbs liquid and the silver complex releases ionic silver into the wound. There are currently two Arglaes™ products available in the UK—a polyurethane film dressing and a postoperative dressing. The alginate powder described above is only available in the U.S. Mepilex Ag is a silver foam on top of a silicone layer, so it is non-adherent and absorptive.

## The Expert Speaks

Cynthia A. Fleck has an alphabet behind her name: RN, BSN, MBA, ET/WOCN, CWS, DNC, FACCWS and is very qualified to write about wound care and types of dressing. She is President and Chairman of the Board, The American Academy of Wound Management, Director of the Association for the Advancement of Wound Care (AAWC), President, CAF Clinical Consultant, and Vice President, Clinical Marketing, Medline Advanced Wound and Skin Care. Her areas of expertise are acute and chronic wound and skin care and education. She is licensed in the states of Missouri and Illinois, but she consults all over the United States and provides legal expert witness review and testimony on wound and skin care issues. As a graduate of MD Anderson/University of Texas Wound, Ostomy, and Continence Nurse (WOCN) education program, Cynthia is board certified as a Certified Wound Specialist (CWS) by the American Academy of Wound Management (AAWM) and as a dermatology advance practice nurse (DNC) by the Dermatology Nurses Association.

Cynthia has graciously agreed to address some of the latest innovations in wound care especially regarding diabetic foot wounds. We will go into detail about immunopathy, inflammation and infection (Triple "I" Brothers) in the next chapter, but for now, let's begin with the types of dressings available to treat foot wounds and infections.

## Silver Dressings

*Silver dressings* continue to be the number one advanced wound care product choice available. These innovative dressings persist in gaining widespread usage, not just for the worst wounds and sites but also for safe, broad spectrum prophylaxis of infection and increased healing outcomes across the spectrum of wound care. Perhaps one of the safest and easiest ways for clinicians to combat bioburden (the total population of bacteria, fungus and viruses) within a wound is to utilize ionic silver. Ionic silver can often provide the "kick start" that a stalled, chronic ulcer needs to begin healing again.

Dressings that deliver sustained release of ionic silver over a period of three to seven days (or longer) are preferred. Since silver has little chance of developing resistance,[3] very limited sensitivity and is available over-the-counter (OTC), it makes a perfect dressing choice, especially for diabetic/neuropathic wounds. Preventing a rampant infection[3] with silver dressings prevents complications, costs, and discomfort associated with infection. It also allows for potentially less frequent dressing changes and a reduction in professional intervention and time. These advanced silver dressings afford more cost-savings in their ability to stay in place and work effectively over several days. The most versatile silver dressings are recommended since they are able to handle a variety of wounds and their changing needs. Dressings that perform double or triple duty are particularly popular since they offer multiple uses.

## Pain Control

Pain-reducing dressings that combine silicones for gentle no-stick, pain-free dressing changes are a major part of wound care treatment. These include super-absorbent foam materials that pull moisture from a wound, thereby decreasing the chance of ragged edges around a wound. Other pain-free products like alcohol-free, non-stinging prep wipes and sprays to protect the fragile area around the wound are also available.

## Growth Factor Delivery Systems and Skin Substitutes

In the future, we will see an increase in bioengineered dressings (such as bioengineered cellulose) that perform more than one function, offering care for a variety of wound needs, growth factor delivery systems, and skin substitutes. These bioengineered *in-vitro* cultured skin cells begin as harvested neonatal foreskins and are "grown" in the lab. Bi-layered collagen products that contain human fibroblasts work to produce an immediate cover and delivery for key growth factors for healing.

## Educational Packaging

Dressing changes occur hundreds or thousands of times every day. Is each policy and procedure at the health provider's finger tips? Do they even know what kind of dressing they're using and the application process or do they go for basic principles and guess their way through? Do patients know how to change specific types of dressings?

Ground-breaking work has been done by wound dressing manufacturers to develop packaging that addresses this age old problem. Most dressings are removed from the treatment cart or clean utility room and taken to the patient or resident's bedside or from the home care nurses' car, into the patient's home. Usually, all the clinician (or worse yet, patient or family member) has is a paper cover that gives little information about what the dressing's function is and how to apply it. New, innovative educational packaging that provides a quick in-service on each and every wrapper is now available and is revolutionizing the way wounds are dressed. In a recent study, sixty-two nurses were given an advanced dressing in a traditional package to apply and none of them applied the dressing correctly. Seventy-seven nurses were then given the same dressing in the educational package and 88 percent of them applied it correctly![4]

## Antibiotic Ointments and Creams

The base or vehicle material of antibiotics affects the wound. There are ointment bases and cream bases. My experience is that ointments keep a wound moist, and creams tend to dry up a moist wound. Most of the wounds on a foot are already moist, and so in the initial phase of healing, the goal is to dry them out. These wounds include ingrown toenails, abscesses, and ulcers, so a cream-based antibiotic helps this type of wound dry out.

The double or triple antibiotic ointments everyone uses are everywhere in the hospital—like little ketchup packets. None of the components of these ointments cover a Gram-negative infection. I use a drug called garamicin (Gentamicin™) cream, which covers Gram-negative bacteria with a little bit of Gram-positive coverage, too. I like to use the prescription Gentamicin™ cream because it is a powerful antibiotic. Antibiotic creams and ointments that can be bought over the counter are probably not going to be adequate to treat a serious infection.

## Foot Notes: Finding Wound Care Professionals and Products

The American Academy of Wound Management offers a free service to help patients find a certified wound specialist (CWS) in a specific geographic area. This includes physicians, nurses, therapists, board certified podiatrists and vascular surgeons. Their Web site is www.aawm.org. The Wound, Ostomy, and Continence Nurses Society (WOCN) offers a similar consultant registry on their Web site at www.wocn.org.

Traditionally, wound and skin care products were available from providers and local durable medical equipment suppliers. Now, patients are able to procure products from retail stores like Walgreens and CVS, as well as a multitude of Web sites and catalogs. Patients are much better informed and often come to clinic visits armed with research, articles, magazine clippings, and Internet sites that discuss their particular wound issues. An informed patient is more likely to heal and less likely to re-ulcerate.

# Chapter Eleven

## Immunopathy, Inflammation and Infection
### (Triple "I" Brothers)

We are all susceptible to foot problems whether we have diabetes or not. The difference is how patients with diabetes physically respond to these problems. When a patient with diabetes develops a wound, like a foot ulcer or an infection, it takes an understanding of how all our body's systems work together to heal the wound or fight the infection. It also takes an organized, methodical approach by the doctor to treat and heal these wounds. After considering the effect of the vascular and neurological systems on these wounds, the third system to consider is the immune system. The results of how these complex systems function together will determine if the wound will heal or if the patient may lose his leg.

Many people have heard of the immune system (immunopathy) in relation to HIV or AIDS, but few realize that immunopathy is a very serious complication of diabetes. The immune system is a specialized system that is charged with fighting and removing infections from our bodies. It accomplishes this function via specialized cells called leukocytes or as they are more commonly known as white blood cells. Their job is to kill bacteria. They are produced in the bone marrow and help defend the body against infectious disease and foreign materials as part of normal immune system function. White blood cells may be divided into subcategories, each with an even more specific function. These defenders of health include:

- *Neutrophils.* Usually first responders cleaning up bacterial infection and other small inflammatory processes like a vacuum cleaner (phagocytosis). Their activity and death in large numbers forms pus.

- *Eosinophils.* Primarily deal with parasitic infections.

- *Basophils.* Chiefly responsible for allergic and antigen response by releasing the chemical histamine causing inflammation.

- *Lymphocytes.* More common in the lymphatic system. The blood has three types of lymphocytes: 1) B cells, which make antibodies that bind to pathogens to enable their destruction; 2) T cells that coordinate the immune response (they become defective in an HIV infection) and defend against intra-cellular bacteria; 3) Natural Killer (NK) cells who have the ability to kill cells of the body (that fail to display a signal not to kill them) that have been infected by a virus or have become cancerous.

- *Monocytes.* Share the "vacuum cleaner" function of neutrophils, but are much longer-lived as they have an additional role: they present pieces of pathogens to T cells so that the pathogens may be recognized again and killed, or so that an antibody response may be mounted. The impaired defense system of the patient with diabetes to infections appears to occur at the cellular level. Here, impaired white cells fail to kill the bacteria because of elevated blood sugar levels.

Immunopathy also plays a role in immunizations. According to Lee C. Rogers, DPM, diabetics don't keep an antibody response as long, thus they aren't immune as long as non-diabetics. This is especially important with tetnus, since a foot ulcer can be a portal of entry for tetanus. The mortality rate is 33 percent in those with diabetes versus 18 percent for those without.

A person with a weakened immune system, or immunopathy, has a diminished ability to heal a wound or fight infection on the cellular level. Deficiencies in the immune system not only leave the body vulnerable to infections, but also create problems that can complicate healing. When wounded, your body responds automatically with both systemic and local reactions to protect itself. Once bleeding is under control, the body begins the process of removing damaged tissue through the inflammatory response. Next, more fluid gets to the site with special cells whose mission is to repair the damaged tissue. This process results in swelling of the area and may stimulate nerves that can cause pain.

At this point, white blood cells start the process of removing the dead and dying cells and blood clots from the wound site. Most wound care authorities believe that because the immune system of patients with diabetes is compromised, the wound fails to enter the inflammatory phase of healing. As a result, there is the potential for a long, drawn-out fight between the forces that heal wounds and infections and those that complicate and delay the healing process.

## The Immune System's Toolbox

Your immune system quietly and constantly guards your body to detect and destroy the ongoing attack of bacteria, viruses, fungi, and parasites. Each year, around 215,000 people in the United States die from a severe bacterial infection known as sepsis, which is more than the number who die from breast, colorectal, pancreatic, and prostate cancers combined. Infectious diseases such as bird flu and severe acute respiratory syndrome (SARS) claim lives around the world. And, researchers believe that the aging process somehow leads to a reduction of immune response capability, which in turn contributes to more infections, more inflammatory diseases, and more cancer. Older people tend to be deficient in some essential vitamins and trace minerals that are obtained from or supplemented by diet.[1]

Eating healthy foods and maintaining an exercise program is one of the best ways to give your immune system the support it needs to keep you healthy. Every part of your body, including your immune system, functions better when protected from environmental assaults and bolstered by healthy living strategies. These will be discussed in the chapter on nutrition.

## Inflammation

Inflammation is a response of the immune system to infection, irritation, or trauma. It is characterized by redness, heat, swelling, and pain. The inflammatory stage results in heat, swelling, and pain. The inflammatory stage of wound healing results in swelling and ironically is of benefit because it dilutes any irritants in the injured area, brings proteins called fibrinogen to form a mesh to cover the wound, traps foreign particles, and forms the scaffolding for new tissue to be laid down to enhance the effectiveness of the immune system.

In the early stages of a foot problem, it may be difficult to know whether a patient has an infection or an inflammatory problem like arthritis or gout. The four cardinal signs of an infection include: redness, warmth, swelling, and pain. Since the symptoms are similar, any type of inflammatory process can be misdiagnosed as an infection and vice versa. To determine which it is, we need to put on our Sherlock Holmes hats, take out our magnifying glasses, and analyze all the information to resolve the problem.

## Infections

In the late 1600s, Anton Von Leeuwenhoek, who invented the microscope, discovered bacteria and called them "wee beasties." Today, in informal medical jargon, we call them "bugs." In most cases, bacteria are the cause of infections in the foot, while in other cases, fungus, mold, yeast, or viruses can be the cause of a foot infection.

Infections occur when bacteria penetrate the protective envelope that covers our body, in other words, our skin. They can range from mild to potentially serious. Often infections in the foot start out small and are relatively easy to treat, like an ingrown toenail or small, localized superficial abscess.

When a patient comes in with an infection, the doctor must evaluate the wound and determine the extent of the wound in terms of size, the condition of the tissues, and what vital structures may be affected. We must first determine the cause of the infection. For example, if the patient has an ulcer, the wound should be probed to see if it extends to the underlying bone. In most cases, a wound that probes to the bone or is exposed to air should be considered infected.

Next, the doctor should identify the severity of the wound by measuring the width, length, and depth, and by documenting the condition of the wound in terms of color, skin condition, and whether the wound has an odor. It takes all of our senses to do a good wound evaluation. To identify the bacteria that may be infecting the wound, a culturette, which looks like a Q-tip with a holder, is often used to swab the wound. Most pathologists feel that a swab culture does not give a true reading of which bacteria are causing the infection. They prefer a tissue sample, but sometimes it's a challenge to find a piece of tissue to send for analysis because the wound is not in the condition where a piece of it can be cut. The tissue sample is sent to the microbiology laboratory for a Gram stain and culture and sensitivity (C&S) test to determine which antibiotics are needed.

## Testing and Knowing the Players

My dad was an avid Pittsburgh Pirates baseball fan. As a child growing up, I would ask him who was playing a particular position or who was at bat. He would always say, "Ya can't tell who the players are without a scorecard."

And so it is with bacteria that are in an infected wound. We need a scorecard to know who's on first. This is why we use the bacterial C&S. In the C&S, the tissue sample is analyzed to identify which "bugs" are in the wound and provides information on which antibiotics might be used most effectively to treat them. There can be, and usually are, multiple species of bacteria in a chronic or longstanding wound, and a different antibiotic may be needed to treat different bacteria. The idea is to find the antibiotic with the highest potency to kill the infection at the lowest dosage. This is called the Minimum Inhibitory Concentration (MIC).

The C&S report helps us make decisions about the patient's treatment regimen. This can be a challenge, because with multiple bacteria and multiple drugs to choose from, the decision-making process may become complex. The "art" of medicine comes into play here. We must consider other aspects of the patient, like his overall health and the functioning of his kidney and liver, as one or the other of these organs usually metabolizes and excretes medications through the urine or feces.

## Gram Stain

In treating an infection, the doctor would want to identify the specific bacteria causing the problem in order to choose the antibiotic that would be most effective. A preliminary test on the tissue specimen sent to the lab is called the Gram stain. Danish bacteriologist Hans Christian Gram invented this test in 1884. The Gram stain categorizes bacteria into two groups: Gram positive and Gram negative. These somewhat large categories help the physician determine which antibiotic would be most effective and the best method for the patient to receive the medication.

A C&S report tells us which bacteria are sensitive to which antibiotics. In the report, all the antibiotics are listed on one side and the bacteria are listed on the top. A grading system identifies the ability of the antibiotic to kill the bacteria. There is an "S" for sensitive, an "R" for resistant, or an "I" for inconclusive. Before prescribing antibiotics, the physician must also consider the kidney function by noting the serum creatinine and liver function by checking the ALT, AST, and Alkaline phosphatase levels. The kidney and liver metabolize and excrete the antibiotics. Poor organ function can lead to toxic accumulation of antibiotics in the body.

While the Gram stain is being done, another amazing test that takes one to two days to complete should be done on the tissue sample that was sent to the lab. It is the culture and sensitivity (C&S) Test.

Before a doctor uses antibiotics to treat infections, he should review the patient's medical history to know if the patient is allergic to any antibiotics. We need to consider other medications and allergies to medications that the patient may already be taking that might interact with the antibiotic we are considering. An example of this is a relatively common drug called Coumadin™. It is used for patients with heart and circulatory problems to keep their blood a bit "thinner" to avoid clotting. Patients taking Coumadin™ must have the dose adjusted to prevent bleeding tendencies while taking certain antibiotics.

Armed with this information, the doctor decides which antibiotic would be best and which method would be most appropriate to dispense the antibiotic: topical, oral, intravenous, or intra-muscular. The method of administration of the antibiotics will depend on the antibiotic itself. If the patient has a fever, an elevated white cell count, and an elevated sedimentation rate, we know he is in dire need of antibiotics and that we need to get antibiotics into his body quickly.

> Bacteria are opportunists ready to infect a wound, even when they're not the primary cause of the infection. Once there is a "portal of entry" (opening in the skin) into the body, any bugs can set up shop and contribute to the infection. Personal hygiene is critical to keep other pathogens out so they don't complicate the situation.

The fastest way is through a vein (intravenous) followed by injecting into a muscle (intra-muscular), usually in the arm or the buttocks. There are some antibiotics, though, that can only be given intravenously no matter what the patient's condition.

## Appropriate Antibiotics

It is critical to use antibiotics correctly. When we do, they can provide miraculous results. When they are inappropriately prescribed, they can cause worse problems because the bacteria develop a resistance against these antibiotics, making existing antibiotics ineffective. This forces us to use newer, more powerful, and more expensive antibiotics, and some that can only be administered intravenously.

A classic example of using inappropriate antibiotics is the use of an antibiotic named Ciprofloxacin (Cipro™). This antibiotic has outstanding coverage against Gram negative bacteria but only fair to poor coverage on Gram positive bacteria. Over-prescribing Cipro for Gram positive bacteria has caused some strains of Gram positive bugs to become "resistant" to it. Thus, we are losing a tremendous tool for fighting infections.

Bacteria can be good or bad. They put the tang in yogurt and the sour in sourdough bread. They produce antibiotics such as streptomycin and nocardicin. Others live symbiotically in the bodies of animals (including humans) or on the roots of plants converting nitrogen into a usable form. Bacteria also help break down dead organic matter and make up the base of the food web in many environments. The oldest fossils known, nearly 3.5 billion years old, contain evidence of bacterial-like organisms.

Despite medical folklore that tells us that most wounds in the foot are colonized by Gram negative bacteria, the most common bacteria that infect foot wounds is a Gram positive organism named: staphylococcus aureus. This bacterium is easily recognized by the creamy golden color of the discharge that it produces in the wound. Fortunately, we have several excellent oral antibiotics that can fight "staph" aureus.

Two of the common Gram negative bacteria found in diabetic foot infections and ulcers are E. Coli and Pseudomonas. Everyone has E. Coli in his colon, which is a bacterium necessary to digest food. It's user-friendly. It can, however, become a pathogen (the cause of disease) if it gets through a break in the skin like a foot ulcer. E. Coli can get into a wound not because we are dirty, but because, when we shower, gravity causes all the body dirt and soap to run down our legs and can get in the foot wound. To avoid this problem and a potentially dangerous complication, you might want to use a special moisture proof protective dressing to cover your foot wound while bathing. Many patients use a large plastic bag secured at the ankle to prevent contamination during bathing. If you do this, please use an aluminum lawn chair or special bath seat in your bathtub to avoid falling.

Pseudomonas is easily recognized by the unmistakable odor that emanates from a wound that it colonizes. It smells like a gymnasium or old athletic shoes. To kill the pseudomonas bacteria, we can use a combination of topical and oral antibiotics and a local treatment for the foot using a recipe of ingredients that are found in most kitchens: mix half a cup of white vinegar (a diluted acid) in a pan of room temperature tap water and soak your foot in this solution for twenty minutes twice a day.

If the problem is between the toes, soak a piece of cotton or gauze in the vinegar solution and put it between your toes to help kill the bacteria; or place the cotton or gauze between the toes while soaking. This separates the toes and assures the solution is reaching all of the infected skin.

The Gram stain test is done to test for not only E. Coli and pseudomonas, but for all bacteria, because infecting organisms cannot be identified by physical examination alone. The Gram stain may also tell us the total quantity of bacteria in the wound. Early diagnostic information obtained from Gram stained smears often allows a prescription of narrow-spectrum antibiotics, thereby reducing the risk of toxicity, super-infection, and the expense of broad-spectrum or multiple antibiotics.

## MRSA (Methacillin-resistant *staphylococcus* aureus)

Patients often ask me why I take a tissue sample for culture of the wound. Obtaining a proper wound culture specimen allows the clinician to identify the bacteria in the wound and as well as the proper antibiotic to treat it. But this method is not used by all physicians when they treat wounds. Due to the time involved in obtaining results of the culture, some clinicians select a broad-spectrum antibiotic likely to treat the problem. If the patient fails to respond to the initial antibiotic treatment, the decision for an alternative treatment may be more difficult.

With bacteria becoming more resistant to antibiotics that are used to treat foot wounds and infections, the choices for antibiotics are becoming more difficult. Now, there is a growing problem in treating infections due to MRSA. Not too long ago,

MRSA was acquired only in hospitals, but now it is frequently acquired in the community and some healthcare facilities. In some communities, other highly resistant bacteria, including pseudomonas aeruginosa and enterococcus species are being found in diabetic foot wounds.

A newer antibiotic named Zyvox™ is as efficacious as intravenous antibiotics for treatment of MRSA skin and soft tissue infections. Zyvox™ can be taken orally, decreasing costs by keeping the patient out of the hospital while on appropriate antibiotic therapy.

To keep from picking up an MRSA in public, keep your personal things to yourself; don't share towels, shoes, socks, makeup, or other toiletries and personal items. Keep wounds covered. Sterilize linens, wash your hands often, and use an antibacterial cleaner like Lysol™ to keep surfaces clean.

## Cost Considerations

The reality of twenty-first century medicine is that the expense of some medication has gone beyond people's ability to afford it, and then healthcare plans do not want to pay for them. So, unfortunately, cost is one of the primary considerations for a doctor when prescribing medication to treat the patient's medical condition. Some healthcare plans have placed restrictions on certain expensive antibiotics and mandate that a doctor select the antibiotic that they approve and for which they are willing to pay.

The best manner to treat the wound or infection must be decided based on the tests and the experience of your physician. Some wounds can be treated with a topical antibiotic or a combination of topical and oral antibiotics. Other wounds that are more advanced in the soft tissues, or worse, in the bones, may initially require intravenous or intramuscular injections of antibiotics to be followed with oral antibiotics for up to six weeks.

Some types of antibiotics can only be given intravenously and may require the patient to be initially hospitalized to receive them. The blood is monitored to be sure the level of antibiotic is sufficient to treat the infection but not too high so as to cause damage to the kidneys or liver. Some patients will have a special indwelling catheter inserted into a vein before leaving the hospital called a "peripherally inserted central catheter" (PICC line), so they may continue to receive intravenous antibiotics outside the hospital setting.

Generally, certain wounds require particular types of antibiotics and applications.

- Deep wounds that have pus and do not respond well to oral antibiotics may need to be surgically opened, drained, and have any infected tissue deep in the wound removed in order for the antibiotics to do their job.

- Superficial soft tissue infections usually respond more quickly to fewer antibiotics in a shorter time. Complex soft-tissue infections that reach deep into the muscle, fascia, and tendon, usually have multiple bacteria in them and can be difficult to treat. This type of infection may require the use of multiple antibiotics taken simultaneously.

- A bone infection will require a different amount and variety of antibiotics, and in some cases, we will need to remove the infected bone surgically.

## Viral Infections

In addition to bacterial infections, there are viral infections. The most commonly seen viral infection is a verruca or as it is more commonly called, a wart. Warts are part of the human papaloma virus family. They are parasites that take nourishment and oxygen from our bodies and excrete metabolic waste products into our bodies. Warts are considered infectious critters. Patients with diabetes should not use over-the-counter preparations for treating warts. They contain salicylic acid and can cause chemical burns, destroy tissue painlessly and become a trigger that can lead to an amputation.

Antibiotics should *not* be considered an everyday treatment. They are powerful medications and can be risky in patients with allergies, decreased kidney or liver function, or those who are on anticoagulant therapy such as Coumadin™. If an antibiotic doesn't heal a bone infection, patients risk complications such as blood poisoning. A worsening infection may place the limb at risk, and patients may need to have the infected bone removed.

## Mold, Yeast, and Fungus Infections

This trio of troublemakers all depend on a dark, moist, and warm environment to prosper, and that is exactly the conditions that are found inside your shoes. We often see these types of infections on the nails, between the toes, or on the sides and bottom of the foot. These dermatophytes are usually responsible for superficial skin infections on the foot that often are referred to as "athlete's foot." This can cause whitish, inflamed, itchy, and peeling skin on the foot that is often misdiagnosed as dry skin. Scratching can spread the infection to other parts of the body via the hands. So good hygiene is paramount.

## Gout

Gout has traditionally been characterized as a disease of the rich. It has a fondness for the big toe joint but can affect any joint. Gout is a genetic disease that reveals itself as an inborn error of metabolism that prevents patients from metabolizing certain proteins. All proteins are classified as being either purines or pyrimidines. It is purines that cannot be metabolized by patients affected by gout. In ancient times, only the rich and royalty had gout because they ate meat that is high in purines while those who lived and worked outside the castle walls did not suffer from this malady. Where do you find purines? In red meat, organ meat, beer, wine, and liquor (clear spirits gin or vodka are usually okay to drink without causing a gout attack).

When the level of uric acid builds up in the body, it causes crystals with sharp points to deposit in the joints resulting in an inflammatory process. Patients report joint pain, swelling, redness, heat, and stiffness. I have seen patients with this affliction and they have pain and functional disability that most people cannot imagine. Some patients have skin wounds from where the uric acid crystals or tophi are literally "escaping" through the soft tissue. I have operated on several patients with this disorder and to my surprise when we opened the big toe joints, we removed a chalky white material that looked like crushed blackboard chalk.

Colchicine is a drug that has the ability to stop the pain of an acute gout attack. Unfortunately, in the process of accomplishing its mission it may make you wish you hadn't taken it. Patients take one pill hourly until they either vomit or have diarrhea. It can be a nasty drug. In an acute attack situation a posterior tibial nerve block can put the foot "to sleep" providing pain relief for eight to twelve hours. It is a good alternative to the traditional treatment and podiatrists perform this procedure well. If you stay away from foods containing purines, you can stop the accumulation of uric acid and prevent gout. In fact, if a person limits their purine intake, they will almost never have a gout attack. A drug named Allopurinol can be used in combination with diet modification to control uric acid levels. With patient cooperation, gout is almost 100 percent preventable.

## Cancer

Primary malignancies on the foot are rare but the foot can be the site of metastasis, the spread of cancer from its original location to a distal site like the foot. One of the only cancers that has a predilection for the foot is named Kaposi Sarcoma. I have also seen malignant melanoma—a very deadly cancer on the foot.

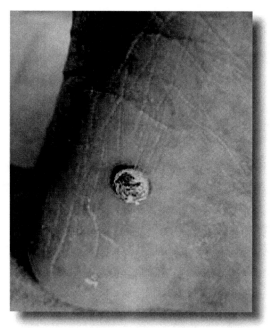

**Cancer on Foot - Kaposi Sarcoma**

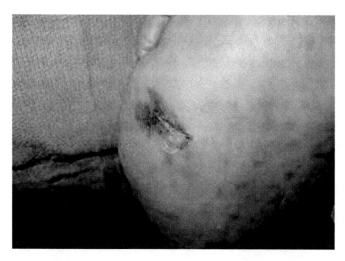

**Cancer on Foot - Malignant Melanoma**

## Protect Yourself, Keep Clean!

Patients with poor hygiene are the most vulnerable to infections, and many times without even realizing it they are their own worst enemy due to their behaviors.

Many of the patients I treat have a fungus infection, or what's more commonly called athlete's foot. Often these patients think their problem is dry skin. They may even have used skin lotion for long time periods without alleviating the problem. This problem requires better personal hygiene and appropriate medication. For this, I give patients a surgical scrub brush with instructions that they vigorously scrub their feet to get all the dead skin off, rinse and dry them well, and apply a topical anti-fungal powder or cream.

Like the swimming pool where you can pick up the virus that causes warts, if you have an infection and walk barefooted in the house, you leave bacteria or fungus on the floor for family or friends to pick it up through an opening or a crack in their feet. This is how infections get passed from person to person in a home. The germs can live in a shower or bath tub. Therefore, it is very important to keep your home environment clean. Lysol™, bleach, or an antibacterial cleaner should be used wherever a person with an infection has stood.

Hygiene is critical to preventing infections, getting rid of infections, preventing recurrence of infections and not picking up a new infection. People who don't practice good hygiene tend to have more infections than those who do. We find that most people who have foot infections bathe infrequently, or not at all. Many people feel that because soapy water ran over their feet while in the shower their feet are clean. There is no substitute for actually washing the feet and in between the toes with soap. Some people cannot see or reach their feet and the reason can be different for each person. The list includes patients with arthritis, the obese, someone who's had a stroke, those who may have only one leg, those who can't see well or those who have either mental disabilities or behavioral issues. These people will usually end up with a bacterial or fungal skin infection. Caregivers can be of immense service in this issue by keeping an eye on the feet of the patients they are providing care for and supporting preventive foot health behaviors.

There are people who don't put clean socks on in the morning, and may use a sock that is damp from perspiration or from exposure to wet conditions from the previous day. Just as they continue to use wet or moist socks they may also continue to wear their shoes when they get wet.

Having dry feet is as important as bathing them because having damp feet can contribute to infections. I have seen many patients who do a good job of washing their feet but fail to dry them adequately. All those at risk for foot ulcers must dry their feet after bathing, especially between the toes. For those unable to reach their feet, a hair dryer may be used only if the temperature is set to the cool setting.

Clean your shoes! If you have a foot infection, so do your shoes. A lot of people do not wear socks, so they are re-contaminating their feet each time they put their dirty shoes on again. Spray your shoes with an antifungal or antibacterial application such as Lysol™. Throw the shoes away if they cannot be washed or disinfected.

## CB's Story

CB came to my office complaining of itching feet and an infection that showed itself by a series of small "bubbles" that opened on the bottom of both feet and oozed a clear to straw-yellow fluid. He said, "Sometimes it seems to get worse, then it gets better, but it never really goes totally away." He reported that he had these symptoms over the past several years with some exacerbations and remissions, and no one had been able to successfully treat his foot problem. We reviewed CB's chart and noted that he had a back injury and walked with a cane. He reported that he was not able to reach his feet, so he did not wash his feet with soap, rinse them well, nor dry them, especially in between the toes. He just let the water from his shower run down his legs and over his feet. He didn't make the effort to dry his feet, so when he placed his moist feet in his shoes, he created an environment where his shoe acted like an incubator and he literally "cooked" his foot inside his shoe.

We took both bacterial and fungal cultures to identify the bug(s) that might be causing the problem. We also had CB throw out all of his socks and shoes since they had been contaminated by the infection, and clean his bathing area at home to be sure he eliminated any further source of the infection. To allow him to properly bathe his feet, we provided CB with a sponge on a plastic stick, an antibacterial soap, and a combination of both oral antibiotics and a topical antifungal cream. With a session of patient education and CB's cooperation, we were able to eradicate his infection.

KEEP THE LEGS YOU STAND ON — Dr. Mark Hinkes

## CK's Story

CK was a retired farmer who spent most of his time at home on the porch, watching TV, or enjoying his family, especially his grandchildren. He had long ago turned the keys to his tractor over to his son, but old habits are hard to break. He had such a love of the soil that he still kept two acres for himself for his personal garden. According to his wife, he would go out to the garden and work on all the vegetables and fruit trees despite that fact that his feet were numb.

CK's eyesight was poor and his feet were so numb he needed a cane for balance. When he came to the office, he had an ulcer on the bottom of the left foot that had been there for several months. He had no previous professional treatment but preferred to use peroxide and bag balm, a moisturizer used to prevent cow's udders from cracking. The medical history for CK noted that he controlled his blood sugars with an oral medication, was taking the blood thinner Coumadin™, and had some mild kidney disease. As was our usual treatment protocol, we took a history and performed a physical exam, got an X-ray, debrided and dressed the wound, replaced his street shoes with surgical shoes, and sent a tissue specimen to pathology for Gram stain and culture and sensitivity (C&S) testing.

We ordered a blood test called a sedimentation rate that is a non-specific test to identify if there was an inflammatory process in progress, or if he had an infection that was not visible. We also ordered a complete blood count to get a baseline evaluation on his blood. When the reports returned, there were three bacteria populating the wound: two Gram positive and one Gram negative. We evaluated the antibiotic choices and prescribed a combination of oral and topical antibiotics. When I asked CK to stay off his foot, he looked at me with his head cocked, and with only one eye open, he responded in a thick southern drawl, "Only if you all come out to the farm and tend my garden."

We saw CK over the next several weeks debriding his wound and taking additional tissue cultures. By the second week, there were different bacteria in the wound, so I changed his antibiotics. By the fifth week, we saw no real improvement. I learned that CK had not stopped tending his garden, and he was still on his feet. His wife told us privately that some days he would return to the house with dirt inside his socks contaminating the dressing on his foot.

We reached a point where no oral or topical antibiotic could be used to effectively treat the infection due to the conflicts of his diabetes medication, his kidney function, and the type of bacteria in his wound that had become resistant to most oral antibiotics. Unable to treat this wound without intravenous antibiotics, our next step was to refer him to an infectious disease (ID) specialist. This physician would have skills and training and could manage CK's intravenous antibiotic treatments. I worked with the ID specialists over the next several months, and we provided ongoing care for CK's wounds. Even though the infection apparently was under control, CK was having many health, behavior, and compliance problems, and eventually he underwent a below-the-knee amputation. Not long afterward, his situation deteriorated and CK's non-compliant behavior cost him his life.

## Foot Notes: Preventing Infection

To prevent infections, patients must change the way they think about their feet and the way they tend to their foot health. Here are some tips.

- Inspect your feet daily, especially between your toes, for sores or cuts. If you cannot see your foot directly, you should use a mirror on the floor or a long handled mirror. If you (the patient) cannot see your feet, ask your caregiver to check them every day. Any changes, even small ones should be evaluated. A locally red, swollen, or warm area on your foot should prompt you to call your physician for an evaluation.

- Bathe feet daily using soap and water. Check the temperature of the bath water with your hand, elbow or thermometer.

- Use a clean towel to dry your feet thoroughly, especially between the toes. A hair dryer set on the coolest temperature can be used with caution. Use powder if necessary after drying.

- Wear well-fitted, clean socks every day.

- Don't walk barefooted. Use shoes around the house, clogs in the shower, swim sneakers at the pool.

- Be sure your shoes are fitted properly to avoid friction or pressure. Inspect shoes daily for foreign objects or irregularities such as loose stitching that can cause foot wounds.

- Lotion should be used on the legs and feet to avoid dryness and cracking of the skin.

- Toenails should be trimmed with the contour of the toe and rough or sharp edges should be filed with an emery board. People with peripheral neuropathy should not cut their own toenails and a podiatrist should evaluate and treat their feet regularly.

- Exercise, proper nutrition, and smoking cessation are important in preventing foot ulcers. If you practice these preventive foot health behaviors, the chances of developing a problem will be minimal. You will identify problems early on and resolve them promptly.

Inspecting your feet everyday is a cost-effective way to prevent infection and reduce the cost of healthcare. Remember that people with diabetes and prolonged high blood sugar levels are linked with damage to the nerves of the feet. Nerve damage can cause loss of protective sensation as well as deformities of the feet. With loss of sensation, people can damage their feet either by repetitive micro trauma, prolonged standing or walking, or a single major trauma by mechanical, thermal, or chemical means.

If you are not practicing preventive measures, the odds of getting a foot infection or ulcer increase. The infection could become so dangerous that you may need to be hospitalized for appropriate diagnostic work-up and therapy to alleviate the infection. The costs of this level of care can become serious (usually between $10,000–$20,000). Prevention pays big benefits in these cases by reducing the cost of care and permitting the patient to continue with their normal lifestyle.

Patients with diabetes and sensory neuropathy may not feel pain. If they have an episode of silent or painless trauma, they may not know they have been injured or have an infection. Many patients think that since they have no pain, they do not have a problem. Nothing could be farther from the truth. If the patient fails to visually examine their foot, they will not know they have an infection until they see blood or pus on their socks. It only takes ten seconds per day to check your feet. Visually inspecting your feet cost nothing, but it could save your foot.

# Chapter Twelve

## Sock It to Me!

We previously talked about the circulation and how critical adequate blood flow is to healing a wound. We also talked about loss of protective sensation that makes the diabetic patient vulnerable to painless trauma. Now, let's look at some preventative behaviors you can adopt to keep your risk as low as possible.

Caring for your at-risk feet can be difficult if you don't have current information. I want to provide a brief source of information to help you purchase socks that will assist you in maintaining good foot health.

### Clean Socks

There are people who don't put on clean or dry socks in the morning, and they may also continue to wear their shoes or socks when they get wet. Dry feet are as important as clean feet because damp feet can contribute to infections. Even if you are unable to reach your feet or bring your foot up to clean it, you must make an extra effort to be sure to dry them, as well, especially between the toes if you are at risk for foot ulcers.

Some people don't put on socks at all. Socks are important to preventing corns, calluses and blisters that can form next to bunions or digital deformities and infection. Socks act as a protective barrier between the shoe and the foot.

## Seams to Me

Never wear open-toed sandals, flip-flops, or any type of shoe without socks! But, not just any old sock. The smartest, safest choice when it comes to protecting your feet is wearing the right type of socks.

Any ridge, seam, or wrinkle can cause pressure points on the bottom of the foot. Your socks should protect from irritation and be free of seams to reduce discomfort and ulceration that seam edges can cause. Toe seams in socks can increase pressure on the toes that may cause blisters or abrasions. Patients with diabetes and peripheral neuropathy are at the greatest risk because they cannot feel developing blisters or abrasions as they are developing.

You might think that cotton or wool socks would provide the best protection for your feet, but that is not the case. Cotton and wool do absorb moisture, which is something a sock should do. However, moisture creates a suitable breeding place for bacteria and actually promotes infections. Wool and cotton fibers keep the moisture they absorb right next to your foot. Additionally, their fibers can be abrasive and cause blisters, which patients with diabetes should avoid. Cotton and wool fibers lose their shape much faster than synthetic fibers. Without elasticity, these type of socks bunch up and wrinkle which cause pressure points on the foot.

Hi-bulk acrylic and stretch nylon are a good choice because they draw moisture away from the skin where it can evaporate, and these fibers are less prone to wrinkling on the bottom of the foot. They range in price from about ten to fifteen dollars a pair.

Ideally, you want to get socks that do not have elastic or only have minimal elastic at the top. Elastic can decrease circulation. There are some stretchy, non-binding socks on the market that create uniform compression that actually promotes blood flow. Since circulation is always a concern for patients with diabetes, these non-elastic socks are a safe choice for foot health.

Select latex-free fibers that contain no harmful dyes or additives. Socks used to be dyed with colors that caused people to break out with allergic reactions. So to remedy this, conventional wisdom recommended that patients wear white socks to eliminate the problem. There are new socks on the market with copper that is blended into the threads that reduce perspiration and decrease bacterial and fungal infections. (www.cupronsales.com)

Bleach should be used on socks. It now comes in two varieties: good old chlorine bleach and new "color safe" bleach. By the way, I also recommend the use of bleach to clean areas in the home environment that may be contaminated with bacteria, mold, yeast, or fungus.

Be sure to replace socks if they begin to show signs of wear.

## Diabetic Socks

Socks may seem rather insignificant in the big picture

of foot ulcers and amputations, but they are actually very significant. Improperly fitted socks, or a poor quality knit can trigger a foot ulcer.

One of the several brands of socks on the market for patients with diabetes is SensiFoot™. Their Web site says that they use an acrylic multi-fiber blended knit, which offers greater protection because it wicks moisture away from the skin to the outer surface where it can evaporate. SensiFoot™ socks are made specifically for patients with diabetes or arthritis. They combine comfort and protection with an antifungal and antibacterial finish, and are machine washable.

All socks have seams somewhere; even tube socks have a seam at the toe. Specialty companies have designed socks with special features for the at-risk patient. These include seams that are flat and non-irritating, and socks with mild compression for venous support.

Wearing the right socks is your first and best defense for your at-risk feet.

## Compression Stockings

Compression stockings are used to keep fluid from collecting in the legs and to limit edema. The stockings are graded by the amount of pressure or compression they exert against the skin and depending on the patient's needs can be used in a below-the-knee or above-the-knee style. The most commonly used configuration is the 20-30 mm Hg compression in a below-the-knee stocking. Higher pressures such as 40-50 mm Hg pressure are sometimes not tolerated well by patients due to the tightness and pressure of the stocking. One of the issues associated with compression stocking is that they can be difficult to put on and to take off. I had one patient tell me he felt like he just went ten rounds of boxing trying to put on his stockings. Some patients refuse to use the stockings because of the difficulty of getting them on. However, there is an aid called a stocking butler that can help.

## Case Study ~ Freeman

Mr. Freeman came to my office with a referral from his PCP for a diabetic foot evaluation. He told me that because of his venous disease and the chronic swelling of his legs (edema), he had been prescribed below-the-knee compression stockings. He said, "Every time I put on the stocking, my toes hurt."

After a thorough examination, I was at a loss to determine why he was in such pain. Finally, I asked Mr. Freeman to put on the stockings. Bingo! I could see that even though the stocking was correctly fitted for the leg, it appeared to be at least two sizes too small for his foot. The heel area of the stocking was located at his arch. Mr. Freeman was referred back to the prosthetics department for refitting of the stocking and the problem was resolved. All patients must be their own advocates and be sure their shoes, and in this case stockings, fit correctly.

## Foot Notes: Sock Tips

- Put on clean and dry socks in the morning
- Wear socks at all times
- Never wear open-toed sandals, flip-flops, or any type of shoe without socks
- Make sure your socks are not folded over, wrinkled,

or have rough edges
- Choose hi-bulk acrylic and stretch nylon socks that do not have elastic at the top
- Select latex-free fibers that contain no harmful dyes or additives
- Use bleach when washing socks
- Replace socks if they begin to show signs of wear.

# Chapter Thirteen

## Walk a Mile in My Shoes

Everything about our bodies is suited to our survival or most efficient function. Our feet were designed to walk on uneven surfaces, like rocks, sand, or grassy turf—not on tile, concrete, asphalt, or linoleum. Wearing shoes is one of the most unnatural things we do. But walking around today without protective footwear is dangerous, particularly for those at risk for ulcers and amputations. The modern convention of wearing shoes occurred for purposes of fashion and ease of commerce and locomotion. Can you imagine trying to shop and push a grocery cart on an uneven surface of small hills and valleys with rocks or debris in the path? Of course not, and yet we take walking on hard, flat surfaces as "normal" with little or no thought about it. Curiously, it is the physics involved in walking that gets us into trouble with our feet.

Each of us responds relatively the same to physical forces that act upon our bodies. Gravity is gravity; but it is these "reactive forces of gravity" that affect our foot when we stand and walk. Patients with diabetes may be at greater risk to the effects of friction and shear physical forces because of their special circumstances—neuropathy, vascular disease, and joint deformities—that can interact with shoe gear and create problems that can lead to amputations. Bone and joint abnormalities (normal anatomy that has changed into an unnatural state or position) such as hammertoes, tailor's bunions, or the loss of the protective fat pad on the bottom of the foot that leaves the metatarsal heads without protection interacts with our shoes. A poorly-fitted shoe that is either too loose or too tight, will rub against the foot, or cause a blister, corn, abscess, or an ulcer. Often, patients who lack protective sensation will buy shoes that are too tight because they cannot feel their shoes unless the shoes are very tight. When wearing ill-fitted shoes, the patient may not know there is a break in the skin until they see blood or pus on their sock.

Humans have been trying to make comfortable and protective foot covering for thousands of years. Some of the earliest evidence of this was discovered with the mummy Oetzi the "Iceman" who lived 5,300 years ago. Exposed by the melting ice on a mountaintop in the Alps, Oetzi was found wearing footwear made of plant materials.[1]

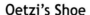

Oetzi's Shoe

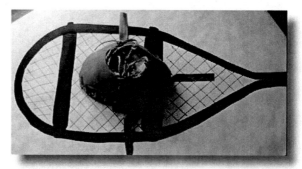

For more images and historical information of shoes, see http://tinyurl.com/6m5aq.

Our landscape presents no fewer hazards for poorly clad feet than Oetzi's did. But in spite of our history of foot coverings and all the years of experience that humans have had at making and wearing shoes, I still have patients who say things like, "I have a closet full of shoes and none of them fit me right," or "my shoes make my feet hurt." Patients from the Depression era recall shoes being passed down from brother to brother and sometimes from brother to sister, and the shoe usually did not fit well. The results ranged from pain and functional disability, to the formation of corns, calluses, and perhaps nerve or heel pain.

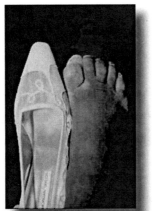 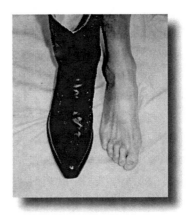

Improperly Fitting Shoes

In a survey done by the American Podiatric Medical Association, it was found that approximately 75 percent of those interviewed felt it was normal for our feet to hurt. Nothing could be farther from the truth. I have had many female patients come to my office saying, "My feet are killing me."

"Did you have your foot measured when you bought those new shoes?" I ask.

"No. I just asked for a size 8A because that's what I've been wearing since I was in high school."

Upon closer inspection and measurement, her correct shoe size was closer to 10B. No wonder she is in such pain!

People have 100 percent control over their shoes and foot gear. We can buy a pair that fits well and are comfortable!

Aside from the obvious fashion issues associated with shoes, the real function of shoes is to cover, support, and protect the foot. Whatever else we attribute to shoes is secondary to those functions. In the at-risk patient, shoes are one of the most important issues. Properly-fitted and well-maintained shoes are essential for the patient with diabetes.

A patient's need for footwear can vary throughout the day according to his activities, but patients with diabetes must use footwear even at home when they might consider walking barefooted, sock-footed, or in house shoes or slippers. This type of foot gear is not protective enough for the patient with diabetes to prevent silent trauma that could lead to an amputation. The question a person should ask is, "If I stepped on a sharp object, or if an object falls on my foot, or if I bump my foot against a door frame, table, or chair, will this house shoe or slipper provide enough protection to prevent an injury to my foot? If the answer is no, replace the foot gear with ones that will protect your feet.

## Case Study ~ Shoes Too Tight

RC was a 62-year-old type 2 diabetic. He had been admitted to the hospital with a fever of 101.1 degrees and a red, swollen, and painful area on the left foot and lower leg. Upon questioning this patient, his history revealed that he had bought a new pair of shoes the previous Saturday. On Sunday, while wearing the new shoes, he took a short hike with his family. On Monday he developed a red, swollen, warm, and tender area on the top of his left foot. By Tuesday the redness had extended to just below the knee in a cord-like fashion.

On Wednesday, when he was admitted to the hospital, RC had chills and fever. Since he was admitted to the medicine service, he was being treated with intravenous antibiotics and other medications necessary to control his blood pressure and blood sugar. No consultation to any surgeon/surgical sub specialty was written, except for podiatry, and that was only to trim his toenails.

On physical exam, RC's circulation was noted to be diminished and he was not able to feel the monofilament testing device when it was applied to his foot. He had a callus below the fifth metatarsal of the left foot and adjacent to the callus there was a hematoma (a collection of blood under the skin that is a usually a breeding ground for bacteria). Upon notifying the admitting physician that the hematoma needed to be drained, he asked me if I could do that. I assured him that I was capable of performing the procedure and it was medically necessary to do it promptly. I got the green light to do the debridement, which consisted of using a scalpel and cutting away the infected tissue (in this case the callus and a portion of adjacent skin). After the skin was opened, a collection of blood and fluid was noted in the soft tissue on the bottom of the foot. In the process of the debridement, we took samples of the material in the hematoma for Gram stain and bacterial cultures. As per the wishes of the infectious disease specialists, a portion of tissue (skin and deep soft tissue) was also submitted for culture. As it turned out, the patient had been given the correct antibiotic but we only learned this following the culture and sensitivity report.

I suggested several local treatments be done to augment the treatment established by the medical service. First was to start moist evaporating dressings of Domeboro® every three hours on the foot. Domeboro® is a drying agent and is very effective in decreasing the heat and local inflammation and in reducing the pain associated with the infection, thus making the patient more comfortable and speeding the healing process. To accomplish this, we placed the affected leg on three pillows lengthwise to elevate the foot. We placed a waterproof pad under the foot and leg. The foot was dressed with a fluffy gauze dressing and secured with white plastic tape that only touched the dressing and not the skin. The dressing was moistened every three hours with the Domeboro® solution and allowed to evaporate to dryness.

We placed a heating pad under the patient's lower back to help increase the circulation from the larger arteries in the trunk to the smaller arteries in the area of the infection to help get more antibiotic to the affected area. The patient was given a surgical shoe that was to be used only while going to the bathroom; otherwise he was on complete bed rest. Within three days, the patient had an excellent response to the treatment and was discharged. The patient was sent home with oral antibiotics and continued the topical treatments.

RC returned to my office the following Wednesday, and to my delight, the infection had been completely eliminated and only a small ulceration remained at the site of the previous debridement. We continued the wound care and the ulcer totally closed. The patient was fitted for prescription biomechanical orthotics (custom insoles made from a cast of the patient's foot) with an accommodation to the area of the previous callus under the fifth metatarsal. This treatment effectively off-loaded the abnormal pressure from the area, reducing the likelihood of a recurrence of the callus and the ulcer.

This case illustrates several areas of risk to the patient with diabetes:

- This patient apparently had not received diabetic education concerning the risks to his feet.
- He was not aware of the benefits of periodic professional foot care for the callus.
- He was unaware of the need to examine his feet periodically while wearing new shoes.
- RC wore the wrong type of shoes for hiking, and failed to visually inspect his foot after the hike .
- The patient developed the infection because his foot was "insensate," and was not able to feel the pressure from the new shoe against the already existing callus. The pressure against the callus from the shoe was enough to create the hematoma that lead to the infection.
- This patient did not visually inspect his feet daily. A visual inspection would have identified the area of the redness and swelling and may have prompted him to seek care earlier and possibly avoiding a hospitalization.

If you are a patient with diabetes and have sensory neuropathy or are at risk for lower extremity amputation, shoes are a most serious issue for your foot health and using diabetic shoes should be a priority in your overall healthcare strategy.

## Types of Shoes

Everyday footwear that has a closed toe box creates an environment that is warm, dark, and moist. Bacteria, mold, yeast, and fungus just love that. Some professionals, like policemen, firemen, and military personnel wear patent leather shoes on occasion, or even frequently. They look great and are low-maintenance—just wipe the mud off, and they're shiny again. The disadvantage is that they're made from plastic, so they keep perspiration and heat in the shoe. The shoe acts like a miniature incubator or oven and can worsen your foot infection. I've seen many patients who wear this type of shoe who believe that their foot problem is dry skin when it is actually a fungal infection of the skin, which is a common problem with these shoes. Leather shoes absorb perspiration and dissipate the heat generated from our feet. Therefore, they are a much better choice.

If you have a foot infection, you shouldn't wear the shoe that you wear everyday—you should wear a surgical shoe. Surgical shoes cover, support, and protect the foot while providing an environment conducive to healing a foot wound. They can also accommodate bandages or dressings that will not fit into regular footwear. Surgical shoes have a flexible sole with nylon uppers and Velcro® closures. Your primary care, family medicine, or internal medicine practitioners may not always be aware of the value of surgical footwear. Any patient who has switched from regular shoes to surgical shoes for a foot problem will usually tell you that his foot feels much better.

There are two types of shoes used by the diabetic or at-risk patient: the extra-depth shoe, and the custom-molded shoe.

Both styles are available through the offices of a prosthetist or physician who may prescribe them for you. In some cases, medical insurance may cover either type of shoe. With the appropriate documentation, Medicare will cover the cost of extra-depth shoes, custom-molded shoes, and insoles. Extra depth or diabetic shoes may also be purchased directly from a shoe store or a pedorthist. Some podiatrists even have shoes available through their offices.

The extra-depth shoe is the one most often prescribed. It is one-quarter to three-eighths of an inch deeper than the average shoe. This provides room for either custom-made insoles like biomechanical orthotics or over-the-counter inserts, and they can accommodate mild to moderately deformed feet caused by bunions or digital deformities.

Many patients with diabetes have partial loss of muscular function of their legs due to diabetic motor neuropathy, low back problems, and other medical conditions. These patients may have difficulty walking. They may trip over their own feet and have a high risk for falling. Another advantage of the diabetic shoe is the ability to have it modified to accept a hinged drop foot brace that stabilizes their foot and leg and helps these people walk with better function and reducing the chances of tripping or falling.

**Custom Molded Shoes**

Custom-molded shoes, made from a cast of the patient's feet, are prescribed for more extreme cases of deformities when other shoes won't appropriately fit the deformed foot. These shoes can accommodate specialized insoles like biomechanical orthotics or arch supports. They can also be modified regarding the style, color, and type of closure. This feature is especially important for patients with arthritis who usually prefer Velcro® closures to laces.

Not only can we modify the inside of a shoe, we can also modify the outside. A common exterior modification includes rocker soles, which are used to return lost mobility to the foot and to relieve or reduce pressure. A rocker sole is applied to the bottom of a normal shoe and permits the shoe to "rock forward" to assist in the push off phase of gait. It is especially helpful for patients who have arthritic changes to the big toe joint that prevent normal function of the toe when walking.

Other exterior shoe modifications include:

- Extended steel shanks, which are pieces of steel are embedded into the sole of the shoe and travel the length of the shoe making the rocker sole more stable.
- Stabilization involves adding material to the medial or lateral portion of the shoe to stabilize a part of the foot.
- Cushion heels add shock absorption where there is a loss of fatty tissue.
- Wedges help redirect the weight-bearing position of the foot and stabilizes a corrected position in a deformity. Wedges are triangular pieces of cork-like materials inserted between the shoe and the sole.

- Extensions increase the thickness or height of a shoe. This material is used to compensate for a limb length discrepancy by making one shoe higher than the other.

## Crocs™ Shoes

Just when we thought there was not a better choice for diabetic footgear, along came Crocs™. On a Caribbean sailing trip from Islas Mujeres, Mexico, to Miami, Florida in May of 2002, three Boulder, Colorado natives began dreaming about the perfect boat shoe. They wanted a shoe that incorporated function, fashion, and fun, was slip-resistant and waterproof, didn't smell and would be the most comfortable shoe in existence. There are many people who have enjoyed wearing Crocs™ and especially folks in the diabetic community. The Crocs Cloud™ model is suggested for patients with diabetes, impaired circulation, impaired sensation, or who have ultra sensitive feet. This shoe is touted to have a super-soft foot bed that provides a gentle environment for sensitive feet, while the roomy toe box allows for use of a heavy sock without creating any tightness or pressure points on the foot. The protective front toe cap and elevated heel rim protect the diabetic foot from stubbing and bruising. This style will accommodate an orthotic. Here is a letter I found on their Web site that sums it all up for Crocs™. It's from satisfied diabetic Crocs™ user Lisa Weisenbach of Jonesboro, Arkansas:

*For many years, I have been searching for a comfortable shoe, without any luck. I am a diabetic with severe neuropathy. I have so much pain in my feet that wearing shoes or socks causes a great deal of pain and discomfort. I am also a Registered Nurse and many of my friends wear the Crocs™ and they all rave about them. One day, I visited the Crocs™ Web site. I discovered the Crocs™ prescription version, which is designed for diabetics. I was so excited. I purchased a pair immediately. When they arrived in the mail, I put them on. I haven't worn another pair of shoes since that very day. They are so wonderful. The comfort is amazing. They are everything that the description states and more. My feet now have room to breathe. There is no part of the shoe that rubs or pinches my foot. When my feet swell, I still have plenty of room. I absolutely adore the Crocs™.*

Shoes are made for style not for health and usually do not conform to the shape of the foot. Crocs™ are a distinct departure from that. Thank you all so much for these amazing shoes. As long as Crocs™ are around, I will never wear another shoe. I wear them year round.[2]

## Do I Need Prescription Footwear?

Prescription footwear can provide a variety of benefits to patients depending upon the nature and extent of their foot problem. For example, patients who have bony deformities such as a bunion or digital deformities and have difficulty wearing standard shoes can walk almost pain free with a shoe that is appropriate in size and depth for their foot. Patients who have lost the protective fat pad on the bottom of their foot, as is seen frequently in rheumatoid arthritis, can get relief of friction and shear forces with prescription footwear. Patients who have had partial amputations of their feet run higher than normal risks of subsequent amputations. They benefit from prescription footwear, especially custom-molded shoes. Some patients have limited ranges of motion in the joints of their feet and standard footwear doesn't let them walk without pain. Prescription footwear can be a part of the solution for these patients permitting them to walk longer distances with less pain.

When a patient has compromised biomechanical function, such as the case of a patient with diabetes with Charcot arthropathy, a molded shoe with a built-in orthotic support may be more practical than trying to provide accommodation and support through the use of an in-depth shoe with a custom orthotic. The main disadvantage of the custom-molded shoe is that it is extremely expensive, often running between $400 and $800 per pair. However, these shoes are a bargain when compared to a $50,000 amputation. Some patients with diabetes can receive shoes from the VA. To see if you qualify for shoes, ask your primary care provider to order a consultation to the orthotics and prosthetic department for an evaluation.

## The Medicare Therapeutic Shoe Bill

In 1993, the Medicare Therapeutic Shoe Bill was passed. It extended coverage for footwear such as extra-depth shoes, custom-molded shoes, or shoe inserts to patients with diabetes. Medicare guidelines state that pedorthic devices include:

therapeutic shoes, shoe modifications made for therapeutic purposes, partial foot prostheses, foot orthoses, and Subtalar-Control Foot Orthoses (SCFO).[3]

Those who qualify for part B of Medicare may receive 80 percent reimbursement (varies from state to state) for one pair of extra-depth shoes and three pairs of multi-density inserts per year. Separate inserts may be covered under certain criteria. Shoe modification is covered as a substitute for an insert, and a custom molded shoe is covered when the individual has a foot deformity that cannot be accommodated by an extra depth shoe. The amount paid by Medicare will go either to the supplier (if the supplier accepts assignment) or reimbursed to the patient (if the supplier does not accept assignment).

The Medicare program encourages the use of therapeutic shoes to reduce "the incidence of complications in the diabetic population." At present, Medicare will reimburse patients with or without a history of foot ulcers.

To be eligible for the Medicare Diabetic Therapeutic Footwear benefit the primary care provider must certify that the individual:

1. Has diabetes
2. Has one or more of the following conditions in one or both feet:
   - history of partial or complete amputation of foot
   - history of previous foot ulceration
   - history of pre-ulcerative calluses
   - peripheral neuropathy with evidence of callus formation
   - foot deformity
   - poor circulation

3. Is being treated under a comprehensive diabetes care plan and needs therapeutic shoes and/or inserts because of diabetes. Therapeutic shoes are medically indicated and include temporary use healing/post-op shoes, modified over-the-counter shoes, depth (added depth shoes) and custom-made shoes.

Shoes that don't fit properly may cause the patient to injure their foot because of poor biomechanics/function or foot deformities. Ill-fitting shoes should prompt a consultation with a pedorthist for a professional evaluation. The patient's feet should be measured and fitted for the appropriate shoes, and all other shoes should be discarded.

A patient with diabetes or someone who is at risk for lower extremity amputation because of other factors such as peripheral vascular disease, peripheral neuropathy, arthritis, low vision, or is unable to self care, shoes are a most serious issue and should be a priority in your overall healthcare strategy. If a patient cannot have his needs met in commercially manufactured shoes, he should see a professional for a fitting for a diabetic shoe or insert.

## But I'm Already Wearing Diabetic Shoes

Most physicians and patients believe that diabetic shoes are the magic solution to all foot problems and that once a patient uses them, the foot is well protected. This is not always true. It is most critical that patients with diabetes have both feet measured and receive proper fitting of their diabetic shoes.

Like all shoes, diabetic shoes also cover, support, and

protect the foot. They are constructed with an insert (or insole) usually made of multi-density materials with a pink insole section called Plastizote® that contacts the foot. This material offers a relatively frictionless surface so it can protect the foot from the forces of friction and shear. It also provides a cushioned platform for the foot. One drawback is that it does have the tendency to "bottom-out," as the material compresses under the sites of the most pressure and loses its ability to protect the foot.

Once Plastizote® breaks down, the corresponding area of the foot becomes vulnerable to the forces of repetitive micro-trauma. Then a protective thickening of skin (a callus) can form on the bottom of the foot. Left untreated, these calluses can lead to abscess or ulcers forming underneath them and can ultimately lead to bone infections.

I recently had a patient with diabetes come to my clinic and complain of an ulcer to the outside of his small toe that literally happened overnight. And just to complicate the problem, this patient's wife was a nurse and felt she could take care of the problem without the patient needing to see a doctor. So, he waited three weeks before seeking professional attention. By then, the ulcer had gotten "out of control" of his nurse/wife's expertise.

He denied any history of trauma, and was upset that he "spontaneously" developed this ulcer. I noted he was wearing diabetic shoes and inquired about them. He told me he had gotten the shoes three weeks earlier during a morning appointment and just started wearing them the day before he noted the ulcer. He never considered the shoes to be origin of the problem. After all, they were diabetic shoes, dispensed by the prosthetics department of the hospital, and those folks should know what they are doing, right? My evaluation of his foot revealed that he had a narrow rear foot and wider forefoot with a bunion deformity, contracted toes. and a tailor's bunion.

An X-ray revealed that he had a prominent portion of bone called a condyle or exostosis in the affected toe. This normally would not have caused a problem; however, the ill-fitting shoe had caused an increase in pressure against the skin in the corresponding area against the toe which led to an ulcer. Then the entire scenario became clear. Even though he had been dispensed what both he and the hospital prosthetics department thought were the appropriate shoes, they were inappropriate for his foot type and were dispensed at the wrong time of day. No one could have known that he had a prominent condyle (portion of bone) that would rub against the shoe. But, the prosthetics clinician should have recognized his foot type, and either provided him with a combination last diabetic shoe, (one that has a narrow heel and wider toe box) or a custom-molded diabetic shoe. Had this been done, the ulcer would not have occurred.

The evaluation of footwear and insoles should be a standard part of the lower-extremity examination. Up to 82 percent of foot ulcers are related to pressure from footwear or narrow or otherwise inadequate footwear.

## Pedorthists

Because of this universal concern about shoes and shoe fitting, a relatively unknown and under-utilized profession has steadily grown in popularity over the past few years. Many medical professionals like podiatrists, physical therapists, and orthotists—people who already have advanced educations—have taken additional training to become specialists in evaluating a person's foot and making recommendations for proper fitting shoes. Though the intention of a shoe is to cover, support, and protect the foot, there are two sides to footwear. It can contribute to or exacerbate existing foot problems especially if not fitted correctly, and it can be part of an amputation prevention strategy when fitted correctly and used to cover, support, and protect the foot.

It is the job of pedorthists to provide the best-fitting footwear to patients with foot problems. They are part of the inter-disciplinary team of educators and clinicians who can help prevent an amputation. They can provide information to patients about every facet of proper footwear and fit. They can also alert patients to the significance of follow-up visits to make sure their shoes continue to fit correctly and to serve their purposes.

Though education for pedorthics started in 1961, podiatrist, Stephen Albert says, "Some podiatrists have taken it upon themselves to become more knowledgeable by doing the necessary course work to become certified pedorthists...... podiatry schools have developed pedorthic training programs that prepare individuals for board certification in the field."[4]

Board certified pedorthists must pass a comprehensive examination that includes knowledge of anatomy and physiology, pathology and injury, and examination and evaluation of the foot and ankle; footwear and orthoses including fit, design, construction, materials, modification, adjustment, and follow-up; and management techniques. Pedorthists understand the anatomy of a shoe, what modifications can be made, and what type of shoe would be best for the problem the patient has. In addition to assuring that a patient's shoe fits well, pedorthists prescribe footwear and all modifications to footwear. The evaluation and recommendations for footwear by a pedorthist can be a vital part of the overall management strategy of patients at risk for amputations and benefit both patients and their entourages by preventing triggers that can lead to amputations.

If a patient is in the early stages of sensory neuropathy (loss of protective sensation), wearing the right shoes is very important. By working with your podiatrist or pedorthist, you may be able to prevent serious diabetic foot complications by simply wearing well-fitting shoes that protect your feet from injury. The shoe should be made of soft, natural materials with a shock-absorbing sole in the right size that does not put pressure or friction on any part of the foot. In order to get the right type of shoes for the diabetic foot, it is best to have a specially-trained Board Certified pedorthist assist you in finding the proper fit.

## Dennis Janisse, C.Ped

Dennis Janisse is a certified pedorthist with his national pedorthic services office headquarters in Milwaukee, Wisconsin. With seven offices in two states, Dennis has been in business for about forty years. He began his career as a pedorthist while doing shoe repair in a small town north of Milwaukee when three doctors began referring their patients to him for prescription footwear. At that time, orthotic work did not exist; a precursor to orthotics was done by cobblers who were trying to modify regular footwear to suit the foot care needs of patients with diabetes. These three doctors brought Dennis brochures for some courses being offered through Ball State University (Muncie, Indiana) and Northwestern University (Evanston, Illinois), which were the only places offering any type of study on pedorthics. Since these doctors were going to send him more business, Dennis and his wife took the courses at both colleges and became certified as pedorthists.

In their little shoe repair shop, they started taking impressions of people's feet and making foot insoles and custom shoes. Dennis enjoyed doing pedorthics because it was really helping people and making a difference in their lives. Over a short period of time, he and his wife started doing pedorthic footwear exclusively and the business grew relatively quickly.

Because most of their referring physicians were in Milwaukee the Janisse's moved there and bought a building where they set up a major facility. Over time, they produced a fabrication shop and with the exception of custom shoes, began to fabricate everything—shoe modifications and braces—in-house. Then came the remote offices where they were able to contract to create elaborate fabrications. However, these offices, located in Texas, were too far away for them to retain control of the quality, so they brought everything back in house. They created a standard operating procedure which gives a consistently quality product that the patients and the doctors could always count on.

Dennis is the past president of the Pedorthic Footwear Association, and the director of pedorthic education for PW Minor—one of the primary orthopedic shoe companies. He is the current director with ABC (The American Board for Certification in Orthotics, Prosthetics and Pedorthics).

Diabetes is Dennis' primary interest from a pedorthic patient standpoint. He says it's all about helping people. He has done quite a bit of work in Taiwan and China and is doing some volunteer work in Mali, West Africa this year. He has done a lot of teaching internationally, working with doctors in Thailand, where they are opening a pedorthic school. He was the overseer on a similar project in Australia. Dennis says, "I can get more people excited about pedorthics, and teach them how to properly take care of their patients. More patients can be helped through teaching than by seeing patients. When I'm in Milwaukee, I still have my own patient load consisting of people who are specifically referred to me."

## What is Pedorthics?

Pedorthics is to footgear, what a pharmacist is to drugs. They don't diagnose or prescribe, but they do fill prescriptions and offer evaluations for shoes, shoe modifications, insoles, or braces for footwear. Pedorthics includes the services of an orthotist and prosthesist. An orthotist can make braces for any part of the body. A prothesist makes artificial limbs for the body. The pedorthist is limited to the foot and ankle.

Pedorthics is still a very small profession. There are somewhere between 2,500 and 3,000 pedorthists in the United States. The best way to find a pedorthist is to go to ABC's Web site (www.abcop.org) and type in your city and state. It will give you the name and contact information for a pedorthist in your neighborhood.

Many major insurance companies now provide coverage for pedorthic services such as foot orthoses or some other partial foot prosthesis, but a majority of them do not cover the footwear. For example, Blue Cross/Blue Shield has fairly good coverage, but there are so many different policies within Blue Cross/Blue Shield, that the coverage can vary depending upon your policy.

Physicians may identify patients who are diabetic and at risk, which means they have neuropathy plus a deformity. They may prescribe diabetic shoes and believe that their job is done. However, they should see the patient wearing the shoes and they should look at the insoles six months later to see how they fit. Without a proper fit of accommodative PPT or Plastizote(R) insoles, a patient may re-ulcerate while wearing diabetic shoes. In these cases, three people are at fault: the physician, who didn't have the patient return to take a look at the fit; the practitioner or pedorthist who dispensed the prescription shoe; and the patient, who did not check the insole on a regular basis. A patient with diabetes with an at-risk foot does not have protective sensation. This patient should always be followed periodically and seen to monitor his situation. Dennis' company actually sends out reminder cards to get patients back to take a look and see what shape the shoes are in after six months. The reimbursement with Medicare isn't that great, so people aren't getting the real sophisticated biomechanical orthotic device they may truly need. Instead, they're getting three cheaper insoles or devices that are not designed to last for a year. The first one gets put into the shoe when it is dispensed, and the patient takes the other two home where they sit in the closet. We definitely need follow-up from the physician, but the practitioner or the pedorthist needs to follow-up as well.

Most of the patients Dennis sees have significant diseases. If a patient's foot is not too terribly compromised, and has some relatively normal biomechanics, then a more functional device probably makes sense. If a person has rigid feet or severe deformities, the functional device is usually inappropriate. When it comes to the elderly population, the diabetes patients, and the arthritis patients, that particular device is not appropriate because it's not going to be able to do much correcting. Therefore, the biomechanics are pretty much lost. Forty- and fifty-year-olds are more active and want to participate, not only in athletic activities but in life, yet they've got prescription shoes that are totally inappropriate.

Because it is a referral-based practice, some patients have problems getting the referral they need. Many physicians, including orthopedists, are not taught about the benefits of pedorthics or conservative care. The only way an orthopedist can learn what a pedorthist does is to do a fellowship with a doctor who recognizes and uses pedorthics. Obviously, a podiatrist does. If they do a fellowship that's surgically oriented, they're not going to get any training in pedorthics there. But, that's because surgeons are doing amputations and various kinds of wound care.

Education is really needed in this area. The issue with pedorthics is very much like the greater issue with the diabetic patient—patients and providers are not educated enough about the benefits of pedorthic care. Therefore, when these kinds of problems show up at the office, providers don't know what to do with them. Dennis does a good job of informing people about the benefits of his profession and the services he offers. He's been fairly successful in his local area. One day, he will have lunch with a physician group; another day, he will teach a Medicare group, or he may go to a diabetes or arthritis support group or organization. He is also an assistant professor at the Medical College at Wisconsin. He is able to include some pedorthic training into the curriculum when he teaches residents, but the vast majority of physicians out there, even podiatrists, are not getting any training. They don't know what a pedorthist does, so they definitely don't use their services. They're anxious to have some exposure to it.

Pedorthics is a wonderful profession. Some of the new materials they are working with include silver, copper, antifungal, and antibacterial materials. There's a self-adhesive material called shear band designed to decrease shear forces, which in some cases, is as important as pressure when we're trying to unload things. Check the appendix for a list of Web sites that are helpful for patients and providers.

People wear shoes that are inadequate. They will spend all kinds of money on clothing, but they don't really respect how important footwear is to their feet, to their entire body and their health. Some people expect their feet to hurt, but the truth is people should not have foot pain. They may have tired feet at the end of the day, but for all the pedorthists in the world Dennis reminds you that your feet do not have to hurt! "I've got some very significant flexible flat feet," he says. "Somebody once told me I was going to be in braces by the time I got to my present age, but I'm telling you, my feet never hurt! They are tired sometimes at the end of the day but I'm not walking around all day with my feet hurting."

The solution to foot pain can be very simple; it doesn't have to be as involved as prescription or orthopedic shoes. It may require only a few modifications. Sometimes, finding the proper fitting shoe is all it takes to make people feel better. There's never been a better time to be a pedorthist than today.

## Orthotics

*I'd rather lose my wallet before losing my orthotics.*
~Patient comment

Foot orthotics are medical devices that fit into shoes to treat a variety of foot problems. Orthotics range from over-the-counter, mass-produced types sold in retail locations to custom-made devices prescribed by medical professionals like podiatrists. Orthotics sold in retail markets or on TV "infomercials" might better be known as arch supports.

When you get orthotic devices from a podiatrist or other medical professional, you usually get custom-made insoles known as prescription biomechanical orthotics. These are used to treat a wide variety of foot problems ranging from bony and soft-tissue problems of the forefoot to heel pain, nerve pain, tired-feeling feet and legs. In some cases they can provide relief of low back, knee or leg pain by controlling the function of the foot and legs. The success of orthotics is based on the practitioner understanding the patient's biomechanical function. A foot that has limited range of motion or a high arch needs a more shock-absorbing type of orthotic. A foot that has a lower type arch or a larger range of motion will benefit from a more controlling type of orthotic. Orthotics can be used to offload the site of a keratosis and to prevent ulcers under the forefoot. For patients who have foot deformities, arthritis or pain with walking and surgery is not an option, orthotics oftentimes offer relief that cannot be provided by other treatments.

Issues of gait and ambulation are in a gray zone when it comes to what type of medical practitioner might be the best to treat these vexing problems. There are many people who suffer with tired feet and legs, and joint pains in their low back, hips, knees, and feet caused by faulty foot function. Too often, the symptoms are attributed to the patient's diabetes or not acknowledged at all, and left at that, without treatment. Most patients and practitioners do not know that custom-made insoles, called biomechanical orthotics, can resolve these musculo-skeletal issues. Working in harmony with the way nature intended the foot to function, orthotics control and permit the most efficient foot function. Since very few MD or DO medical students have training in such issues, they generally are ignored. Podiatrists are specially trained in biomechanical (how structure affects foot function) theory and are the best practitioners to see if you feel you might benefit from a "biomechanical tune up" on your feet.

## Arthritis

You don't necessarily have to be a patient with diabetes to suffer from one of a wide variety of foot or leg problems. With over 300 diagnosable problems in the foot and ankle, unequal limb length and arthritis are equal opportunity villains. Forty-million Americans suffer with this painful and debilitating disease. Osteoarthritis affects twenty million while rheumatoid arthritis affects about two million patients. The painful result of arthritis in the foot is related to inflammation. Instability in gait and loss of balance with fear of falling is not uncommon when the thirty joints in each foot are affected.

Complaints of musculo-skeletal pain are common for many people. The pain can be anywhere up and down the skeletal tree. Some folks have low back pain, some have back pain that radiates down their leg, some have back and knee pain and the permutations are endless; all the way to the big toe joints.

If all musculo-skeletal pain were caused by arthritis, it would be a snap to diagnose the reason for everyone's musculo-skeletal pain. But it's not that simple. When I see patients who have complaints of musculo-skeletal pain in their feet or legs, I want to know if they have had any joint replacement or implant arthroplasty procedures done for their hips or knees. The ankle joint implant has not been perfected to the point that it is commonly used at this time. If the patient has vague musculo-skeletal pain in his low back or up and down his legs and has had a joint implant, I will be highly suspicious that his legs may not be the same length. A hip or knee implant procedure can leave one limb longer or shorter than the opposite limb. Most times the patient is unaware that his legs are not the same length, and the price he pays is musculo-skeletal pain.

How do we figure out if this is your problem? We put the patient on their back in the supine position. We then use a tape measure and check the distance from the anterior superior iliac spine or ASIS (a bony prominence of the hip) located just in front of the pocket on a pair of jeans) to the bisection of the distal tibia or as we call it, the inside of the ankle. It is not unusual to find limb length differences of one-quarter to one inch on some patients. A limb length difference is a common cause of faulty biomechanical function that can change the gait of a patient resulting in new pressure points and vulnerability to blisters, keratosis, and pain that was not present before the implant procedure.

There are several options to treat the problem. The

easiest method to treat a limb length difference of up to one-quarter inch is to use a versatile custom-made device called a biomechanical orthotic that can be modified to accommodate a limb length correction for the short leg. In cases where the difference is one-half inch or more, we usually look to spread out the lift between the sole of the shoe and the orthotic.

While treating people's foot problems may not be perceived as glamorous, many people have real pain that leads to functional disability and even bad moods. In too many cases, I have met people who have had previous treatment for their foot problems, only to be disappointed with the results. When I listen to their stories, I always feel bad for them, and hope to solve their individual puzzle about their feet and restore them as close as possible to normal and pain free function.

## Ginger's Story

Ginger was in her late forties and worked in the food service industry. She stood for long periods of time and had experienced pain in her feet for most of her life. "I had to stop doing the serving, carrying the trays because my feet and ankles hurt so much," she told me. "The trays are heavy, maybe sixty pounds, including the plates. I try to work at the bar or seated if I can."

On her initial consultation, I diagnosed her with heel pain due to inflammation of soft tissue and forefoot pain due to a nerve entrapment, both problems typically seen in people in the food service industry who work long hours standing on hard, unyielding surfaces. Ginger had two different types of pain in two separate areas of her feet and both were bad.

After we performed our history, physical exam, labs, and x-ray evaluations, we gave her several steroid injections for treatment of the nerve pain in her forefoot and the pain was totally relieved. She still was plagued with heel pain. As an integral part of her examination, a biomechanical exam was done.

It revealed abnormal foot and leg function, or faulty biomechanics. We looked to control her abnormal foot and leg function with biomechanical orthotics. Ginger was hopeful that the orthotics would help her, but she was quick to point out she has used orthotics before and they barely helped at all.

On her follow-up visit, she was wearing orthotics in her black New Balance shoes, tuxedo pants, and starched white tuxedo shirt, ready to go to work. She was still having pain to the inside of her ankle and heel. She had a sad look on her face and told me how she was dreading going to work that day because she knew her feet were going to be hurting that night. We discussed all the options including heat and ice, stretching exercises, no barefooted walking, oral anti-inflammatory medications, and night splints.

I reviewed her chart and talked a bit about where her foot was hurting. I looked at her feet and her orthotics and thought to myself, perhaps the orthotics were under-corrected. To modify the orthotics, I placed a specially trimmed and beveled small piece of three-eighths-inch adhesive felt on the bottom of her orthotic to increase the correction. In front of my eyes I saw a woman transformed. She took a few steps and became a different person.

"It's gone!" she said, "the pain is gone. After twenty years, it's gone."

Walking in what appeared to be disbelief, she held her head high and smiled as she walked around my office. I have never experienced a patient's response quite like this. It was a good day to be in service to my fellow woman. It made me feel great as a doctor and as a person.

## Types of Orthotics

When additional biomechanical control is needed, post-orthosis shoe modifications and/or ankle-foot orthosis (AFO) may control distribution of forces during stance and ambulation. Patients requiring more permanent devices for unstable Charcot or neuropathic foot may use custom-molded footwear, insoles, inserts, and walkers such as Charcot restraint orthopedic walker. Let's look at a few of these devices that can be used for accommodating and controlling foot function.

## Custom-molded Footwear

Custom-molded shoes are expensive, often cosmetically unacceptable and require expertise to cast and fit. In addition, custom-molded footwear is seldom necessary today because of the wider array of last sections (a last is theoretical model of a foot that is used to create a shoe) now available in depth footwear. Wide "last" shoes accommodate various insoles and orthosis. These shoes also can be altered to include rocker soles and other modifications. Many patients have difficulty using their hands due to arthritis or may have visual problems. Custom-molded shoes should be reserved for patients with severe foot deformities that cannot be accommodated in standard footwear. These include Charcot foot, partial amputations, bunions, or deformed and contracted toes, amputations, and where there is a large variation in size between feet, that cannot be accommodated in standard footwear.

## Insoles

Simple insoles protect the at-risk foot structures through cushioning, shock absorption, shear forces reduction and padding. After wearing certain types of insoles, the pressure from the foot can cause the insole to bottom out and the insole will not fulfill its mission to redistribute the forces/pressures against the foot and the patient may re-ulcerate.

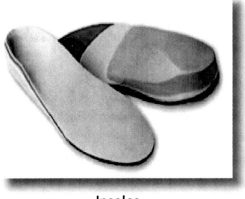

Insoles

Over-the-counter insoles are inadequate for the needs of the at-risk foot. At minimum, insoles require customization by a pedorthist or a podiatrist to provide appropriate pressure distribution.

## Rocker Soles

Rocker soles are standard care for offloading the forefoot

in footwear and accommodating a fixed ankle brace. They can also be used for patients who have limitation of movement or pain in the big toe joint when walking. Rocker soles effectively reduce forefoot pressures. However, they present a tripping hazard when caught on carpets or uneven floors.

## Shoe Inserts

There are a variety of inserts or insoles that may be placed inside a shoe. Everyone has seen the over-the-counter variety sold at retail stores whose function is not specific but rather is vague with no medical purpose in mind. Often, we can see on the packaging claims such as "helps to relieve stress" or "provides foot comfort." While this type of insole can provide comfort my patients have told me that in the longer run they really have not benefited from using this type of insole.

There is another type of insole that is fabricated to custom fit the patient's foot and shoe. It is designed to serve a specific medical function such as protection from sheer forces and stress, extra support, shock absorption for the heel, arch, or the full foot or to control foot function.

While generic insoles often are helpful for some patients, others require an insole that is custom tailored for their particular foot and foot problem. Sometimes, patients have trouble getting a proper fit from over-the-counter insoles, and, after all, with each one of our feet being just a bit different in size and configuration, how could we expect to be successful getting a proper fit from a mass-produced generic product?

As opposed to the mass-produced over-the-counter insoles, custom-made prescription biomechanical orthotics are one of the tools that can help prevent foot ulcers. There are two types of specialized shoe inserts, or orthoses, that are available: customized, and custom-made. A customized insert can be either accommodative, to accommodate the foot; or functional, to control the foot. It starts with a prefabricated base. A pedorthist can adapt it to the patient's needs by adding a metatarsal pad, wedge, or heel cushion. A custom-made insert, or biomechanical orthotic, is typically for patients with more critical foot problems. It is made from an impression of the patient's foot that is taken with the foot in a specific position to assure not only proper fit but also proper function.

## Orthotics vs. Arch Supports

The philosophy behind an arch support is that the function of your foot is solely to support your weight. Typically, arch supports have a higher arch than the foot of the person trying to use them. The arch support literally tries to out muscle your arch by pushing it up. Ask anyone who has ever tried to use an arch support, and more than likely you'll hear a response close to, "I could not wear them. They hurt my foot."

But, there is another philosophy about the function of our feet that is based on the discipline of podiatric biomechanics: our feet do more than just support our weight. We live in a three-dimensional world and our feet move and function in three dimensions. We walk, run, dance, and jump; we move in three dimensions. We do more than just stand in one place and a normal functioning foot facilitates our ability to make these movements. That's why arch supports usually fail and biomechanical orthotics usually work.

## Making the Orthotic

The first step in fabricating a biomechanical orthotic is a thorough biomechanical evaluation of each of the patient's feet. This will reveal any functional or structural abnormalities of the foot so a prescription can be written for the orthotic to address the individual needs of each foot. As peculiar as it may sound, I have seen patients whose feet appear to be mismatched in terms of structure or function. One foot may have a high arch while the other has a low arch. Or perhaps one foot has a deformity like a bunion while the other foot appears totally normal.

The next step is taking an impression of each foot. This is done by taking a cast impression of each of the patient's feet usually in plaster or a sock impregnated with a resin-like fiberglass. In this case, the foot is held in a position called subtalar joint neutral that places the foot in the position it should be in the mid-stance phase of gait. Orthotics prepared in this fashion work in harmony with the way nature intended the foot to function. Some physicians like to take an impression of the patient's foot using a shallow box that is filled with pressure sensitive foam. The foot is pressed into the foam, and the resulting imprint is used to create the orthotic. I have not been successful in capturing a good mold of the foot by this method. Therefore, I do not use it. The latest technology uses a computer to scan the bottom of the patient's foot. This data is sent by the Internet to the laboratory. The data is decoded and used in a CAD-CAM (Computer-Aided Design-Computer-Aided Manufacture) machine to create the orthotic. Whether a mold is made of the foot or computers scan the foot, both the foot information and orthotic prescription are usually retained by the orthotic manufacturer. Should the patient desire a second or subsequent pair of orthotics, it can easily be manufactured without re-casting or scanning the patient.

Orthotics can be made from various materials, depending on the patient's foot needs. For example, the most flexible orthotics are made from cork and leather and are used for patients who have limitation of joint function. Patients who require more control of their foot function and less shock absorption can benefit from orthotics that are made from firmer thermoplastic materials. Specialized materials such as leather, pigskin, and neoprene rubber can be used for the top covers.

Biomechanical orthotics can control abnormal function as well as help relieve pressure from the bottom of the foot. This is done by relieving (or "offloading") areas of high pressure with specialized padding incorporated under the orthotic top cover itself. I have found the use of biomechanical orthotics to be a very important part of my prevention strategy for diabetics as well as a valuable treatment for patients with a variety of foot problems. Often, the use of orthotics can relieve pain or functional disability and prevent the reoccurrence of a foot ulcer or the need for surgery.

### Foot Notes: Tips for Buying Shoes That Fit Correctly for Patients with Diabetes

- Measure both feet and fit the larger foot. Very few people have the exact same size on both feet.
- Do not rely on the size of the shoe to be the proper fit for your foot. The shoe industry has undergone radical changes over the past twenty years and for the most part,

shoes are no longer manufactured in the United States. The manufacturing plants are now located in South America and Asia. Shoes are made from a theoretical model called a "last." The last is made from a copy of a real person's foot. It is clearly obvious that the morphology or body characteristics of the Asian model are going to be different and smaller from our bodies in the West. Therefore, it is best to use the numbers only as a guide. One day I was looking at a shoe that was manufactured in Europe and the sizes ran from 38 to 46. I thought to myself, Who could have feet that big? Not even the legendary basketball superstar Shaquil O'Neil, who wears size 22, could fill those shoes. Then, I learned that the European sizing system is quite different from what we are used to. Be sure to ask for help if you see strange sizes on the shoes you might like to buy. A size 9 in Western countries might not really be the size 9 you are used to wearing. In fact, it might really be an 8½ or 8. And if you're buying European shoes, they use a different sizing-system than Americans. Instead of women's sizes from 5-11, European sizes range from 38 to 46, and they run wider.

- Do not rely on a size that you may have been wearing for years. Have both feet measured and fit the larger foot. Your shoe size may change as you get older, and the shoe industry has changed over the past twenty years, as well.
- The best time to buy shoes is late in the day. Gravity pulls fluid down toward our feet and as the day progresses, there is likely to be more fluid collecting towards the

feet and ankles. Shoes bought late in the day will be comfortable all day. Shoes bought in the morning may well be uncomfortable by day's end.

- Be sure to wear the appropriate type of sock or stocking for the shoe you are buying. Be sure the shoes fit comfortably, immediately. There is no such thing as "I'll take them home and break them in." The only thing that might get broken is your foot. Some people have a wider front of the foot and a narrower back of the foot. This type of foot needs a special type of shoe called a "combination last" shoe. Not all manufacturers make this special type of shoe and therefore the styles of shoes that fit you correctly may be limited. If a patient needs this type of shoe, you may have to ask specifically for it. New Balance shoes are made in widths and this may offer the patient with diabetes a better fit.

- Shoes should be constructed from natural materials, such as leather or other natural fibers. Natural materials permit the foot to "breathe," that is to dissipate heat and so stay away from plastic shoes.

- Shoes should have an adequate sole for shock absorption and protection of the foot. Many people have difficulty using shoe laces and prefer a Velcro® closure. There are variations on lacing shoes (such as elastic shoe laces) that can change the pressure against the foot and make the foot more comfortable.

For definitive information on shoe lacing, visit www. fieggen.com/shoelace/lacingmethods.htm.

Having several pairs of comfortable shoes will make your feet happy.

## Foot Risk Categories

Shoes have a significant impact on everyone's foot health, but more so if you have diabetes. Selecting the right shoe and visually inspecting your feet daily or more frequently when wearing new shoes should be a critical component of your overall amputation prevention strategy. Before you even step foot into a shoe store there are several questions you should ask yourself.

1. When is my foot at special risk? Patients who are in Evaluation and Management Category 0 (see Chapter 2), or who have protective sensation and no foot deformity probably have more flexibility about the shoes they can wear without increasing their risk for a foot problem. However, you are at a higher risk for developing ulcers, infections, and the triggers that can lead to amputations if: you are in category 1, 2, or 3; have neuropathy or peripheral arterial disease; have bone, soft tissue, or nail deformities; or have had previous amputations.

2. For what activity will the shoes be used? Clearly, one of the most preventable tragedies I have seen with my patients is that they wear the wrong shoe for the wrong activity. Walking shoes are designed for walking, not hiking or sports activity. Patients with neuropathy are particularly vulnerable to trauma caused by their shoes. Remember the case study of our patient who ended up hospitalized with an infection that required intravenous antibiotics because he wore the wrong shoe for the wrong activity?

3. If I wear an arch support, accommodative insoles, or prescription custom biomechanical orthotics, will the shoe I am buying have enough room for my insoles? In order to answer this question, bring your insoles with you while shoe shopping so you can "test" them in the shoe store.

4. Diabetic shoes are expensive. Can I get a quality pair of shoes at a discounted price on the Internet? While bargains seem to be everywhere on the Internet, there is no substitute for actually going to the store, having both feet measured while standing, fitting the larger foot and physically wearing the shoes before you purchase them.

5. I've heard of cars being recalled for defects; can that happen to my shoes? Remember that shoes, like any other mass-manufactured product, can be defective. In some cases, it is a defective shoe that can lead to sprained ankles, pain, or functional disability. In the patient with diabetic neuropathy, a defective shoe can become a trigger for bigger problems. No, you are not crazy, if you feel there is something not quite right with your shoe. There actually may be something wrong with the shoe you just bought. When in doubt, return it and try a different pair.

After you get your new shoes home there are a few simple rules concerning shoes and amputation prevention.

- Inspect the inside of the shoes for loose stitching or rough spots in the shoe lining before you put them on.

Also check for foreign objects. Patients have reported finding things such as pins, keys, coins, a peanut, a screw, and even a bottle of nail polish in their shoes.
- Wear the appropriate sock for the shoe you are wearing.
- Keep your shoes in good condition. Shoes with worn heel or soles should be repaired or replaced. Shoes with damaged uppers should be replaced.

## Foot Measurements

The Ritz Stick and Brannock device are the two most common types of measuring devices used to measure foot size. In addition to providing overall length and width measurements, the Brannock has the advantage of measuring the heel-to-ball length as well. The heel-to-ball length is a relative measurement of the length of the patient's arch to the overall length of the foot.

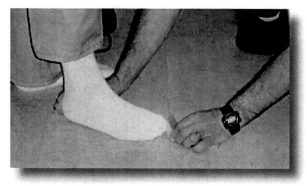

**Ritz Stick-Length**

The Brannock device and Ritz Stick measure the linear width across the foot. This width measurement can be inaccurate because it does not take into account the circumference or thickness of the patient's foot.[5] The last determines the heel height, toe box shape, and volume of the finished shoe, as well as the flair, such as an inflare, outflare, or straight last shoe.

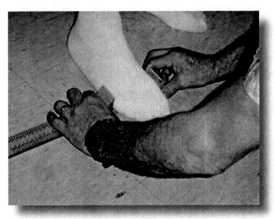

**Ritz Stick-Width**

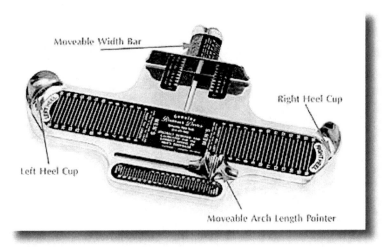

**Brannock Device**

# Chapter Fourteen

## Depression and Diabetes

If diabetes is so dangerous, and yet manageable with proper care, why do so many people not follow their doctor's advice? Why do they continue to deny that they are the person solely responsible for what they eat and how they care for their body?

Patients with diabetes should know that maintaining optimum health with appropriate behaviors is the best method to assure they will not have to deal with a limb loss and the personal costs associated with it. Some patients seem to have a disconnect between their disease and the behaviors that are best for their health. They may see their health failing in front of their eyes and not have the power or desire to change their habits and behaviors toward an attitude of prevention. If a patient's behavior is critical to preventing an amputation, *why* do they behave this way?

Perhaps the most costly part of being diabetic is the behavioral issues that accompany the disease. Medical literature on diabetes has identified several reasons why patients may not be compliant in managing their diabetes or wounds.

> Which came first, the chicken or the egg? Depression triggers diabetes and diabetes can trigger depression.

Many patients behave this way because they are in denial—especially when first diagnosed—because they feel there is nothing they can do about their condition. Some patients see diabetes as a death sentence, and decide it's not worth trying to overcome it. They may think the disease is going to get them and there is nothing they can do about it. Denial or avoidance is a very normal reaction. It is the mind's way of protecting itself in extreme circumstances. Who wants to deal with one's mortality every second, especially if all those threats are described as inevitable unless you are more than perfect? Unfortunately, once in denial, many people stay there with no blood testing, no attention paid to diet and exercise, no adjustments made to insulin dosage (they may "forget" to take it), and avoidance of doctors or anything related to diabetes. This makes the very scary consequences of uncontrolled diabetes that much more possible. This is one of the things that drive people into denial in the first place.

People don't change just because we tell them there is a better option, and fear has not been shown to modify a patient's behavior. Some people have to be "scared" into actually taking action. How many people do you know who did not stop smoking until they had lung cancer? It's the same way with diabetes; people don't expect diabetes to harm them, and it's easy to ignore until it's too late. People change when they conclude that they have no other option. Another school of thought about changing behaviors is that people change when they see someone else doing well. While I have high regard for these theories, they don't always seem to hold up when we apply them to the patient with diabetes. On an almost daily basis, I see patients with diabetes who have lost a limb sitting in a wheelchair in the hospital smoking area lighting up cigarettes. I see patients with chronically elevated blood glucose levels who have neuropathy yet they fail to change their habits. Some are still drinking sugary soft drinks or alcoholic beverages and eating unhealthy foods without regard to their diabetes. It is truly amazing and at the same time sad.

Some patients may feel they have enough of other things to worry about that seem more important than their diabetes. They are given an even longer list of the serious complications of blindness, kidney failure, heart attacks, ulcers, infections, amputations and decreased life span if the person strays one iota from the prescribed plan. Without considering the emotional impact of this information, the fear that it inspires is very hard to deal with. Patients may leave it up to fate to decide what happens with their diabetes.

Some patients are exactly the opposite. When they are told how to take insulin, given a diet of foods to eat, and a long list of foods not to eat, they try their best to eat healthy foods and never cheat. It takes huge amounts of energy and dedication to maintain strict control over diet, insulin, and exercise, only to have their diligence rewarded with blame and condemnation from their doctor or those they love. "What have you been eating? Your sugar level is still too high! You have to try harder!" To be expected to watch every mouthful of food, monitor every movement, and account for stress level everyday for the rest of your life, is just too much for some. The work it takes to stay healthy, and the sometimes thoughtless people who hammer away at the patient's best efforts causes patients to feel isolated and that no one cares about them. Diabetes does not always react the same way to the same event, and the patient may soon find that their action plan is unachievable. A sense of helplessness takes over.

## Case Study

During our interview, Dr. Larry Lavery told me about a patient he had worked with for the past seven years. She is forty-three but looks like she is sixty-three. She does not have a lot of money and she is not very well-educated. She lives with her mom, who looks younger than she does. Dr. Lavery has observed her system fail. He tries to give her positive pieces of information, explain to her why different steps need to be taken, why she needs to focus on her hypertension and blood sugar control and how all of this information translates to what is going on with her legs. She has fractured her tibia, and has countless other problems. Her mom once pulled a little piece of skin off her foot which created an ulcer, and she ended up having an amputation of her fourth and fifth toes. All of the referral slips, medication, and little pieces of encouragement did not help, as she is still in the hospital with blood sugars of 400. She has serious depression. A lot of people in this situation get clinically depressed and can't see out of the pit. Their body is betraying them. They need to be active for the disease but cannot because they have a wound on their foot. Depression and giving up is a keystone for people with diabetic foot problems.

Dr. Lavery also worked with a 38-year-old Mexican-American patient who lost his right leg after a foot infection. He then came back with an ulcer on his other leg. He had severe sensory neuropathy and had given up. His kidney functions were horrible but he refused to go for a workup that might put him on dialysis. Dr. Lavery believes that people do not understand why they get foot ulcers. Even some physicians believe that it is just spontaneous.

Dr. Lavery's story reminds me of the time when I was driving home one night from work with the windows down, enjoying the fresh air and early evening sunlight. Not really thinking about anything special, just enjoying nature. In my line of work, I am rarely outdoors during the day. I suddenly began to wonder just how many patients I have served in my career.

When I got home, I sat down at my calculator and punched in the numbers, just for fun—fifteen patients a day, twenty days a month, twelve months a year for thirty years—that total was well over 100,000 patient visits! I have seen many people and encountered a variety of personalities. I have met people from every part of the world, and have served their foot care needs, sometimes successfully and sometimes not. The patients I have not been successful in treating causes me to think hard about their cases and why we were not successful. I have tried to learn from those cases so I could be a better physician for other patients.

My background is in psychology and I am a continuing student of human behavior. I have always wondered what makes people tick and I guess am still trying to understand the process. Being a podiatrist and in the "people" business has really given me wonderful insights into patient behavior. While most of my patients with diabetes act just as normally as you or I do, some patients just don't seem to get the program. They fail to understand the issues of blood glucose control that results in vascular and neurological disease. Some fail in adhering to a treatment plan and some go on to lose limbs and lives. This issue is not just about their foot; this issue is about their entire body and every aspect of their lives.

All this has made me wonder if the small vessels in the brain can be as affected as those in the back of the eye, in the retina, or deep within the kidney? We know that chronically elevated blood glucose levels contribute to vascular disease. Could this vascular disease also affect brain function as it does other organs? If so, what effect might this have on a patient's behavior? Perhaps it causes a brain chemical imbalance or a psychological depression that influences why some patients cannot or will not adhere to a treatment protocol.

## Diabetes and Depression Are Interrelated

Depression is a risk factor for anyone with a chronic illness, but the risk of depression is increased for patients with diabetes. It is one of the tragic complications of the disease.

For centuries, physicians believed there was a link between diabetes and depression. Most thought the emotions actually caused diabetes. In 1679, a British doctor named Thomas Willis went so far as to write, "The cause of diabetes is an emotional state I will call extreme sorrow."[1] Only within the past twenty years have doctors begun to notice the psychological distress in people with diabetes and how it affects their ability to manage their illness and cope with the stress of living with the disease.

KEEP THE LEGS YOU STAND ON — Dr. Mark Hinkes

Because it interferes with the patient's ability to self-care and function well in life, depression associated with diabetes increases the risk of death. Depression can create poor self-discipline and a lack of willpower. Depressed people can't seem to get motivated, organized, or understand the need to take good enough care of themselves. It also contributes to poor adherence to medications, diet, and blood sugar control, which creates a reduced quality of life and increased cost of healthcare. Many go on to experience complications in their eyes, kidneys, and extremities.

## Jack's Story

Jack is a patient with diabetes. I have seen him for ongoing foot care over the past year, but he looked different to me on his last visit. He was not very animated; he shuffled his feet as he walked into the treatment room, moved slowly, and did not look me in the eye as he usually did on previous visits.

"Jack," I asked, "what's up?"

He only raised his drooping head to say, "Doc, I feel lousy."

We talked for a few minutes and through the conversation Jack confided to me that he recently had not been able to maintain his blood sugar levels in the normal range for him and this had a very depressing effect on him.

"I have no energy, I don't feel like eating or reading; I just feel bad."

Chronically elevated blood sugars can have a profound effect on patients, not only physically and physiologically, but emotionally as well. Jack could remember a time when his blood sugars were more in control and during that time he felt much better.

I encouraged Jack to visit with his PCP for evaluation and management of depression. Additionally, we suggested that Jack make an effort to return to tighter blood sugar control, to take his medications, eat right, and exercise with hopes this would help turn him around.

Weeks later on a follow-up visit, Jack returned in better spirits reporting that he had acted on our suggestions and while he was not totally recovered from his depression he felt better and had discussed the situation with his PCP. He reported they were also working on the problem together and his PCP had placed Jack on an antidepressant medication that was helping him cope better with his problems.

While Jack's case demonstrates how elevated blood glucose levels can affect patients emotionally, it also reminds us that we must not forget to address the psychological needs of our patients, too. Treatment of depression in patients with diabetes can improve their outlook on life, and as a result they may feel more like trying to control their blood sugar level and adhere to their action plan for maintaining good health.

## Foot Notes: Managing the Psychological Aspect of Diabetes

Research studies have shown that a depression management program can significantly reduce mortality among depressed patients with diabetes. The people I know who have not experienced denial have had excellent medical care, which taught both the physical and the psychological/emotional impact of living with diabetes. They have continuing medical care that is non-judgmental, and they have a support system in place that allows for the inevitable human error while emphasizing how important it is to do their best to maintain good control at all times.

Here are a few tips on managing the psychological aspect of diabetes:

- Find a supportive inter-disciplinary team to assist you with all areas of disease management affected by diabetes.

- See a therapist or counselor regularly and talk about your diabetes and your emotions toward it.

- Understand that you may have a period of unexplainable high blood sugar levels. Don't get frustrated and give up. While you are feeling motivated, set up a support network you can rely on when things are not going well.

- Interact with friends who understand your frustration about dealing with diabetes. You will find social networking groups online where you may make friends with other people who have diabetes.

- Continue to educate yourself about diabetes and depression. A good source of inspiration and support is the Internet. There are several mailing lists and newsgroups where you can get the latest information. Read books or join a local discussion group.

- Stop listening to judgmental voices you hear either internally or from people who try to put you on guilt trips. Find new friends who will not lecture you, but instead will encourage you to start again.

- Become part of a local support group about life with diabetes. They understand that things go up and down, and will take into account the frustration, fear, and anger that occurs when you do everything right, but nothing works.

- Don't isolate yourself from others or avoid social activities. This is a very hard thing for a depressed person to do, but it is so helpful to get out and have fellowship.

- Be in "tune" with your body enough that if you do feel strange, you will do a blood sugar check immediately rather than putting it off.

- Try to be less of a perfectionist and accept "mistakes" as something to learn from, instead of reasons for giving up entirely. Hopefully, the next time things are going badly these things will make denial seem much less attractive.

- Forgive yourself after a slip instead of giving up completely.

You have to do this for yourself because you want to feel better and because you deserve a healthier life.

# Chapter Fifteen

## An International Look at Diabetes, Podiatry, and Amputation

Writing this book has been a growth-filled experience for me. On a daily basis, I have thought of the thousands of patients I have seen. It has brought to mind the cases that stand out and help illustrate points in the book. In this process, I am continually being educated and finding deeper insights into the issues of lower limb amputation in patients with diabetes and other at-risk patients.

I was browsing the Internet looking for resources related to my topics when I realized how my perspective had recently changed. When I started the book, my focus was to educate patients and other interested parties in amputation prevention by sharing my personal experiences both as a treating physician, researcher, and administrator in the PACT Program. The more I dealt with the issues, the more I realized that looking at this problem with a narrow local perspective (what's happening at my hospital, my state, or my country) fails to identify the true magnitude of the problem. That is when I decided to broaden the scope of this book to include an international perspective to show what is happening around the world and who is doing the work.

Worldwide, we are all facing the same problem with diabetes. Whether here in the United States or in China, England, or India, we face a lack of education and awareness as well as limited resources and access to proper healthcare. Every country is trying to solve these same complex problems, each having different resources and limitations. Diabetic foot problems are common all over the world, but the treatment methods vary greatly depending upon legislation, protocol, resources, and availability of medical professionals. Depending upon local laws, podiatrists in Africa, Europe, or Asia may have a DPM degree but they can't do the complex procedures on the deep structures of the foot. If I, or someone who has a DPM degree, were to go to a non-DPM recognized country, we would be limited by the laws and rules of that country.

Everyone, regardless of where they live, should have access to the best technology, education, and medical care. It is up to all of us to share what we know with one another so everyone gets the benefit of what Larry Harkless, DPM, Dean of Western University of Health Sciences School of Podiatric Medicine in Pomona, California, calls the 3-Ms of prevention:

1. Multi-factorial risk: understand all the risks and comorbidities

2. Multi-factorial intervention: treat all of the risks affecting the patient with diabetes

3. Multi-disciplinary staff: each has its own expertise.[1]

With devastating human, social, and economic consequences, diabetes places a severe burden on healthcare systems and economies everywhere, with the heaviest burden falling on low- and middle-income countries. Despite the fact that diabetes is a global epidemic that claims as many lives per year as HIV/AIDS, global awareness remains disturbingly low.

In collaboration with World Health Organization (WHO) in Geneva, the International Diabetes Institute produced an unpublished report of global predictions of the number of people with diabetes for various countries for the year 2025. It was estimated that in the year 2000 there were approximately 160 million people with diabetes in the world. The numbers are expected to rise to over 280 million people by the year 2025. Approximately 85 to 95 percent of all diagnosed cases are Type 2 diabetes.[2]

With nearly one billion people worldwide suffering with foot problems including pain or functional disability to their feet, the availability and level of foot care differs widely around the world. In the United States, there are specialized medical programs, including limb preservation programs, associated with a few major hospitals and medical centers, wound care centers and podiatrists in most major population areas. But, this is not the case in other countries. For example, Italy has no podiatry service; India has a new trend in establishing entire clinics and hospitals dedicated solely to caring for problems associated with diabetes, which includes foot care services.

Despite the presence of these specialized facilities and providers, foot care and patient education is available on a limited basis nationwide and the results for patients with diabetes are close to those in the U.S. There were over 50,000 non-traumatic lower extremity amputations done for patients with diabetes in 2005 in India. Germany ranks close behind India with 30,000 non-traumatic lower limb amputations in their diabetic population in 2005.

## Europe

According to Dr. Robert Frykberg, there has been success with endovascular procedures in Europe, and they are far ahead of America in this regard because they've been doing it a lot longer.

The International Diabetes Federation estimates that there are approximately 25 million people with diabetes in the 25-member states of the European Union. Estimates for the region for the year 2025 are likely to increase and reach nearly 30 million. The total number of people with diabetes in Spain, Italy, France, Poland, and Germany amounts to 69.2 percent of the entire population affected in the European Union. Most European countries have international guidelines on diabetic foot care and have multi-disciplinary foot clinics that include professionals such as a podiatrist, diabetes nurse, diabetic specialist, angiologist/intervention radiologist, vascular surgeon, microbiologist, orthopedic surgeon, orthotist, and shoemaker. The main area for concern is the quality of care for patients with active foot lesions while they are in hospital.

Dr. Stephen Morbach is chairman of the Diabetic Foot Study Group of the European Association for the study of diabetes (EASD). He reports that since the implementation of a multi-disciplinary foot care team across Europe, the amputation rates in Denmark have decreased by 40 percent from 1982 to 1993. Much of the success is noted in the areas where Danish people with diabetes are reimbursed for most of their payments for special shoes, insoles, and their visits to the podiatrist. It is estimated that adequate treatment is available for up to 75 percent in a multi-disciplinary setting.[3]

The Chair of the International Working Group on the Diabetic Foot is Karel Bakker, MD, PhD in the Netherlands. A study by the IWGDF was conducted to identify the role of podiatry in diabetic foot care in the Netherlands. All 122 hospitals were asked to answer questions regarding the availability of a podiatrist, the method of financial reimbursement for their services, the existence and arrangement of a specialized foot team, and a functioning foot clinic for patients with diabetes. The results from that 1995 survey revealed that thirty-nine out of the total 122 hospitals had a podiatrist specifically for the care of patients with diabetes. Twenty of the hospitals had a specialized diabetic foot clinic with a podiatrist working next to an internist for more than two hours a week. When compared with an earlier study, the presence of a specialized foot clinic or podiatrist did not affect the rate of diabetes-related lower extremity amputation.[4]

## Asia

Data regarding diabetic foot problems in Asia is sparse. The International Working Group reported that there are only five specialist foot care clinics in China and no podiatry services at all.

Dr. Bob Frykberg spent many years in Boston before he came to the Carl T. Hayden VA Medical Center in Phoenix, where he is now the chief of podiatry. He has been involved in a number of major and minor investigator-initiated studies. During the thirty years that his work has been published, he has taught podiatry to students and residents. The diabetic foot community across the world is a small, tight-knit group of people. Therefore, Dr. Frykberg is in regular contact with a lot of international colleagues across the globe—many who specialize in diabetic foot problems.

His travels have taken him to China to learn and to share. I've asked him to give us his perspective on what's happening with the diabetic foot in China. I'll let him share in his own words:

> Issues with the diabetic foot in China is a growing problem because China as a whole has westernized their diet. It's more of a problem, obviously, in the industrial or metropolitan areas as compared to the rural areas. China is taking an aggressive approach to diabetes and diabetic foot problems. I've been there four times with the Beijing International Diabetic Foot meeting and I'll be going back there next month for my fifth trip. They are a very interested and dedicated group of people who are by no means backwards. They are much more cognizant of our literature than we are of theirs. They're taking a very strong interest in this area. In fact, they are training general surgeons to be diabetic foot surgeons, and nurses to be what they would call podiatrists specializing in diabetic foot problems. They don't have podiatry as we know it in the United States. This is also the same situation that is present in India, the second largest country on earth, which claims to be the diabetes capital of the world with about 40 million or so patients with diabetes.

For the past twenty-seven years Lee Sanders, DPM, has worked as a podiatrist within the U.S. Federal Health Care

System. He has also traveled to India and China to help establish the LEAP program (Lower Extremity Amputation Program). In the program, providers were given kits, including diabetes literature written in simple language as well as a piece of monofilament used to identify the loss of protective sensation on the foot.

With an estimated 35 million people amounting to 8 percent of the population, India has more people living with diabetes than any other country. Patients with foot ulceration, most frequently associated with neuropathy and infection, seek treatment late, and as a result, more than 200,000 amputations occur each year.

Born in the United Kingdom, Dr. Paul W. Brand was an orthopedic surgeon who went to India to work with medical missionaries after World War II. He anticipated being there a year or two but stayed for twenty years working with people who had leprosy. In post-WWII India, if you thought your family member had leprosy you dropped them off and ran. Brand was taking care of people no one wanted. The insensitivity of the tissues that accompanies this disease is similar to diabetes. For instance, people with leprosy would wake up and part of their nose or their finger would be gone. At the time, people thought it was spontaneous. But, Dr. Brand was a great observer and he stayed awake to watch at night. He noticed that people had such severe neuropathy on their face, hands and feet that rats would eat the affected body parts while the patient slept. To address this problem Dr. Brand made a bed with a rail around it so the rodents couldn't reach his patients.

He was not willing to accept that people would just get leprosy and lose their life. He developed a total contact cast to take pressure off the wounds, which was challenging in hot and humid India. Dr. Brand came to the United States and worked at the Carville Hanson Disease Center in Louisiana and for several years put on a workshop at a leprosarium. When Dr. Lavery was a first-year resident, he went to a foot workshop at the leprosarium. The building was a big public health estate with moss-covered trees. At breakfast, Dr. Lavery was the first one in the cafeteria. An elderly man shuffled up and asked if he could join him. This man was Paul Brand, who then shared information with Dr. Lavery on his life experiences and his work with patients with neuropathy.

Paul Brand has written several books. His most famous is *Pain: The Gift Nobody Wants*. Dr. Brand has written other books about his experience in India.

## Africa

The region of Africa that lies south of the Sahara Desert contains thirty-three of the fifty poorest countries in the world. It is expected that this area will experience the greatest risk in the prevalence of diabetes over the next twenty years. Diabetic foot problems, particularly neuropathy, are an increasing public health problem, which are already a leading cause of admission to the hospital, lower limb amputation, and death in patients with diabetes. Early diagnosis, education, and treatment are crucial in this area, as you will note in this story about Laura Roehrick, RN.

About fourteen years ago, Laura Roehrick was a diabetic foot nurse for Kaiser Permanente. RNs in the U.S. are rarely taught foot care. In fact, she was taught that she was not to cut toenails and did not know that she could provide this care for her patients. She was told this care was up to the podiatrist or family only. The truth is RNs may provide high-risk diabetic foot care but cannot diagnose, prescribe, or perform surgery. The more she learned, the less thrilled she became with the way foot care was provided to the patients, so Laura quit Kaiser and started her own independent foot care practice in California. She is a second-generation pioneer in the field. Teresa Kellachi is her mentor. Laura took Teresa's training, expanded upon it and created her own way of doing things that will help save feet in a way that is uncommon in this country. She uses sterilized burs from non-medical industries such as woodworking, lapidary, or a dental drill and converts them into a tool that she uses on calluses, and corns, or to sculpt toenails that are too thick and hard to cut. These cordless drills/tools are battery-operated and have the potential to be used in rural areas without electricity.

Laura's is an unusual degree, and with the need for diabetic foot care being so great in the U.S. you may be wondering why more nurses do not specialize in foot care and begin their own private practice. Nurses in the U.S. do not know they can operate a private practice. Those who do know are flocking to it because they can make money and help people in a tangible way. However, many physicians are not thrilled about having nurses entering their turf. In contrast, Canada has five to six thousand nurses who have been through foot care training offered via technical colleges. In addition, insurance companies in Canada cover foot care provided by nurses in private practice.

Tired of fighting the bureaucracy surrounding nurses doing foot care in the United States, Laura chose to take her skills to an international level. Politics abound everywhere, but at an international level, especially in developing countries, there is more acceptance for nurses taking an active role in foot care. She taught in Canada on two occasions and considers herself a foot care nurse ambassador. She feels very strongly that the nurses in Canada and the U.S. should pool their collective resources to create universal foot care guidelines based on best practice act. Unfortunately, neither country seems to share her enthusiasm. She feels that each country is preoccupied with their own bureaucracy and red tape and too busy to see or think outside the box.

She presented educational lectures in England, but Africa drew her attention. Along with approximately 15,000 people (several hundred were podiatrists and doctors), she attended the International Diabetes Federation (IDF) 19th World Diabetes Congress. She was the only American foot care nurse who attended the meeting held in Cape Town, South Africa in 2006. She brought a photo album of before and after shots of feet she had worked on. When she spoke with African healthcare providers and showed them what she was doing, they begged her to come back and teach them more about her techniques for reducing calluses and thick nails. These are the skills necessary to save limbs and lives.

With no sponsorship from any organization, she knew she would have to find a way to purchase her supplies and get them to Africa. In July of 2007, she cashed in a small retirement account and used her credit card to purchase plane fare and shipping costs for one hundred pounds of medical equipment. Her 19-year-old daughter went with her to Dar Es Salaam, Tanzania, where she worked with an African doctor to train the staff of his private diabetic foot clinic to use the drill and various burrs that she donated and to make the herbal foot salve she created to help soften calluses and keep the skin smooth and free from fissures and cracks, which can be a portal of entry for infection. The fact that many Africans go barefoot poses special problems when it comes to preventive foot care for people with diabetes. There are also problems caused from the calluses formed on the feet from being in the prayer position.

There are 13 million diabetics in Africa. By 2025, this number is estimated to increase to an astounding 25 million diabetics. That's a 98 percent increase. Treatment clinics are scarcely available in African cities. While having coffee one morning in Zanzibar, Laura spoke with the elderly native man sitting on the bench next to her. When she found that he was diabetic and suffered from dry skin and calluses, she proceeded to give an impromptu educational in-service program right there on the street. The outdoor coffee stand suddenly became a diabetic foot education class where about forty people listened carefully to her advice about the importance of proper hygiene, using a foot file or pumice stone to smooth calluses, to check regularly for any cuts, blisters, sores or signs of infection or fungus. Many of these people had friends or family members who suffered from diabetic foot problems, amputations, and even died due to gangrene. This experience inspired Laura to develop a preventive foot care program that could reach people before they got the first wound. She knew she needed to come back to Africa, once again, with more equipment and more training materials.

Laura's primary concern is to prevent foot wounds from ever happening and advancing to life-threatening stages.

She plans to do this by educating people on the streets with literature published in Swahili language, giving out packets of salve and foot files, setting up training and treatment clinics, and teaching nail clinicians how to care for the diabetic foot. Nail technicians are another underutilized source of help in preventing amputations. Laura's plans include recruitment of nail technicians into a more advanced foot care course aimed at amputation prevention. Three of laura's American women friends are currently enrolled in a certified nail technician program and will be taught how to treat feet using Laura's method once they have completed their certification. Then, Laura will take them with her to help train nail technicians in Zanzibar. When the Zanzibar program proves to work effectively in Africa, she hopes to take the model program to other developing countries.

Laura and a Swahili doctor named Fadhill Abdalla started a project that involves the local Rotary chapter. Rotary president, Stephanie Hill, from Colorado, has been in Zanzibar for eight years. These three are currently in the initial stages of a grant application process. It may take one to two years to complete the preparation and planning, but the initial stages have begun. In the meanwhile, Laura is forming Preventative Diabetic Foot Care Alliance—her own non-profit organization to assist with this project. She is in the process of obtaining her 501c3 status, which will allow her to write grants to get funding for foot care in Africa. She wants to set up a teleconferencing TV-type station so she can teach the African practitioners without having to travel there.

Due to the poor quality of water, Africans consume eight to ten sodas per day, along with a Westernized diet containing a lot of high-fructose sugar. Like many Americans, Africans get little or no exercise. In addition, many of the anti-viral medications used to treat the high-volume of HIV in Africa can actually *cause* diabetes. Very little is done to prevent foot wounds; the streets are dirty and the people walk barefooted. When they come to the medical clinic for a foot wound, they are usually in bad shape—many have gangrene. Amputation is not a routine treatment because most patients with diabetes with a foot wound die from infection, before they have a chance to be treated. There is no regulation on healthcare practice. Africans do not have extra funds or medical insurance to help pay for treatment.

In March 2008, Laura, was awarded with the American Red Cross Everyday Medical Hero for Northern California. She hopes this will create awareness for better foot care in patients with diabetes.

## Canada

Howard Green, DPM, has a unique perspective not only on medical issues affecting patients with diabetes, but also on the politics associated with them. Originally from Halifax, Dr. Green stopped in Philadelphia to get his DPM degree before heading on to Vancouver for his postgraduate medical and surgical training at Vancouver General Hospital. It was on that part of his journey while interviewing for a residency program that I met him. In 1993, he opened his private practice and today he is the director of the podiatry surgical residency program at Vancouver General Hospital.

Dr. Green feels that podiatry has been accepted into the mainstream of medical care in Canada; however, there are issues of great concern in British Columbia. In 2002, BC had a reversal of policy concerning foot care. Heretofore, foot care was a covered service, but the new rules have changed and the patient is now financially responsible for their foot care. This poses some problems because diabetic feet are expensive to treat. It could be simple, on-going care or it could be long-term ulcerations which require surgical intervention, followed with shoes, boots, and bracing. Podiatrists in Canada can see a patient and tell him what is going on with his feet, and what needs to be done, but when the cost is explained, he may not get treatment due to financial concerns. If he is hospitalized, a patient is covered for all services except that of the podiatrist. Outpatient care in an office, regular follow-ups every few weeks perhaps for ulcer monitoring, debridement, shoe modifications, orthotics, walkers, or ankle-foot orthoses—are not covered. If the government would cover the cost of podiatric care, more people would enroll in preventive programs. Unfortunately, the global diabetic population for the most part is in a slightly lower socioeconomic bracket and sometimes they defer treatment due to the cost.

In the United States, podiatric treatment is covered through Medicare, Medicaid and HMO's. In both the U.S. and Canada, it is a struggle to get acceptance of podiatry as a mainstream care for foot conditions. Once podiatry practice becomes accepted by doctors and patients, and insurance companies cover it, better care will be available for everyone.

The laws in Canada appear to be similar to many states in the U.S. when it comes to scope of podiatry practice. Podiatrists are able to perform surgical procedures that include both soft tissue and bone in the foot. They can diagnose and treat disorders related to the foot and ankle. What is not being realized is that foot problems are accompanied by multiple postural symptoms—back, knees, hips, and ankles. When it comes to surgical treatment, podiatrists have to focus on the foot since they don't have privileges above the ankle. Surgically, podiatrists in BC can go as deep into the foot as needed; they can even do amputations of the foot.

Patients with diabetes can receive genuine amputation prevention care in Canada by qualified podiatry providers. This is not available in a lot of places around the world. In some countries, foot care is considered to be routine care. Therefore, patients with diabetes don't have access to podiatrists who can do amputation prevention care. In BC, the diabetic foot and ankle clinic is run by a group of orthopedic surgeons interested in limb salvage and diabetic foot care. There are podiatrists involved, but due to the financial aspect, not many wish to participate without compensation for their services. The medical community in BC recognizes the importance of podiatry. Whether it's the diabetic population and their potential problems or general education of patients on overall foot health, Dr. Green tries to improve his skills and knowledge and do as much as he can to treat patients in the best way possible. He pushes for education of the general public and general practitioners by giving lectures at the local hospital and to groups that want information about podiatry.

Within the native Inuit Indian population in Canada there is a high incidence of diabetes. The Native Affairs branch of the government provides some health benefits coverage to the tribes for certain appliances and things such as custom orthotics, shoes or braces. If a patient applies for coverage and documents the need for it, Native Affairs will often approve it and fabricate or prescribe whatever appliance is needed.

## Central and South America

The prevalence of diabetes in the Central American region ranges from 5 to 20 percent. As a result of globalization and urbanization in Latin America, the disease has reached epidemic levels with prevalence particularly high in Mexico, the Caribbean, and certain countries in Central America.

According to IDF, there were about 19 million (or 6 percent of the population) diagnosed cases of diabetes in Latin America and the Caribbean in 2003. That number is expected to reach 36 million (7.8 percent) by 2025.

The World Health Organization reports that the average cost of diabetes care in Latin America is $703 per person. At $1,219 per person, Cuba has the highest average cost of care in Central America, while Colombia has the lowest ($442). Not surprisingly, Mexico has a diabetes rate of 10.7 percent among people between ages twenty and sixty-nine. The government has begun to address the problem through launching several education programs and awareness campaigns that highlight obesity as a risk factor for diabetes. The Mexican Diabetes Federation (FMD) still finds it hard to reach Mexicans, particularly the poor, because they cannot afford to take time off from work to attend diabetes workshops and learn how to maintain their well-being. They are yet to realize that diabetes exists because of their diet and the lack of exercise. Diabetic foot care in Brazil is well organized, thanks to the excellent cooperation between healthcare professionals and the ministry of health. More than sixty foot clinics are in operation across the country. This is having an effect on amputation rates.[5]

This is by no means a complete list, but you may find worldwide statistics regarding the prevalence rate of diabetes listed by country at www.cureresearch.com/d/diabetes/stats-country.htm.

# Chapter Sixteen

## Footing the Bill for Diabetes and Amputation

Until someone has experienced a foot wound or lower extremity amputation—either themselves or by witnessing a loved one's illness—it is difficult to fully understand the degree of suffering it causes or the many levels of costs that exist. The costs of dealing with a foot wound (or in the worst cases, an amputation) are substantial, varied, and devastating. By varied, I mean there are costs that go beyond financial to include social and psychological elements. These costs can affect your daily routines, your pastimes, and your ability to work and to be self-supporting. They can also affect your family and friends' lives. All of a sudden your life is not about getting out of bed each morning to enjoy your independence, but it is about adapting to an altered set of circumstances that hopefully lead toward healing.

Let's review the financial, social, and psychological costs for amputation. Unless otherwise stated, the figures for the financial aspects section are from www.hospitalmanagement. net.[1]

## Financial Aspects

Professor Pierre Lefèbvre, president of the International Diabetes Federation, says, "Foot problems are the most common cause of admission to hospital for people with diabetes. In developed countries, it is estimated that foot problems account for 12 to 15 percent of total healthcare resources. In developing countries, they may account for as much as 40 percent of the total resources."

Annual healthcare expenditures are 2.3-fold higher for people with diabetes. In fact, one in five healthcare dollars was spent caring for someone with diabetes. One in ten dollars spent on healthcare is attributed to diabetes-related complications.[2]

In 2007, the cost of diabetes care in the United States was $174 billion. Medical expenditures accounts for $116 billion of it; medical costs for directly treating diabetes was $27 billion, $58 billion to treat diabetes-related complications, and $31 billion in general medical costs. And, those numbers are only increasing. The other $58 billion in this figure is accounted for in the loss of national productivity while these patients were being treated.

Men with diabetes aged 60-64 have eight times the number of hospital inpatient days, seven times the number of emergency visits, and six times the number of physician office and outpatient visits for heart failure compared to men without diabetes. Just think of all the indirect costs associated with this: days absent from work, reduced job performance, less productivity at home, reduced labor force participation, reduced earnings capacity due to permanent disability, and loss of productivity from death. Diabetes also imposes intangible costs in terms of reduced quality of life, pain and suffering, and family members' loss of productivity as they devote their lives to caring for loved ones with diabetes.

Research estimates that up to 70 percent of all lower-limb amputations are related to diabetes. Annually, 2.5 million patients are treated for foot ulcers in the United States. Medical literature will show a variety of figures on the costs of treating foot infections, ulcers, and amputating a leg, but most sources agree that the care of an infected foot ulcer can cost between $8,000 and $10,000 per hospitalization. Hospitalization accounts for about one-half the medical costs for diabetes. Almost half of all healthcare expenses come from higher rates of hospital admission and longer lengths of stay each time.[3] Healing a complex and deep ulcer costs as much as $70,000. That is not counting the estimated cost for three years of subsequent care once the patient leaves the hospital. The cost for those individuals whose ulcer healed without the need for amputation is estimated to be between $16,000 and $27,000. Now, let's look at those who were not as fortunate and had to undergo an amputation.

A foot amputation can cost close to $30,000; a leg amputation can cost $60,000 or more depending upon what other complications and comorbidities go along with it. The costs increase when the severity of the amputation increases, the length of hospitalization increases, the need for rehabilitation increases, and the need for home care and social services increases. I remember seeing data for one patient who was hospitalized for over 400 days. The cost of his care was the most expensive I had ever seen based solely on the number of days he needed to stay in the hospital. These statistics do not include the care that must be provided after the patient leaves the hospital. The estimated three-year cost for home care and social services ranges from $30,000 to $60,000.

In addition to these direct costs, there are the indirect costs due to loss of productivity. If cost estimates are broadened to include cost to the individual and loss of quality of life, then the estimated cost of diabetic foot care rises dramatically.

Additionally, two million diabetic people in the U.S. do not have medical insurance coverage. About 50 percent of people with diabetes have medical insurance funded by the government—primarily through Medicare. Society as a whole pays for this in the form of higher insurance premiums or raised taxes to fund government programs that treat diabetes and its complications. Therefore, this disease touches nearly everyone in some way.

## Why Is Hospitalization So Expensive?

Some of the first financial costs of healthcare come from meeting the regulations of the Joint Commission on Accreditation of Healthcare Organizations or JCHAO. Their mission is to continuously improve the safety and quality of care provided to the public through provision of healthcare accreditation and related services that support performance improvement in healthcare organizations. Next, we have federal, state, county, and municipal rules and regulations that must be met and the facility maintained to those standards. Other costs of institutional healthcare include insurance, legal matters, community support, and millions of dollars of "free care" resulting from uncollected fees that ultimately get written off, especially in hospitals that provide care through their emergency room facilities.

Inflation also affects healthcare costs. Most drugs, supplies, salaries, and equipment costs continue to rise, and healthcare costs seem to generally rise faster than everything else. There are a large number of hospital services that don't seem to be directly related to patient care, nevertheless, they are figured into the cost of your hospital stay. Here is a partial list of what expenses might be incurred during the treatment of a patient with diabetes.

**Maintenance/Control**

Diabetes medication - oral
Insulin and supplies
Glucose monitor and strips
Blood pressure medicine

**Testing and Laboratories**

Medical consulting services
Nuclear medicine/radiology
MRIs, CT scans, X-rays, ABI, MRA
Testing, non-invasive venous
Duplex doppler and ultrasound
Blood count
Blood glucose level tests
Hemoglobin A1c test
Liver and kidney function tests

**Wound Care**

Pharmacy services - consultations
Antibiotics

Dressings
Sleeping/pain medications

## Offloading

Shoes- extra depth/custom molded
Insoles/biomechanical orthotics
Canes, walkers, crutches, braces
Prosthetic services

## In-Patient Hospital Services

Maintenance service
Security service
Engineering service
Food service
Housekeeping service

## Rehabilitation Services

Braces, prosthesis, motorized carts/wheelchairs
Gait training
Physical therapy services
Kinesiology

## Home Healthcare

Continued medical services at home include intravenous antibiotic administration, wound care/dressing changes, transportation to and from healthcare appointments, assistance with bathing, dressing, feeding, and medication monitoring.

## Cost-Effectiveness of Prevention

A simple change in diet and lifestyle could prevent many of the new cases of diabetes we see each year. If prevention education and behavior could reduce the incidence of foot ulcers and amputations by 25 percent, it would be cost-effective not only in saving money for patients with diabetes but the entire healthcare system—including insurance companies. Patients with diabetes with risk factors are the ones who really need to receive education to help reduce comorbidities and focus on preventive behavior. But how? Dr. Paul Brand recommended a national campaign to encourage healthcare professionals to remove patient's shoes and socks and examine their feet, and to use a tuning fork, pin, tendon hammer, and a 10-gram monofilament nylon testing device to test for loss of protective sensation. Educational programs should be created to meet the specific needs of the patient. Preventing amputations is cost effective and engenders a better quality of life for patients. It requires *everyone* in your posse to help, and that includes you.

## Facts and Figures on PACT

Data on the PACT Program for 2003 through 2007 at the VA Tennessee Valley Healthcare System shows the overall amputation rate has *decreased* by 40 percent.

Costs for patients with diabetes:

1. Pharmacy          Decreased by 48 percent
2. Labs              Decreased by 32 percent
3. In Patient        Decreased by 44 percent
4. O&P               Increased by 110 percent

Annual Cost/diabetic patient is *decreased* by 38 percent.

Total Costs in 2007 as compared to 2003:

1. Pharmacy          Decreased by  $112,445
2. Labs              Decreased by  $24,718
3. In Patient        Decreased by  $1,796,073
4. O&P               Increased by   $84,718

Total Cost Savings is *increased* by $1,849,073

Based on these numbers, if we could duplicate the results we could have a cost reduction for amputations in the United States of $1.9 billion!

Another podiatrist in the VA system who has had excellent results with the PACT Program is Howard Kimmel, DPM, MBA, FACFAS, of the Department of Veterans Affairs in Cleveland, Ohio.

His poster presentation "The Effectiveness of the PACT Program in Reduction in Limb Amputation Goals and Objectives" was given at the Third Congress of the World Union of Wound Healing Societies in Toronto, Canada. The emphasis was to decrease the amount of lower extremity amputations that are due to vascular and neuropathic complications in United States Veterans. To effectively prove how pro-active screening can decrease the amount of lower extremity amputations, he gave statistics that showed amputation rates decreased from 8.05/1000 patients with diabetes in 1999 to 3.94/1,000 patients with diabetes in 2005.

Next, we will look at the psychological costs of living with diabetes and returning to life after an amputation.

## Psychological Cost of Diabetes

In addition to the physical and financial costs, there can also be psychological challenges. Some patients may become depressed and this can cause them to lose interest in following their treatment plan. Therefore, counseling should be part of the plan to manage diabetes.

It is impossible to put a price tag on what it costs a person emotionally or mentally for living with the diabetic condition and its comorbidities. However, this story will give an idea of how difficult it is to not be able to do what everyone else is able to do.

## Case Study

In order to more extensively discuss the experience of living with diabetes, I met Mr. and Mrs. D outside of the clinic setting where I normally see Mr. D for foot care. At this point, Mr. D had an ulcer on his foot and was required to stay off his foot in order for it to heal. Here's a recap of our conversation that day.

Mrs. D: My husband has always been in charge of everything, you know. I want him to get well so bad. I'm mean. I tell him, "You can't get up. You can't do that." I want him well, but we just can't do the things we used to do. He's really a great cook, so it's kind of hard to take that away from him. He wants to come in the kitchen, but you have to stand up to cook. It is a lifestyle change. Honey, bring me a glass of water. Honey, would you do this? I'm a honey-doer. I don't mind and he knows it.

Mr. D: It's pretty tough sitting all day. I go play cards with the boys in the morning for a few minutes. As soon as they get ready to play golf, I go home and I sit in my chair until I go to bed. But now and then I get up and walk to the kitchen.

Mrs. D: It's so sad because he's been so active. He played golf everyday of his life. When he wasn't working he was at the golf course. Now, he can hardly. . .

Mr. D: I could ride with them, but . . . I bought some new tennis shoes. I bought one pair, and they worked so good that I bought two more pairs. They let you play golf in tennis shoes now, so I played golf in my new shoes and walked a lot. Then, I had a lot of things to do and a lot of people to see. I spent a lot of time on my foot, and as the weeks rolled on, it became sore. One day I noticed swelling. That's when I came to see you. The same thing happened a few years ago. We went to a funeral, and visited some friends while we were there. I spent a lot of time on my foot. When we got home, I noticed that a little ulcer was already worn through, so I went to see my primary care doctor. The doctor did a little bit, and I went home. I came back and I saw another primary care doctor. He was unconcerned, but I insisted that my foot was not right and he had to do something about it. He looked at it again and said, "It's gonna be alright." I lived with it a little bit longer. He kept giving me the run-around until I got mad. He finally popped the blister and that made things worse. We went to another doctor, and another. Finally, we went to the orthopedic surgeon.

Mrs. D: We couldn't get into the hospital. We had waited over a month when I got so mad I finally called him (the physician). I lost my Cajun temper, and they got him in the next day. By then, he had serious problems. While he was in surgery, the doctors called me from the operating room and said, "I don't have any choice but to take his toes off."

And of course I was crying, and the surgeon said, "Get a hold of yourself. It's not the end of the world."

"Well that's *my* husband you've got up there, and you're cutting on his foot. *You* do this every day. I *don't* do this every day. Give me a little time to think about this." I didn't know if he was asking for my opinion or not, but I was getting a little scared because he was so nonchalant about it.

Mr. D: He did the surgery but he didn't take out the bone. I went home and had to go back because it wasn't getting any better. In fact, it was getting worse. The doctor looked at it and said, "You're gonna be alright."

I went back home but two or three days later, it still wasn't better. I went back to the doctor, and the surgeon was there. When I told him what was going on, he said, "You've got to have another surgery."

That time they took the bone out and it healed, and it's been all right ever since. Shortly after that, I had a heart attack, and had to have bypass surgery. They had to debride the foot where it was hurt before they got any veins from that leg. They took the vein out of the other leg. That healed up good, and I never had any problem.

When I was diagnosed as being diabetic twenty-five years ago, I was never told about my blood sugars or the risks. Shortly after that, I got a divorce. I moved and didn't see the doctor.

Mrs. D: When we got married I asked him to take his medicine. I'm a mother. When you've got kids—you do everything for them. He would say, "This is my sickness. I handle my own medicine. I don't need to be told what to do."

My grandmother lost both legs to diabetes, so I knew diabetes was bad. But his wasn't bad because he took pills.

Mr. D: I never did take the pills serious.

Mrs. D: No, we didn't; neither one of us.

Mr. D: Then the pills started to affect my kidneys and my liver, so I had to come off the pills.

Mrs. D: Now he takes insulin. He can't keep his blood sugars in check because he does not eat right. If there's a pie, he'll take a little piece, and then another little piece until it's gone. I don't know why it's so hard.

Mr. D: My doctor said if I want to eat a piece of pie, then I should go on and eat it because sometimes it's worse not to. He told me to just take more insulin if I eat something sweet. Sometimes I give myself my shot when I'm supposed to and it doesn't work. I can tell in the morning. My eyes are blurry. Then when it gets low, I get nervous and shaky. I test my sugars four times a day and sometimes more than that. If it goes down low, then I have to eat something to bring it back up. I watch it pretty close, but it's hard to keep it under control. It never gets over 300— sometimes it'll get to 200 (It shouldn't get over 130).

Mrs. D: One night he woke me up and the bed was soaking wet. He was sweaty because his sugar level had gotten so low.

Mr. D: It was 38 when we tested it.

That was the end of our discussion that day, and I am sorry to report that just a few months later, Mr. D lost his battle with diabetes.

Mr. D mentions he was not able to play golf with his friends once he developed a foot ulcer. Let's explore in more detail the social aspects of patients with diabetes with foot problems.

## Living with an Amputation

Of all the costs an amputee must deal with, the personal costs in terms of life changes are the harshest of realities. Because of the inability to pursue normal activities in the same way (if at all) after an amputation, the patient may feel a loss of self-worth. These patients may benefit from seeing a psychological counselor to deal with these life-altering experiences.

Many patients return to their former lives virtually unaffected by losing a portion of their foot. But for patients with more proximal amputations returning to their life with their new handicap may be the most difficult of all their adjustments. The loss of a digit usually permits most patients to return to their normal life, hopefully more respectful of their disease, while the loss of a limb can have profound repercussions making return to a normal life almost impossible. The loss of a limb is a life-changing event not only for the patient, but also the friends and family members who provide care and support. The negative impact of ulcers and amputations on the physical, social, and emotional aspects of life can be profound. The patient sees himself losing his independence while caregivers see the deterioration of a loved one.

While most patients are able to adjust to a medical condition such as a cold, the flu, or a more complex condition like a fracture, dealing with diabetes or an amputation is an entirely different experience. A patient once told me that being an amputee was like participating in a triathlon in which he never wanted to participate.

Patients who undergo an amputation eventually ask themselves, "What's going to happen to me? What's my life going to be like now that I have lost a leg?" The state of a patient's health and their mental determination will significantly influence the quality of their life when they return home after an amputation. Younger amputees, those who lose a leg to trauma such as in war or auto accidents generally seem to adjust and respond better to their situation. Many can be seen competing in athletic activities such as playing wheelchair basketball and even running in competitions using the most advanced prosthetic legs. It is usually the older patient who loses a leg due to neuropathy and complicated by PAD whose life is most changed. Some patients seem to continue where they left off in their lives. They accept their situation and work through it, while others, not as healthy or determined may experience significant changes in their lives.

## Social Aspects of an Amputation

The most life-changing effect of amputation is the loss of personal liberty—the opportunity to choose how to spend one's time. In most cases, patients become dependent on others during their adjustment back to their normal life. Until the patient has adjusted to his new life as an amputee, and before the fitting of a prosthetic leg, his life may be totally disrupted. After an amputation, most patients see the world from the vantage point of a wheelchair. Some never get out of that wheelchair. For example, the small things we do around our home like hobbies, tinkering in the garage, gardening, cooking, taking the trash out, or running to answer the phone all become difficult experiences to the amputee.

Even after adjusting to his new life, it is more difficult for the amputee to do something as simple as going grocery shopping. For transportation, he may have to use a van or small truck outfitted with a motorized hoist to travel with his wheelchair or motorized scooter. Even with handicapped parking and preferential seating, attending a sporting or cultural event is much more complex for the patient with an amputation. Much of it is certainly doable, but it takes patience and a little extra time.

Some diabetic amputees may not be able to return to their former work position and may lose their ability to earn a living severely affecting their families. It is not unusual for other family members to work longer or have multiple jobs to support the members of their family who cannot work.

To better understand the issues concerning amputation and amputation prevention, I have attended an amputee clinic, where patients with recent amputations are evaluated for their needs, and especially for prosthetic legs. In speaking with these patients who have experienced an amputation there are two universal thoughts they share. The first is "I thought this would never happen to me." The second is, "If I had known this was going to happen to me, I would have taken better care of myself."

## Case Study

Sam was a bit overweight. When I hit the up button on the foot pedal of my blue power chair, I heard a groaning noise as the chair struggled to lift him up about four feet from the floor, so I could take a peek at his foot.

"Doc, I'm on the comeback trail. I've lost sixty pounds in the past year and my blood sugars have been pretty much

KEEP THE LEGS YOU STAND ON — Dr. Mark Hinkes

under control." A quick inspection of Sam's foot revealed he had lost the distal part of his right first toe. "I really wasn't paying enough attention to my feet until I suffered an ingrown toenail that got out of control," he told me. "It ended up with an infection that got to the bone really fast."

He came to my office because of a callus to the amputation site and was concerned that this might lead to losing more of his foot. When Sam shared his family history with me I was astonished to hear he had lost a brother, a sister, and both of his parents due to the complications of diabetes. I took extra time with Sam to discuss the benefits of controlling his blood glucose levels and practicing preventive foot behaviors.

"Johnny was just plain hard headed," Sam explained. "He didn't care what he ate or how much he drank. I don't know why he didn't care about himself. Doc you scared me about my diabetes and I am grateful for it."

I thought about that for a few seconds and realized that my intention was not to scare him, but rather to share knowledge so he might have a better chance of keeping his leg. So here is a guy—the only one in his entire family—who seems to understand his diabetes and is able to cope with it.

## Foot Notes: Common Questions about Amputation

Common questions asked by amputees include: How long will I be in a wheelchair? Will I ever be able to walk again? What needs to be done to my home so I will be able to live there?

After an amputation, patients are vulnerable to complications such as infection, blood clots, pulmonary embolisms, and ulcers to the remaining foot or sacral area. Long post-operative stays due to complications can keep the patient in the hospital for longer than anticipated.

401

An amputation injures the patient's body, mind, and soul. Every patient should be offered an opportunity to discuss the amputation procedure with a mental health professional-psychologist or psychiatrist both before and after the event. Counseling may also be helpful or necessary in the post-operative transition phase as well. Attitude makes a tremendous difference.

Post-op wound care is especially important to be sure the site heals without breakdown or infection. After the incision from the amputation site is healed, there can be edema to the stump that can go on for six to eight weeks. To address the issue of edema (swelling) and to prepare the stump for a temporary prosthetic limb, patients wear a special elastic dressing called a "shrinker." When the swelling is reduced to a satisfactory level, the patient can be fitted with a temporary prosthetic limb.

Many people live in homes that are not friendly toward disabled persons. There are steps in front or back of the house; the bathroom and bedrooms are upstairs; hallways and door frames are not wide enough to accommodate a wheelchair. Furthermore, bathrooms are not handicapped friendly and the house may need to be remodeled to accommodate the patient's new needs. Falling is always a fear for someone learning to balance and walk with only one leg. Phantom pain does happen, but I have not had much exposure to patients with this problem.

# Chapter Seventeen

## Complementary Medicine

We have the good fortune to live in a time when traditional medicine and alternative healing methods are proving to benefit mankind in unimaginable ways. But no one knows everything, and not everyone is trustworthy. There are practitioners in both traditional and alternative medicine who are there only to make a buck in the easiest and most lucrative way they can. Far too many times that means removing a leg when it could have been saved. Therefore, it behooves a consumer to learn all they can about both traditional and alternative healing methods to make an informed decision about how to proceed with healing. Read everything you can in books and on the Internet. Seek out consumer watchdogs who give you the other side of the story. Balance your findings, and go with your gut instinct.

There are new remedies that may have sounded suspicious on first hearing. Some of them now have proven records of helping with various aspects of wound healing. These include machines, electronic devices, and both internal and topical medicines. But beware—not all do what they claim.

In this chapter, we will discuss traditional and non-traditional methods that have proven to heal in specific areas and under specific circumstances.

## Complementary Therapies

I have an open mind about holistic and complementary alternative therapies. That said, whenever I hear of these issues I always ask myself, "What does the medical literature say about this?" Most times I will do a PubMed (www.pubmed. com) search to see if I can find any studies in the subject.

There are several complementary therapies that work well with modern Western medicine. Let's look at one therapy that is an ancient modality that has been used for thousands of years to treat the whole person—body, mind, and spirit.

In the January 21, 2008, the *U.S. News & World Report* ran a cover article titled "Embracing Alternative Care, Top Hospitals Put Unorthodox Therapies Into Practice." The magazine explores the controversies and benefits surrounding complimentary and alternative medical care (CAM). Therapies mentioned are massage, Reike, or "healing touch" that is used to rebalance the energy field that practitioners believe surrounds the body and flows through it in defined pathways, affecting health when disrupted. Another CAM treatment is acupuncture. To my surprise and delight, the article lists academic medical centers where acupuncture therapy is practiced: Children's Memorial Hospital in Chicago, Mayo Clinic, Duke University Medical Center, the University of California in San Francisco, and Vanderbilt University.

## Acupuncture

As part of traditional Chinese medicine, acupuncture is among the oldest healing practices in the world. It is based on the concept that disease results from disruption in the flow of energy (qi) and imbalance in the forces of yin and yang. Acupuncture restores the flow of qi as well as the yin-yang balance through the stimulation of specific points on the body. A variety of techniques may be used, including the insertion of thin metal needles through the skin.

In the United States, acupuncture is considered part of complementary and alternative medicine (CAM); these practices and products are not considered part of conventional medicine. CAM is used with conventional medicine, and alternative medicine is used in place of conventional medicine. However, ten years ago, an National Institutes of Health (NIH) Consensus Development Conference assessed acupuncture's effectiveness in treating various diseases and conditions.[1] Although some clinical trials showed the effectiveness in treating specific conditions, findings are reported as inconclusive due to challenges in devising appropriate controls and blind studies.

## Dr. Chongbin Zhu

Dr. Chongbin Zhu is a special person in my life because he's been taking care of a portion of my health. I was taking a nap on my parent's couch last year. I rolled over and fell off. As a result, my shoulder and knee were in bad shape. Through his wonderful work and rehabilitation, I'm feeling better than I have in a long time.

Dr. Zhu came to the U.S. from China ten years ago with training in both Chinese and Western medicines. With his Masters Degree and PhD in acupuncture, he picked traditional Chinese medicine as his career. He integrates acupuncture with traditional medicine and modern science in the medical field to treat a variety of chronic conditions. Most people understand the basic aspects of acupuncture in terms of balance, ying and yang, and equilibrium, but I've asked him to talk about acupuncture in terms of the diabetic patient.

Balance is a key word in Chinese medicine and especially in acupuncture. He sees diabetes as an imbalance between yin and yang; it shows a deficiency in yin. This is why a patient usually manifests the condition by feeling thirsty or hot, by losing weight and not feeling well in general. Acupuncture helps to regain balance in the whole system. It causes the organs, immune and central nervous systems to gain control of the imbalance so the patient can create a better condition or balance. This includes major symptoms and their consequences such as peripheral neuropathy and ulcers. It also assists with the mental and emotional aspects (psychosocial depression) of the illness. In general, acupuncture treatment can help patients rebuild their confidence, not just their physical health. Acupuncture helps a person gain the confidence needed to help their body heal.

When social interaction is interrupted by a diabetic condition, not only the diabetic or insulin part of the patient is affected, but also their brain chemicals are dramatically changed. When insulin is decreased, people develop depression or anxiety. This creates an imbalance in the network of the body and things start falling apart. Acupuncture repairs the broken network and directly stimulates the mechanism in the peripheral areas and also activates the central nervous system to promote a signaling of the serotonin and peptide synapse—a key event in the central nervous system which controls our emotions and immune system. The return of balance generally causes people to feel calmer, more peaceful, and more confident in all the things they are doing to help their body heal. This positively impacts their social interaction. The increased level of serotonin can be proven by a follow-up CAT scan.

No matter how much medicine we use, no matter what treatment we give, no matter how much time we spend with the patient, if the patient doesn't have adequate circulation it's going to be tremendously difficult to heal a wound. Acupuncture directly affects peripheral circulation as well as the central control of the vascular system. In terms of the peripheral part, an acupuncturist may insert needles into the points along the meridian pathways to reach blood vessels and the nervous system. While acupuncture applies to those points, it also directly stimulates the nervous system and the linked vessel system. If a blood vessel contracts too much, acupuncture helps it expand to give more blood flow. If the blood vessel is not contracting enough, acupuncture helps regulate it and give a sufficient supply of blood. Either way, acupuncture is beneficial in the regulation of proper function in the blood vessel at the site where the function needs improvement. It also helps regulate blood vessels via the central vascular system. The brainstem is the center for the heart and the blood vessels. It contains a key neurotransmitter known as norepinephrine. When acupuncture is applied, that center is activated to work in a very coordinated way to balance brain chemicals and enhance blood circulation in the peripheral extremities from your trunk.

Dr. Zhu says:

>*You take your medication, but it can't get to the end of the extremities due to lack of blood flow. That's why Chinese medicine combined with*

*mainstream Western medicine is so beneficial— each one complements the other. So, when acupuncture plus medication is used, a patient with circulation problems may have his hands return to normal after one or two months of treatment. This was the case with one of my patients who had extremely poor circulation in her hands. She had ulcers on her fingers. She said, "I suffered for five years. Now, within two months, it is healed."*

## Massage

Massage improves circulation, stimulates muscles, reduces tension, and often alleviates pain. It also provides a time for you to examine your feet, giving you the chance to notice a problem before it gets worse. Gently rubbing sore muscles and joints can often provide needed relief. But don't massage a foot that is inflamed or that you think might be injured.

Any reason, including massage, that focuses the patient's attention to their feet is a good thing. If the massage is for comfort, I have no problem with that; but if it is done *instead* of consulting a physician for appropriate diagnosis and treatment, then it is inappropriate.

## Viagra

Speaking of complementary practices, maybe we should take existing technology and apply it in new ways. I'm referring to Viagra, which is a very hot topic in scientific and social circles. Yes, you read that correctly. Viagra is known as a cyclic guanosine monophosphate (cGMP) and has the potential for healing chronic wounds due to the enhancement of nitric oxide (NO). Here's how it works on a biochemical level; NO stimulates an enzyme called guanylyl cyclose to synthesize more cGMP, which activates PKG to help blood circulation. Viagra helps peripheral blood circulation in a similar way. It facilitates relaxation of smooth muscle tissue dilating the blood vessels and increasing blood flow to the tissues. Cyclic GMP is a messenger that regulates the NO pathway. NO is made from the amino acid L-arginine and is considered the ideal biochemical balance to promote wound healing through oxygenation, better blood flow, neovascularization and wound healing.[2]

Obviously, Viagra is the social circle topic, but recently the *Journal of Wound Care* carried an editorial about the benefits of Viagra and how it works chemically to enhance circulation in the hands and feet. Where there is a constriction of the blood vessels, people have blue or dark extremities. The hands and feet are very cool. A patient may say, "My hand is so cold, I cannot touch anything because it hurts, or is tingling."

Viagra really helps peripheral blood vessels expand so they can move blood through the circulatory system. But Viagra also has some central nervous system side effects. People taking it report depression and headache, probably from vasodilatation (widening of blood vessels). However, this would be a good treatment for patients who have Reynaud's phenomenon or scleroderma.

In 2004, Dr. Zhu published a paper about Viagra in the *Journal of European Pharmacology*. Viagra makes Serotonin transporter (uptake) activity too high, leaving the patient less serotonin available to do the work, thus leading to depression and anxiety. So, in this situation we might use something to block the serotonin uptake pathway so the patient can benefit from the serotonin they naturally produce. That is exactly the research area Chongbin is in now—serotonin transporter regulation. Who would have thought that Viagra could end up having a wonderful benefit for people's mental well-being?

Regarding the neurological aspects of acupuncture and the diabetic patient, there are three subcategories of neuropathy or nerve systems: sensory, autonomic, and motor. In neuropathy, the first thing that is affected is the central nervous system because that's the first thing a patient feels. Maybe the motor neuron too, but the motor activity is okay with most folks. So, let's take the sensory part. When the sensory nerve endings get affected, the protective shield (called the nerve sheath) surrounding the nerve is affected. With neuropathy, those sheaths peel off like tree bark; it's like a frayed electrical power cord with slits that expose the wiring inside. When that happens, people develop constant numbness due to demylenation of the nerve, and eventually the conduction alters significantly in the nerve ending or trunk, resulting in loss of normal feeling. But, in the early stage, it's easy to use acupuncture to regulate or regain the normal function.

When the demylenation (loss of nerve sheath) occurs, it's much harder. In other words, functional rather than structural abnormality is easier to treat with acupuncture. Acupuncture activates the peripheral nervous system and sends a signal to the central nervous system, which in turn sends a signal back to peripheral nerves to repair those abnormal parts and return the sheath to normal health. The symptoms will be gone in less than ten treatments, which will take about two months.

In the late stages, acupuncture still helps, but in a different way. Acupuncture can help repair the injured sheath.

After one month, we clearly see the sheaths growing back along the nerve. Nerves grow slowly at about 0.1 millimeter per day. Given time, the nerve might grow fully, but it takes a really, really long time; so, both the doctor and the patient must be unwearied in the wait.

The patient may feel like their stress level has been reduced, their legs may feel more functional, without as much tingling (40 to 60 percent better). They may still have problems, but they are more manageable. This is without any internal medication or any other treatment, just with the acupuncture. When combined with medicine, the results may be achieved faster—almost half the time.

Most medical literature seems to say that changes in the patients with diabetes happen about ten to twenty years from the onset. I asked Dr. Zhu, "Are patients who have had diabetes for longer time periods still able to use acupuncture to benefit them in the area of neuropathy? Does it matter how long the blood sugar has been out of control? What's the defining parameter on that?" To which he replied:

*I must say that's a very key point. Early stage refers to the condition when they start to feel neuropathy symptoms usually within a year. So, that's what I refer to as early stage. However, the diabetic condition might be longer than that; but, if you can find the diabetic condition as early as possible, that's an extra benefit. In late stages, most patients with neuropathy have had their symptoms for over a year. Currently, I'm treating a patient. He's not diabetic, but his neuropathy has been bad for five years. Tingling all the time. I treated him probably four or five times and saw a little improvement, but I don't expect healing to occur fast.*

Dr. Zhu and I both see people with very dry skin, who have fissures and cracking in the skin. He tells me that acupuncture is able to treat this condition because the autonomic nervous system is part of your internal organs. "That is why you sweat; it's an acetylcholine system. And that's the system in enterogastric (gut track). So, does acupuncture have any effect on acetylcholine or autonomic nervous systems? The answer is 'Yes.'"

Dr. Zhu has used acupuncture to treat, with some extent of success, people who have very dry peeling skin also having rashes, chafes, and ulcers. Still, the earlier you start treatment, the better and faster results you will see. The late phase is generally hard because it takes so many treatment times without showing much improvement. Both doctors and patients may get frustrated with trying.

Does acupuncture have any benefit in helping patients control blood glucose levels? As we all know, blood sugar is regulated by insulin. The production of insulin is controlled by other organs and systems—the thyroid for one. And other systems are growth factor, leptin, estrogen, testosterone, and of course the nervous system. It has been long established that those are regulated by acupuncture.

The one particular group of people working with acupuncture regulating hypothalamus, pituitary, adrenal, and/or sex gland have done a great job. What happens there is really amazing stuff and fun. For example, when the growth factor or thyroid secretions decreased in some conditions, insulin secretion is also affected. Again, that's the result of insulin level fluctuation. Maybe in the morning it's too high and in evening it's too low. It seems to be related to growth factor and thyroid. Acupuncture can be used to stabilize this fluctuation. Of course, we can use medication, but medication tends to target a single site; not caring about the related network. That's the problem. It would be good if we could find some method to target multiple sites in the network to reduce any side effects.

We explore different ways to treat the fluctuation. We use some herbal medicines (some herbal medicines work great, some don't), but in terms of acupuncture, most of it works great. But, remember, acupuncture helps to re-coordinate different body systems. It doesn't introduce any exogenous substance into the body. We expect acupuncture to regulate in a way that our body system can adapt. So, we can benefit from proper acupuncture treatment, but we don't want to exaggerate. While acupuncture is a safe, natural stimulation or natural therapy, it also has limitations on what it can achieve.

It's easier to find an acupuncturist or acupuncture therapy in some countries than others. In most of the Asian countries (Japan, Korea, Vietnam), acupuncture is very commonplace. In China, where acupuncture parallels Western medical systems, it's very easy to find; almost all of the hospitals have acupuncture. Other countries (Germany, Britain, any European countries) adopted acupuncture as one of the therapeutic modalities. But, in Africa, probably less. Based on the list of licensed acupuncturists from the Division of Health-related Board in Tennessee from two years ago, we have about twenty acupuncturists in Nashville. About 100 acupuncturists are licensed in all of Tennessee, plus about fifty practicing acupuncture and chiropractic together. But, in San Francisco, there are over five-hundred.

They don't have conventional Western medicine in some rural areas of Africa. Chinese medical acupuncture is a good alternative because it is easier to access, and in remote places people with expertise can practice acupuncture without needing complicated equipment. As long as you have a hygienic environment and sterilized needles, you can set up a clinic anywhere. Three or four decades ago, Chinese people had limited access to Western medicine. That is why acupuncture was so popular and is still so common in Chinese medicine; and it has contributed to the health of the Chinese people for many centuries. In the U.S., mainstream is always mainstream. Even those with open minds still see acupuncture as an alternative or complimentary medicine. It is still in trial and experimental phase. Acupuncture and Chinese medicine offer a real alternative to a diabetic patient who may develop a wound or who may be facing an amputation. More people are becoming aware of the benefits of acupuncture and are starting to use it even though medical insurance policies do not cover it.

In China we say, "This is a global village. We are global people." Here in the U.S., we are in the same village. We are very open-minded and want to share whatever we have to benefit the health of our world."

## Alpha Lipoic Acid (ALA) for Treatment of Neuropathy

Diabetic neuropathy is a perplexing problem. It is one of only a handful of medical problems that can paradoxically make your feet feel numb and painful at the same time. In some cases, the symptoms may affect the hands and arms, too. This problem is usually seen in patients who are diabetic who have had elevated blood glucose levels for an extended period of time. Other causes include tumor, medication, and cancer.

Another reason for this problem can be exposure to heavy metals like lead or mercury. Some patients who have worked in the electric utility industry relate to being exposed to PCBs, sometimes up to their elbows, while repairing electrical transformers, who also display symptoms consistent with peripheral neuropathy. It is not unusual to see peripheral neuropathy in patients who have no family history of diabetes who have been in the military and have been exposed to Agent Orange or radiation from nuclear explosions.

One theory about peripheral neuropathy is that it is caused by free or unpaired electrons. These free radicals are caused by elevated blood glucose levels. Free radicals attack the nerves and lead to the dreadful complications we see in neuropathy of pain, tingling, burning, and numbness. In some patients, this problem can affect their ability to stand or walk without falling or may keep them from sleeping. While control of blood glucose levels seems to be the universal first step toward managing peripheral neuropathy, there are others methods that also work.

In my research on peripheral neuropathy, I decided to look up alternatives to the existing treatments. I found a chemical called Alpha Lipoic Acid (ALA). Medical literature contains many references to ALA and its ability to work with the antioxidant vitamins C and E to potentate their ability to rid the body of free radicals. In the United States, ALA is considered a food supplement and can be purchased over-the-counter without a prescription. In Germany, where most of the research has been done on this drug and throughout Europe, it can only be purchased by prescription.

Vitamin C is water-soluble and goes to the water-soluble tissues to grab free electrons, and vitamin E is fat-soluble and goes to the fatty tissues to grab free electrons. If you add Alpha Lipoic Acid to your vitamins C and E regimen, the vitamins grab the free electrons, and then the Alpha Lipoic Acid grabs them from the vitamin C and E. Now the vitamins are free to go back again and remove more free electrons. For those patients whose cause for neuropathy is free electrons, this treatment is a home run. Patients will come back three to four weeks later saying, "Doctor, it's a miracle! All the burning and shooting has stopped." But it doesn't work for everyone. Unfortunately, because pharmaceutical companies could not see how to make money on Alpha Lipoic Acid, doctors weren't using it. Recently, some vitamin supplements are starting to include ALA as recognition of its value, and consumer interest is increasing.

I recently saw a patient who returned for evaluation of his neuropathy. He was given a treatment regime of ALA with vitamins C and E. He was astonished to report to me that since taking these medications his neuropathic pain had vanished and his blood pressure was also lower.

If you are having problems with numbness, pain, burning or tingling to your feet or legs and suspect it is from diabetic neuropathy, consult your physician to see if Alpha Lipoic Acid may help you. While there is evidence that ALA can reduce the symptoms of peripheral neuropathy, not all patients will respond well to this drug.

## Hyperbaric Oxygen Therapy

For healing of chronic, stubborn, or postoperative wounds and to minimize the risk of infection, many experts recommend hyperbaric oxygen therapy (HBOT) for their patients with diabetes. In fact, hyperbaric oxygen therapy has been used for many years as an adjunctive therapy in the treatment of diabetic foot wounds. This type of therapy can help heal wounds due to weakened immune systems and poor circulation. It is also a key to healing radiation burns. Healing tissue needs oxygen and HBOT not only increases tissue oxygen levels but it improves the killing ability of white blood cells.

While there are products that claim to provide oxygenation via encompassing the leg in a plastic type container, these units fail to compare to systemic therapy that can be achieved by the patient entering a chamber where the entire body can absorb higher concentrations of oxygen. Data from a preliminary study showed a significant increase in local wound nitric oxide levels during and after treatment. Increased nitric oxide levels are an important factor in promoting wound healing.[3] Hyperbaric oxygen should be considered a pharmacologic application that promotes a proper inflammatory response in the diabetic foot wound.

In a study published in the *Journal of Diabetes* by M. Kalani, the conclusion supported adjunctive HBO therapy as being valuable for treating selected cases of hypoxic diabetic foot ulcers. "It seems to accelerate the rate of healing, reduce the need for amputation, and increase the number of wounds that are completely healed on long-term follow up."[4]

## Vitamins and Dietary Supplements

When a patient presents with problems with their arterial circulation and surgical intervention is not the appropriate choice, there are some herbal and dietary supplements that may help augment the circulation and heal a wound. Aspirin is good for cardiovascular support. Bioflavonoids from citrus fruits support vein and capillary health. The body needs vitamin C for collagen formation and to repair itself, but most of us don't get enough of it in our food. Zinc is a trace mineral (silver) necessary for many enzyme reactions and helps T cells mature. Vitamin B Complex supports the function of most of the body. Vitamin E containing gamma, delta, and beta tocopherols is a great antioxidant.

Supplements made from seeds and leaves of various fruits and plants are thought to have medicinal properties that may be useful to the patient with diabetes for assisting with blood sugar control. Since this is not my area of expertise and this book is not about herbal and dietary supplements, I will simply list some that I found online:

Asian ginseng, bael leaves, beta carotene, bilberry, bitter fenugreek, ginkgo biloba, goosberry (amla) leaves, grape seed extract, gymnema sylvestre, indian gooseberry, indian kino or malabar kino, ispaghula, jambul seeds, lutein (an antioxidant that supports eye health), lycopene, madhuca, mango leaves, neem (margosa), neem leaves, stevia (a natural non-chemical sweetener to use instead of aspartame or accharine), sweet potato leaves, and tenner's cassia. See Appendix D of this book for more references.

If you decide to try herbs and find you feel better, do

not assume that your diabetes is under control and that you should stop taking the medicines your doctor has prescribed. As with any drug or diet plan, you should work closely with your physician to be sure you get the benefits of both natural and medical knowledge. You may also want to consult with an herbalist whose expertise is in this arena.

## Exercise

Moving your body is natural and is essential for good health. A body is not meant to stay in one position for long periods of time. Activity improves insulin resistance, decreases cardiovascular disease and stroke, increases circulation, decreases blood sugar levels, and helps control weight. Exercise can be broken down into three categories.

1. Exercise: walking, jogging, biking. Patients need to decide what to do, when to do it, and how often. A good tip is to wear a pedometer to see if you are walking enough. Set your goal for 10,000 steps per day. The average person should walk 4.5 miles per day, 115,000 miles in a lifetime.
2. Strength: weight lifting, Pilates.
3. Flexibility: both Yoga and Tai Chi lower A1c and lead to weight loss and better control of sugar level in type 2 diabetes by improving glucose metabolism, enhancing immune function, and lowering blood pressure, along with aiding in weight loss.

## Nutrition

Hippocrates said, *"Let food be thy medicine and medicine be thy food."* Food is certainly a factor in all aspects of diabetes. Unfortunately, Americans have quite a sweet tooth. Each person consumes about 100 pounds of sugar per year. No wonder so many Americans—particularly children—are overweight and obese. Added caloric sweeteners, such as high-fructose corn syrup, may be one of the major reasons, according to the October 2006 issue of the *Harvard Health Letter*.[5]

Diets high in sugar, fat, and cholesterol that lack adequate nutrition have a highly negative effect on blood sugar control and wound healing. Wound healing consumes a great deal of energy and requires not only complex carbohydrates and omega fats for energy but also requires proteins and vitamins.

Proper nutrition is the most natural and healthy way to give your body what it needs for optimal function. When the body is nourished at the cellular level, it improves the overall health of the body and all its systems. Here is a quick look at nutrition.

1. Carbohydrates are a rich source of energy for cells to function properly. Carbs enhance white cell activity to strengthen the immune response. However, starchy foods and products containing refined white flour require the body to do nothing to get its energy from simple carbs. They immediately turn to sugar and raise glucose levels whereas complex carbs found in vegetables require the body to break down the carbs in order to get to the source of energy. This process of metabolism causes the body to use what is needed and not store the excess as fat.

2. Protein is a nutrient that is the building block of bones and muscles and is vital for collagen synthesis. Insufficient amounts of protein affect the quality of wound healing. Your body uses more energy to digest protein than it does to digest fat or carbohydrate. Foods high in protein can help slow the digestion process, and do not raise the glucose level. In fact, protein foods actually help stabilize blood sugar. Protein comes from meat (make sure it is lean or fat free), seafood, eggs, dairy products, beans (especially soy beans), legumes, seeds, whole grains, and nuts. Watch out for butter, cheese, and ground beef that contain mostly saturated fat. These can elevate your LDL or bad cholesterol level, which can increase your risk of coronary artery disease.

3. Fats aid in cell membrane structure and help in wound healing. However, not all fats are created equal. If you avoid the kind found in olive, canola, and other plant oils, you may miss out on the very thing you're trying to do: help your heart and health. Look for cooking oils that contain olive oil, omega-3, omega-6, omega-9, and zero trans fats. Avoid man-made trans fats also known as partially hydrogenated oils.

4. Fiber is a friend to patients with diabetes. Fiber can help you manage diabetes in more ways than one. It's good for the intestines, moderates blood sugar response, and helps keep cholesterol in check.

5. Vitamin A is critical in wound healing and absolutely necessary for adequate inflammatory response. You get Vitamin A from colorful fruits and vegetables rich in beta-

carotene such as carrots, spinach, kale, cantaloupe, apricots, papaya, mango, peas, tomatoes, peaches, and red pepper.[6]

6. The cherry is a diabetes super food. A new animal study shows tart cherries as a "super fruit," that may help reduce inflammation, potentially lowering the risk of type 2 diabetes and cardiovascular disease. Sorry, folks, but cherry soda doesn't count!

I came across an article online stating that vegan diets (meaning no meat or dairy) may be able to reverse diabetes symptoms. That's pretty remarkable information in my view—I've not heard of any way to reverse diabetes before—but I think it's worth mentioning. A study from the *Journal of the American Diabetes Association* had doctors at three universities test ninety-nine people with type 2 diabetes. Half were given a vegan diet, and the others were given the standard diabetic diet. After twenty-two weeks, 43 percent of those on the vegan diet lost more weight and were able to stop taking some of their medications or lower the doses. Only 26 percent on the standard diet were able to do that.[7]

**Drinks and Beverages**

Move away from the sports drinks! People think these drinks are healthful, but many sports beverages and juice drinks are sweetened with sugar or high-fructose corn syrup. While these watery-looking drinks seem "light" and refreshing, in reality, they add back the calories you just burned while exercising. Not surprisingly, they can actually make you gain weight.

Sodas do more harm than good. I read an article that cola can take rust off a car bumper. What, then, does it do to *your* body parts? Harvard researchers report that women who drank one or more sugar-sweetened soft drinks per day were 83 percent more likely to develop type 2 diabetes than women who drank less than one a month.

Alcohol adds needless calories and causes blood sugar to rise quickly. This is how the drink gives it "high" or buzz. There is no nutritional benefit to any alcoholic beverage other than an occasional glass of red wine which may have some cardiovascular benefit. These "empty" calories can lead to obesity and a higher risk of developing diabetes.

Drinking too much alcohol can raise the cholesterol levels (triglycerides) in the blood, lead to high blood pressure, and heart failure. Excessive and binge drinking can lead to stroke.[8]

## Foot Notes: Daily Checklist of Healthy Prevention Behaviors

1. Did I wear my pedometer today?
2. How many steps did I walk today?
3. Did I walk/exercise more today than yesterday?
4. Did I take my medication at the correct time and the recommended dosage?
5. Did I get a nutritious intake of foods and beverages today?
6. Did I refrain from smoking?
7. Did I refrain from drinking alcohol?
8. Did I wear my shoes all day, even indoors?
9. Did I inspect my feet today?
10. Did I drink enough water?

11. Did I take time to breathe deeply enough to oxygenate my body sufficiently?
12. Did I observe preventive behaviors for my feet to protect them?

# Chapter Eighteen

## Solutions for Prevention

> *The doctor of the future will give no medicine, but will interest her or his patients in the care of the human frame, in a proper diet, and in the cause and prevention of disease.* ~ Thomas A. Edison

In previous chapters, we looked at the anatomy of the foot and discussed the vascular, neurological, and musculoskeletal systems and how each system must function in harmony with the others for normal function and especially for wound healing. We discussed physically how the bony structures of the foot affect its function and the science of podiatric biomechanics. We also have looked at the issues of diagnosis and treatment of foot wounds and the growing science of wound care. We have touched on issues concerning footgear, insoles, and braces in the overall amputation prevention scheme. We have also tried to educate the reader about identifying risks of the diabetic foot, shared options of prevention, and suggested alternatives of treatment. We have looked at the science involved in the effort to prevent amputations including anatomy, physiology, biomechanics, endocrinology, wound care, vascular surgery, shoes and insoles and the psychological and social aspects of limb loss.

We have dealt with issues of the physical world. These issues are critical in understanding why people develop foot problems and how to resolve them. These factors are under the control of both the patient and the physician. But, there is another dimension to successful amputation prevention and this is the one that only the patient can control. This critical factor necessary for a successful amputation prevention strategy is the patient's behavior. This is number one on the list of solutions for prevention.

A patient's ability to understand a prevention or treatment plan for healing a wound is just as critical as any other part of an amputation prevention strategy. Patient behavior can make the difference between an amputation prevention effort being successful and a limb being lost. This behavioral component may be the most difficult aspect of managing the patient with diabetes. I have heard many patients talk about their experiences and have learned there are recognizable behavior patterns of patients with diabetes.

Dr. Bob Frykberg of Carl T. Hayden VA Medical Center in Phoenix, Arizona says that the most common problem he sees in the VA Hospital is non-compliance. "Ulcers and infections get far ahead of the patients because the patients aren't taking good care of themselves. Drug dependency is also a big problem—especially cigarettes," says Dr. Frykberg. "We see neuropathy, obesity, and severe peripheral arterial disease in middle-aged patients and younger. Many have large, ischemic venous ulcerations. They've got both sides of the circulation impaired, and those are particularly difficult patients.

"Many of them are in denial. They have neuropathy, but it doesn't hurt them. They don't participate much in their own care maybe because they feel that no matter what happens to them, the VA will be there to take care of them. People are non-compliant especially with offloading and offloading devices. Some people fail to keep their medical appointments. Joslin's 1934 article in *New England Journal of Medicine* made a point about how important cleanliness is in managing diabetic foot problems and preventing gangrene. I see a lot of gangrene or necrosis due to ischemia and/or infection. Poor hygiene is often a problem even in a young population."

## Compliancy Issues in the Elderly Population

In my interview with the medical director of the senior care service, and chief of geriatrics at the VA Hospital in Nashville, Jim Powers, MD, told me that his older patients with chronic illnesses have to adhere to many different sets of goals for each disease they have. "Whether it's medication, activity, or safety concerns, they add up," Dr. Powers says. "Making more requests on our patients means it's highly probably that non-adherence to regimen is going to occur. If the patient relies upon a caregiver to assist them with these recommendations, it's even less likely they're going to comply. So, we have to be practical. We work with the patient and the family to decide on appropriate goals and how can we work together to achieve them. Older individuals may be eligible for certain benefits to help them achieve their goals, such as home health or rehab services. We might be able to provide in-home monitoring in the form of technology for functional limitations or perhaps the reporting of physical exam parameters such as oxygen or blood glucose readings. These can be acted upon by the doctor or the home nurse working with the primary care provider.

Blood sugar screening for the elderly has routinely been done only in individuals who have a higher likelihood of having diabetes, such as those who are overweight or have PAD in their family history. In dealing with a frail geriatric patient, we may have to modify the controlled blood sugar. If there are periods of hypoglycemia, dizziness, or symptoms which may predispose the patient to falling, we have to be aware that strict control may not be possible in that individual. As much as we can, we try to follow the ADA guidelines of hemoglobin A1c of 7 percent or less."

## Making Patients our Partners

As much as the responsibility of self-care and preventive behaviors rest on the patient, I believe the current issues with patients who have diabetes is partially the fault of the medical community. We really have not made patients our partners, and *partners* is the keyword because neither the medical community nor you can solve these issues alone. If we work together, no one need lose a leg unnecessarily ever again.

When I see a patient for the first time I am primarily interested in their foot health, but since the foot is attached to the body and not an isolated entity, I need to know about the whole patient. I want to treat the issue that brought them to me, but I also ask, "Do you have any other foot problems you might like to discuss with me?" While the referring physician may have identified an issue that requires the care of a podiatrist,

I have found that patients don't always tell their primary care physician everything about their foot health and foot problems. When they are in my chair looking eye to eye with me, I give them a chance to "tell all." I usually hear a range of problems but there is a universal theme to these patients.

Those patients who have sensory neuropathy usually have chronically elevated blood glucose levels, too. They have pain, or burning and tingling to their feet and legs, usually are taking high doses of medications that have difficult-to-manage side effects, and they are depressed, and have difficulty with mood swings.

Our discussion enviably moves toward the issue of patient responsibility. While other physicians may tell patients that their blood glucose levels are high, and make recommendations for medicines, they fail to educate the patient on the consequences of chronically elevated blood glucose levels to their feet and legs. In my discussions with patients, I always invite them to be my partner.

I explain that there are certain things that only their physicians and providers (posse) can do for them, and certain things that only they can do. If each of us does our best in the area of our own responsibilities, when the patient develops a problem, we probably can get it fixed. However, if the patient fails to do their part, no matter how much technology, medications, time, and resources we use to try to help the patient, our efforts will probably fail.

Patients *must* be our partners, fulfill their responsibility to control their blood glucose levels: do not smoke, do exercise and practice preventive foot care behaviors in order to prevent the dire consequences of diabetes to their feet.

## A Wakeup Call to the Patient

While most patients at least shake their heads in obliged agreement and go on with their daily life routine unaltered by our discussions, occasionally I get pleasantly surprised and see patients make changes for the better. I had such a patient recently and took the time to discuss the risks to his feet and legs due to his diabetes and the benefits of partnership in his health.

## Case Study

As we talked I could see Steve's eyes open wide. He was apparently shocked to learn that his behaviors were in large part responsible for his own misery. "Doc, my feet and legs have burning pain all the time." His blood glucose was elevated that day and his hemoglobin A1c was very elevated. We discussed many of the aspects of his daily life that could be changed to his own benefit. They included a change of diet, losing weight, regular exercise, taking his medications, practicing preventive foot behaviors, and to stop smoking.

The medical literature tells us that fear is *not* a motivator for the patient with diabetes. But, in some cases, education can be a motivation.

On a follow-up visit four months later, Steve was a different person. He told me. " Doc, I don't want to lose my legs, so I decided to try it your way, and you know what? I feel better, I have lost weight, and I have fewer symptoms in my feet and legs. Thank you for taking the time to show me what I had to do to take care of myself."

## Adherence to Medication

One of the issues that deeply affect patients' health is adherence to taking their medications. Adherence is defined as when a patient is taking their medication in a way that is both beneficial and agreed to by both the patient and the prescriber. An article in *Archives of Internal Medicine* found that more than one in five patients were not taking their medications for diabetes properly.

Non-adherence can cause unfortunate problems if not discovered in time because it raises blood glucose levels (A1c), blood pressure, and LDL cholesterol levels. Properly taking your medications can prevent hospitalization and even death if you have diabetes mellitus.

Assessing the non-adherence with medication prescriptions should be an important part of every patient visit. Dose escalation may become a serious problem for patients. It may seem to physicians that the dose isn't adequate, when in reality the medication is not being taken. As the dose is increased, based on faulty information, the results can be catastrophic. The first step to improving adherence is to emphasize the value of the prescription to the patient. For instance, we tell patients with diabetes that the medication will help reduce their blood glucose levels and that will prevent the complications of blindness, renal disease necessitating dialysis or even a kidney transplant, and numbness that can lead to amputations. The ease of taking the medication also influences adherence. A pill is easier to take than an injection.

Next is communication. Patient adherence is ultimately based on their understanding, motivation, and ability to follow through on their portion of the physician-patient partnership. The FDA wants all patients to know the following about their medications:

- The medication's name, strength, daily dosage, and how often it should be taken.
- The purpose of the medication. Providing written information provides patients a resource they can refer to at home.
- The importance of refills and avoiding lapses in doses.

I believe it is important to reassure my patients that diabetes can be managed or is important enough to manage, especially if I detect any behaviors that may complicate the healing of a wound or prevent an amputation. If a patient wants to keep his limbs we need to work together to form a partnership. Diabetes is a medical condition that is an issue between the patient and his body. No matter how good your doctor is, no matter how much medicine we use, or what new high-tech equipment becomes available, the success of your control of your body will dictate the quality of your life.

I cannot monitor what a patient eats, or be sure they take their medication, or if they exercise, or practice preventive foot care. I can educate, examine, and administer professional medical treatment in my office, but the foot and leg are not detachable. Unlike dropping off and picking up dry cleaning, you cannot leave them in my office and come back on Tuesday to pick them up when they are fixed. Healing and preventing foot wounds requires the cooperation, focus, and energy of the patient. Therefore, patients need to help themselves. As the old adage goes, "if you are not part of the solution, you are part of the problem." Make no mistake about this; the quality of your life rests on your shoulders.

## Round Up Your Posse

While practicing prevention is up to the patient, a partnership between healthcare workers and patients will result in better detection of foot problems and the best healthcare for patients with diabetes. Because it requires ongoing attention to medication, blood glucose monitoring, meal planning, foot care, education, and screening for comorbid conditions and complications, diabetes is best managed by a multi-disciplinary care team. This is what I call your "posse." Since *you* are the sheriff of your health, you should "round up your posse," if you have a foot that is at risk. Your posse should consist of a primary care physician, advanced-practice nurses, a diabetes educator, a nutritionist, a podiatrist, a surgeon, a physical therapist, an infectious disease specialist, a psychologist, an orthotist, and a pedorthist.

A multi-disciplinary team for the treatment of diabetic foot ulcers is the most effective way to improve the outcome and long-term prognosis of patients and reduce the risk for amputation. A doctor who is not familiar with the alternative treatments for foot wounds may not realize that a lack of circulation is the reason for the delay in healing.

Each member of your team sees your problem from his area of expertise, and working with a team, you don't have to wait six weeks to see the cardiologist, or another two weeks to see the vascular surgeon. Everyone is at one location. Everyone on your team knows the details of your case and which steps are his responsibility. For example, if you have a deep abscess in your foot, your podiatrist will know that you should have an MRI to show the exact extent and location and that a plain old X-ray will not do. While your podiatrist can treat the local wound, he or she may discover that other health factors may also need attention and refer you to the healthcare worker best suited to address that problem. For example:

- An endocrinologist can adjust medications if your blood sugars are elevated.

- A cardiologist can identify/treat heart problems prescribe medications to control blood pressure.

- A vascular surgeon can order tests like an ABI or arteriogram to identify circulation problems and decide how to repair or replace damaged blood vessels.

- A nutritionist can set you on the right path if you are not eating properly.

- A podiatrist can care for local foot problems like corns, calluses, and nails and cast you for custom-molded orthotics if you have problems with the biomechanical functioning of your feet.

- A pedorthist can evaluate and fit you for proper shoes.

- A prosthetist can evaluate and fit you for custom made braces or, in a worst case, for a prosthetic limb.

- A psychologist can help you stop smoking.

- An infectious disease specialist can recommend antibiotics and monitor your organ functions if there is an infection.
- A radiologist can interpret X-rays, scans, and MRIs.

Multi-disciplinary teams can exist in a private care setting if there is someone dedicated to coordinating the care among the different practices. When someone first hears the diabetes diagnosis about their feet they should:

1. Start looking for a multi-disciplinary team

2. Get an education about what types of things they can do to prevent foot ulcers, infections, and amputations from occurring, and

3. Enlist their family members to help.

Normally, when a patient gets a diabetes diagnosis, their family doctor or the endocrinologist will refer them to a certified diabetes educator who will teach skills in how to manage the disease. The patient can be referred to a podiatrist or foot care provider who can teach him or her how to take care of their feet. Many of the complications can be prevented sometimes by simply obtaining and wearing correctly fitting shoes that protect the foot.

Working with an inter-disciplinary team is rapidly becoming the norm. I realize that not all communities have a multi-disciplinary team, and you certainly can't look them up in the phone book. However, you can search the Internet for American Diabetes Association (ADA) meetings and find out who's speaking. The Internet can help you find someone who has an expertise in your area. The ADA has a professional membership directory where you may look for a listing of foot care providers or vascular surgeons in your area who have a particular interest in diabetes. Your PCP may be able to refer you to a specialist who can provide the tools necessary to achieve your goals.

## Moving in the Right Direction

While this book serves as an educational tool, there is much more to learn that what would not fit into the scope and pages of this book. Education of the patient, caregiver, and medical professionals is a huge step moving in the right direction toward prevention. Steve Kravitz, DPM, Founder and Executive Director of the American Professional Wound Care Association says education can reduce the number of lower extremity amputations by one-third.[1]

From his observations at local and national meetings, as well as working with university centers and people in the community, Dr. Larry Lavery discovered that people who care for the diabetic foot are not usually defined by their degree or training. He believes diabetes is still a stepchild of the medical community. People who end up gravitating towards care for the diabetic foot are driven by a passion to take care of that group of people. For Dr. Lavery, the interest started with family members. For some others, it may be a personal episode or interaction with a patient that triggers an interest. People may see that they can make a difference, or that there is a void or an abyss in the medical care system for patients with diabetes. There is a cross-section of medical professionals who take an interest in diabetes.

"An important way to impact the disease is to reach the common person in language he or she can understand, like Paul Brand's books did," says Dr. Lavery. "Education must be the focus and new technology may provide the opportunity to increase those efforts."

## Education for Patients

Classes for diabetes have a tremendous benefit in prevention. When offered in the primary care setting, a visit to a nutritionist devoted specifically to patient education may be highly cost-effective for the healthcare system.

Presently, you cannot depend upon your doctor to tell you everything you need to know about diabetes and managing the illness with a focus on prevention. It's up to you to educate yourself. With the ever-increasing amount of information available on the Internet and the results of scientific research in this area, there are new opportunities daily to learn about wound healing and preventing amputations.

I Googled the words "amputation prevention" on the Internet when we first started this book and the search resulted in 175,000 matches. As this book was going to publication two years later, a Google search resulted in 767,000 matches.

Dr. Lavery, from Scott & White Hospital at Temple, Texas, is professor of surgery at Texas A&M Health Science Center College of Medicine. He says, "Patients need to be educated immediately when they are diagnosed with peripheral neuropathy. Doctors should test patients, give the results, explain the risk category, and present a plan of action. There is so much information but doctors have failed to implement it in a cohesive, organized,

437

standard method. Eleven percent of patients with diabetes face amputation, and those are the people we need to reach."

A lot of doctors miss the opportunity to understand the information a foot clinic can provide. The clinic can send a report back to the primary care physician and explain that the patient is high-risk due to injuries and that aggressive action concerning education, footwear, and doctor's visits must be taken. Patients really appreciate it, though. A woman who was referred to Dr. Lavery was really impressed by the screening that was done because she was not aware such tests were possible. Dr. Lavery said to her, "Let's get the pressure off this ulcer. You have pretty severe nerve damage and if we can take the pressure off this heel and transition you into a special shoe or insole, things will improve. You can't ignore your feet." At this point, the patient was engaged because she participated in the exam. She enjoyed the Doppler circulation test because she could hear the blood flow and know what the pressure meant. She needed to be reassured that she had good blood flow, but bad neuropathy."[2]

## Education for the Medical Community

Only about half the American population receives the type of preventive care they need, and that includes those who have a known chronic illness. Awareness and prevention begin with education of the patient and his caregivers, but it also extends to the medical professionals who treat him. Education of the primary care physician is a number one priority. They're fairly well educated now—they can recognize a problem and know that the person is going to need intervention, but the MD may not know where to send the patient for treatment. It's becoming better over the last thirteen to fifteen years, but when a patient with diabetes comes in with a foot ulceration and neuropathy, they may not know to send them to see a podiatrist for that.

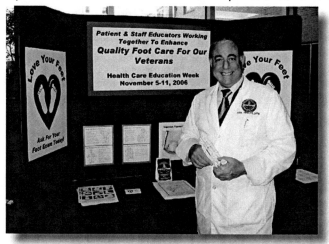

**Dr. Hinkes at Health Fair**

Far too many amputations are being done because many physicians are too quick to amputate. Many of these amputations can be prevented with revascularization (re-establishment of blood supply), proper education, and self-care, and by having a team of professionals working together to treat the patient. David Allie, MD at the New Vascular Horizons Meeting on September 5, 2007 said, "With new technologies of lasers, cryotherapy, and balloon angioplasty, patients are having amputations that can be prevented. Amputation as a first choice is wrong; limbs can be saved; 90 percent can be salvaged with re-vascularization."

Traditional disease treatment programs tend to focus on managing symptoms rather than on improving quality of life by practicing preventive behavior. It is much easier to keep your health than it is to regain it once it is lost. Nowhere is prevention more needed and useful than with those who are showing signs of pre-diabetes and those at risk in early stages of diabetes. Diabetes in many cases can be prevented altogether with proper nutrition and adequate exercise. And, yet, when it comes to evaluation and management of foot problems, there is a lack of education for the medical professionals who provide care for this illness. There is virtually no educational energy devoted to this topic in most schools that teach medical sciences. This is very distressing because it is contributing to unnecessary amputations.

There are isolated schools where medical education includes information on the feet, but my experience over the past ten years working in medical education has been that most medical students, residents, and the resulting medical practitioners have very little knowledge about the diabetic foot.

Once a month, during my lunchtime, I have the pleasure and honor to present lectures to a handful of the residents who rotate through my hospital. I am always curious about their backgrounds, where they got their medical education, and want to know how much exposure have they had to foot problems. Their responses make me feel sad for them and their future patients. A few students may have had a rotation in vascular surgery or endocrinology where they have had cases that required patients to take their shoes and socks off, but as far as learning about the diabetic foot or even about the top ten foot problems that may confront them in private practice, they have had virtually no exposure or experience.

Medical professor and noted researcher, Lawrence A. Lavery (DPM, MPH), is a world-renowned expert in amputation prevention in high-risk patients with diabetes. He says that the standard education concerning the diabetic foot is just a few pages long and usually contains a bunch of dos and don'ts. The educators, while they have a lot of passion, do not really understand the diabetic foot. They sometimes do not tell patients why problems are occurring because the educators need their own education. The foot is a niche study and is still wrapped in mythology and misinformation.

At Dr. Lavery's center, the education program for people with diabetes is a five-part program. There are five sessions of forty-five minutes each. The foot is covered during session four. They start with 100 people in the first session, but the attendance will dwindle until only twenty or thirty people who are really interested in foot education end up in this fourth session.

Traditional medical education has always ignored foot problems and it was precisely this fact that started the first school of chiropody, the M.J. Lewi School at the turn of the twentieth century. That school has grown to nine schools of podiatric medicine in the United States and other schools of podiatric medicine worldwide. Without the appropriate knowledge concerning foot health issues by the primary care community, patients will continue to receive inappropriate diagnoses, sub-standard care, and suffer the loss of a limb as a result. Clearly, medical students need to have education and training concerning the foot, especially in working with the diabetic foot.

There is hope. According to Dr. Jim Powers, there are two recent society actions to help improve the recognition of the diabetic foot and to assess and prevent problems. Vanderbilt

University Hospital has adopted a quality indicator that requires the physician to document in a patient's chart at least once a year that the feet of the patient with diabetes have been evaluated. Another new development relates to the American Geriatric Society. In their third revision of ACOVE (Accessing the Care of Vulnerable Elders), the diabetes guidelines give a recommendation that a patient's foot be evaluated at least once a year by the clinician and as needed depending on clinical circumstances. There is evidence to show that evaluating the diabetic foot helps preserve limbs and improve quality of life. The ACOVE publication gives evidence-based recommendations and statistics.

Aggressive management of the diabetic foot can prevent amputation in most cases. Even when amputation takes place, the remaining leg and a person's life can be saved through good follow-up care from a multi-disciplinary medical team. Education of people with diabetes and healthcare providers is essential. The latter need to be trained to detect problems early and take appropriate action, such as:

- Relieving pressure on the foot
- Correcting for poor blood supply
- Treating of infection
- Maintaining control of blood sugars, blood lipids, blood pressure and cessation of smoking
- Cleaning and dressing of foot wounds and ongoing professional foot care for debridement of keratosis and nails

- Educatiing of people with diabetes and their caregivers
- Preventing recurrence of foot ulcers
- Teaching patients how to check and look after their feet.

Healthcare decision makers have a key role to play in removing the barriers to implementation that still exist in many countries. Reduced amputation rates engender a better quality of life.

There are a number of conferences where medical professionals can learn more about the multi-disciplinary approach to diabetes and amputation prevention. While these are few and far between, they are happening and this is a giant step in the right direction. I will post notices of multi-disciplinary conferences regarding the diabetic foot on our blog www.amputationprevention.com. Be sure to check often as we update information for promoting better healthcare for the patient with diabetes.

## Global Awareness and Education

Next, let's study some of the groups, organizations, and conferences that are moving in the right direction toward amputation prevention through global awareness and educational efforts.

## St. Vincent Declaration

In October 1989, representatives of government health departments and patients' organizations from all European countries met in St. Vincent, Italy with diabetes experts under the guidance of the World Health Organization (WHO) Europe and the International Diabetes Federation Europe (IDF). In this meeting, a unanimous agreement was made about the level of diabetes care these organizations wanted to achieve in Europe during the next five years. The St. Vincent Declaration was signed by all countries and each country agreed to formulate plans and take action at the local level for the prevention, diagnosis, and treatment of diabetes and its complications.

Including healthcare professionals, governments, diabetes associations, the pharmaceutical industry, patients and caregivers, the St. Vincent Declaration stresses the importance of co-operation among all groups concerned with diabetes. It particularly emphasizes the involvement of the patients in their own health management with the monitoring of blood glucose levels at home.

## World Diabetes Day

World Diabetes Day (WDD) is a campaign effort conducted each year by the IDF. Each year, WDD (www.worlddiabetesday. org) has a theme to help educate and create public awareness about the causes, symptoms, complications, and treatments associated with diabetes and its prevention. Not only is the general public the target of this educational effort; much like the purpose of this book, healthcare providers also need to be trained to detect problems early and take appropriate action.

## World Walk Foundation

World Walk (www.worldwalkfoundation.org) an international diabetes initiative—includes the teaching of physicians, nurses, physical therapists, and administrators both in person and via the Internet. The care which can be provided by a temporary visiting team of foreign doctors, nurses and physical therapists is limited. Dr. Cornelius Donohue has found a way to increase the number of patients treated and assure adequate continuity of care once he leaves a mission area. He "teaches the teachers" while he is there and asks that each native caregiver commit to training 100 more caregivers during their professional career, and ask each of them to commit to do the same. By the third generation, 1 million caregivers will be trained from the endeavor of the original caregiver and could result in adequately trained personnel delivered to the most rural regions of the developing world.[3]

## Juvenile Diabetes Foundation (JDF)

The parents and caregivers of children with diabetes need to be aware of the issues that affect the foot of a child with diabetes. Hopefully, their children will grow up with good foot health habits, and enjoy the long-term advantages. Children with diabetes can benefit from early education about their feet and how to identify risks and to protect themselves. The Annual Ron Santo Walk to Cure Diabetes draws people together in a healthy manner. People walk for a worthy cause, while being sponsored by large corporations, small companies, civic organizations, and schools raising money to help find a cure for diabetes. For more information, see www.jdrfillinois.org/walk/walk.html.

## American Podiatric Medical Association

The American Podiatric Medical Association's (www.apma. org) "Knock Your Socks Off" campaign encourages patients to ask their primary care physicians to examine their feet as part of every regular check up. A complete foot examine can detect the effect of diabetes to the foot in the early stages. The primary care provider can refer patients to a podiatrist for preventative education before a problem arises.

The American Diabetic Association wants a resolution from the United Nations on diabetes. Diabetes would be the first non-communicable disease to have such a resolution. The cost of diabetes in the U.S. is expected to be over $400 Billion in 20 years. The UN resolution will

- Increase global awareness

- Bring greater recognition of the burden of diabetes

- Help reposition diabetes as a health priority and to develop effective strategies to treat and prevent the disease.[4]

## CLEAR - Center for Lower Extremity Ambulatory Research

James S. Wrobel, DPM, is an Associate Professor of Surgery and Director of the Outcomes Research Program at the Center for Lower Extremity Ambulatory Research (CLEAR) at the Dr. William M. Scholl College of Podiatric Medicine, North Chicago, Illinois.

Dr. Wrobel's undergraduate background was in kinesiology; he also has a Masters' in Science in outcomes research, clinical decision making, and health policy from Paramus College.

Some of his research involves health services research and the diabetic foot, and he is published in the area of diabetes and foot complications. Jim is one of those people who has a wonderful opportunity to influence the education of the up and coming doctors for the better. He teaches clinical medicine and biomechanics to fourth year students and residents, and runs clinics at the VA hospital of Chicago where he works.

Dr. Wrobel's group looked at a number of issues from the health services research perspective. One of the interesting findings they discovered in the focus of Medicare patients is that their major amputation rate seems to be somewhat variable throughout the country even after accounting for demographics. These rates vary nine-fold over the hospital referral regions throughout the country. This suggests there's a bit of medical uncertainty about how we diagnose and how we treat certain conditions that may eventually lead to major amputations. Jim's research also looked into the high-functioning teams treating diabetic foot conditions within the VA system to see how they coordinated their care among providers (primary care, nursing, podiatry, vascular surgery, orthopedic surgery), and the continuum of care in the rehabilitation, out/in-patient setting. They wanted to see how this type of combined care is coordinated and what strategies lead to successful outcomes and lower amputation rates. What they found was that a patient with diabetes has the best chance of getting well when seen by an interdisciplinary team.

"Unfortunately, patients and doctors aren't thinking ahead in trying to prevent comorbidities from the diabetic condition," says Dr. Wrobel. "Most of the time they're reacting to conditions after they occur. So, if someone has a very bad infection or a foot ulcer that's not healing and they're told they need a major amputation, that's when they seek a multi-disciplinary team— usually in academic settings where a podiatrist is working with a vascular surgeon, endocrinologist, infectious disease specialist, and such."

David Armstrong, DPM, has an endless store of energy. His bio is impressive. He is professor of surgery at the University of Arizona. He is also founder and co-director, with renowned vascular surgeon Professor Joseph Mills, MD, of the Southern Arizona Limb Salvage Alliance (SALSA) at the University and the Southern Arizona VA Health Care System. Armstrong also holds a Master's of Science in Tissue Repair and Wound Healing from the University of Wales College of Medicine and a PhD from the University of Manchester College of Medicine, where he was appointed visiting professor of medicine.

Prior to his tenure at the University of Arizona, Armstrong was professor of surgery and associate dean at the Dr. William M. Scholl College of Podiatric Medicine at Rosalind Franklin University of Medicine and Science in Chicago. During that time of significant productivity, Dr. Armstrong founded and directed the Center for Lower Extremity Ambulatory Research (CLEAR), the first major interdisciplinary research unit at a college of podiatric medicine. CLEAR is an interdisciplinary team composed of clinicians, scientists, and nurses whose focus is to prevent lower extremity complications from diabetes. The CLEAR program is probably the largest group in the world dedicated to amputation prevention.

"I would agree with John Dunne who said that no man is an island. No doctor or nurse is an island; it takes a team to make a difference," says Dr. Armstrong. "One plus one can equal three when you put like-minded people together who really care about health; it can make a really big difference."

CLEAR is headquartered in North Chicago with a diverse group having individual talents with a variety of expertise including a number of bench research collaborations in wound care.

## Research on the Rise

A research group in Bethesda, Maryland announced recently that they believe they can link two current technologies—continuous glucose monitoring and insulin pumps together to accomplish the same function of a normal functioning pancreas. This parley of technologies would reduce the number of times a patient with diabetes would need to stick their finger to obtain a blood sample for glucose monitoring. How would it work? A glucose sensor would be implanted under the skin and transmit blood sugar readings to a monitor. A computer would then calculate the correct insulin dose that would be automatically provided by an insulin pump. This surely is twenty-first century technologies providing a better quality of life for patients with diabetes.

> *There are trials going on,*
> *which means there will be answers soon.*
> —Vickie R. Driver, DPM, MS[5]

Other efforts toward healing the effects of diabetes are on the horizon. One includes the recent transplanting of Islets of Langerhans cells—those are the cells in the pancreas that create insulin—from one person into another person's liver. It worked, and the recipient started making insulin.

There's also, the human genome project, where they're untangling DNA, and there's stem cell research. I think both of these projects have great potential to deal with the issue of diabetes; in fact, it could very well be in our lifetimes that diabetes will become an extinct disease because of one of these projects.

## Training at Georgetown and Inter-disciplinary Teams

The inter-disciplinary or multi-disciplinary approach is the best way to get the most positive results in dealing with patients with diabetes because it offers them a better quality of life, and it costs less. There should be centers dedicated to the inter-disciplinary approach where multiple disciplines of medicine work together.

John Steinberg, DPM, graduated from podiatry school in 1995. This schooling was followed by three years of surgical residency and then, in 1998, he completed a one-year diabetic limb salvage fellowship through the University of Texas in San Antonio. From his fellowship, he developed a strong interest in teaching diabetic limb salvage and wound healing and therefore stayed at the University for another six years to develop his craft.

About six years ago, Dr. Steinberg was recruited to start a comprehensive program at Georgetown University for podiatry and specifically limb salvage. He is also an assistant professor in plastic surgery and a full-time faculty member at Georgetown University. He works exclusively at the Georgetown University Hospital, where he runs an outpatient clinic twice a week and does inpatient work, mostly in the operating room, three days a week. About seventy-five percent of Dr. Steinberg's patients have diabetes, and most of those patients have some type of wound or a history of wounds or amputation. As part of the interdisciplinary team that deals with patients with diabetes, Dr. Steinberg adds his surgical skills to saving feet and legs when surgery is performed. With this skill, he added the ability to deal not only with the ulcerations and prevent amputations but also to correct the etiology of the problem.

The interdisciplinary team with which Dr. Steinberg works is comprised of the specialists necessary to properly manage a high-risk patient with threatening wound-healing complications or amputations. He directs the center along with Dr. Chris Attinger, but knows there are many spokes that make up the whole wheel. Without any part of that wheel, the results just aren't the same. The need for this interdisciplinary approach has been difficult to prove, although there are several good articles that discuss the need and the success of such a limb salvage team. When you see such a team in action and clinically functioning, there is no doubt that this is the correct approach in caring for such a problem.

Dr. Steinberg believes it will become easier to advocate for multi-disciplinary teams in the future. Emerging publications are mentioning multi-disciplinary teams, and researchers are discussing the importance of this type of care for the patient with diabetes. The most important need now is to get hospitals to recognize the efficiency of these teams. They can deliver better care for the patient, and the teams are cost effective as they design a practice around the concept of foot salvage. Rather than running away from multi-disciplinary teams as a financial loss, hospitals are now looking for how they can form such a team.

The treatment technologies have advanced tremendously in the past twenty years, not only for wound care, but also surgical techniques, limb salvage, and revascularization techniques. Particularly in the last ten years, there has been an explosion of devices, tools, drugs, and dressings to use in the role of diabetic foot salvage. While doctors have access to these new technologies, the diagnostics have not kept up with the therapeutics. There is no test at the moment to determine which patients need growth factors, which wound is producing too many MMPs (enzymes that destroy collagen) or which wound is colonized and infected. The diagnostics and their availability have been one of the great limiting steps.

Despite the frustration over diagnostics, there has still been an amazing jump over the last decade in how doctors can topically manage a wound with a true scientific dressing instead of something simple applied to keep the wound moist. Doctors are now able to interact with the wound bed, moderate components that are in too high of a ratio, get a wound balanced and properly prepared for surgery.

In Dr. Steinberg's clinic, the use of debridement is still straightforward with hand instrumentation. If someone's wound is significant enough to require surgical debridement, hydrosurgery or the Versa Jet™ will be used. These techniques allow the doctors to debride a wound precisely without removing excess tissue. At the clinic, Dr. Steinberg also uses two ultrasound technologies—one being a contact ultrasound and the other being a non-contact high-frequency and low-frequency ultrasound. The ultrasounds have proven helpful with wounds being prepared for a graft as well as some of the more challenging atypical wounds such as vasculitic ulcers.

At Georgetown, Dr. Steinberg is very aggressive in his attempts at limb salvage. He has the availability needed for procedures, as the operating room schedule has two rooms five days a week for limb salvage. He is able to get a patient in the room with short notice and not have to fight an operating room add-on schedule that often gives amputations the lowest priority. It is rare for someone to be an inpatient at Georgetown and not go to the operating room for a debridement, biopsy, grafting, or manipulation every three to five days. The doctors are surgically aggressive to debride anything that is not the right color or right consistency but could possibly be viable. The proactive treatments also minimize the patient's exposure to long-term antibiotics, hospitalization time, and re-infection and speed the closure of the wound.

There is an amputation support group at Georgetown that is based on a group Dr. Steinberg started with Dr. Harkless in San Antonio. The group has been in place for three years and meets once a month. One of the most common discussions in the group is from patients who are happy with their below-the-knee amputations and regret that the procedure was not done sooner. Some of these patients have lost six months to a year of their lives in and out of the hospital before the need to amputate was determined. Patients in this situation prefer to get the amputation done and move on with their lives.

Patients with diabetes are complex, medically challenging, and sick patients. At Georgetown, Dr. Steinberg has the benefit of being in a hospital-based center at which twenty people can be in the operating room within three minutes.

Dr. Steinberg believes that a huge part of the success at Georgetown is not physician-driven, but nurse-driven. Some of the key successes at Georgetown come from the communication in referring providers for the outpatient who is discharged to a facility. These referrals are done through an elaborate tracking mechanism run by the nursing staff, nursing manager, and four nurse practitioners.

When treating patients with diabetes, egos of doctors must go out the window. The first contact with the patient is always the nursing staff or practitioner staff. There are not enough physicians to provide contact time for the patient, so a team approach is needed. Dr. Steinberg will often ask the nursing staff to determine the appropriate dressing for a patient rather than dictating that action.

Even with a staff of twenty people at a clinic, Dr. Steinberg believes what takes place in the private practitioner's office is a huge component of success. If the clinic does not get the referral at the right time, or if a private practitioner cannot recognize what needs to be done, then the whole team falls apart. Dr. Steinberg hopes that practitioners make it a goal to keep patients away from his team by properly screening them and considering appropriate surgery ahead of time.

Low-cost prevention and educational strategies such as self-management education are critical to limiting the spread of diabetes and the suffering it causes around the world. The more we do to create awareness and teach prevention, means fewer people will suffer this horrible disease.

## DF-Con - Diabetic Foot Conference

Dr. Armstrong is also involved in DF-Con, the Diabetic Foot Conference, which I had the opportunity to attend this year. It gave me real insight about how the diabetic foot problem is basically the same all over the world, but the way we approach it in terms of our resources, politics, and education is what makes the difference. The central theme is focusing on an area that's been ignored for a long time. Patients don't think about this problem, and most people don't care.

> *Diabetes is like dealing with an evil, angry deity that attacks silently. People die of silent heart attacks, they develop wounds silently because of neuropathy. Then, when the victim dies, people blame the heart attack, or the infection, or the stroke; they rarely blame the real enemy—diabetes. It's a nefarious disease.*
> —David Armstrong, DPM University of Arizona

Co-chair, George Andros, MD, is a well-known vascular surgeon who saw a need for an international interdisciplinary diabetic foot meeting. He and Dr. Armstrong developed and called it DefCon at the time. DF-Con (www.dfcon.com) is now an inter-disciplinary foot conference designed to draw together clinicians from around the world. In the 2007 meeting, more than fifty nations were represented. "It's a meeting dedicated to sharing information across disciplines," says Armstrong. "It's an exciting time when you're able to share information and see that light bulb go on in another clinician's or a patient's eyes."

## Training Courses

These training courses are training grounds for others to go out and train other providers in their communities. A two-day comprehensive, fast-paced course was designed for healthcare professionals within the Veterans Administration who want to increase their knowledge in the education, care, rehabilitation, and management of the veterans with diabetes and limb loss. Enhancing the Care and Rehabilitation of the Diabetic Amputee was presented in June 2008 by Ossur Americas & Advanced Rehabilitation Care via the VA Atlanta Healthcare System in Atlanta, Georgia. Speakers included Robert Gailey, PhD, PT, Jeffrey Robbins, DPM, and Ian Fothergill, BSc.

The course provided a comprehensive review of the latest in the management of foot care, prosthetic fitting, alignment, and physical training for the patient with diabetes. Innovative methods and rehab solutions demonstrated to attendees treatment options that may be implemented with their veteran population immediately upon completion of the course. Participants are now able to:

- Explain the etiology, physiology and pathological changes that occur with Type 2 diabetes and insulin resistance.
- Describe the progression of diabetic foot ulcers and the interventions that reduce the risk of amputation.
- Describe the VA PACT Program and its components.
- Identify the role and limitations of diabetes exercise programs with emphasis on fall prevention.
- Discuss the chronic complication and goals associated with diabetes.

- Compare and contrast orthotic management and shoe wear for the patient with long-standing diabetes.
- Identify functional outcomes and measures commonly employed for the diabetic population.
- Discuss prosthetic socket options, compare and contrast prosthetic foot and knee options.
- Prepare veterans for prosthetic training and implement a functional gait training program.

## Diabetic Limb Salvage Conference

Dr. John Steinberg and Dr. Chris Attinger hosted the second Diabetic Limb Salvage Conference at Georgetown University in September 2008. This conference was started because the two doctors wanted to inspire and create more teams across the country like the one found at Georgetown. The Georgetown clinic gets many visitors who want to do things the Georgetown way. Since everyone cannot visit the clinic, Doctors Steinberg and Attinger instituted the conference. This three-day program featured over sixty faculty members in every discipline from nursing to administration to physical therapy to vascular surgery, infectious disease, podiatry, plastic surgery, general practice to cardiovascular surgery. The participants were about fifty percent physicians and the rest of the attendees were comprised of other healthcare professionals who work with patients with diabetes. The conference does not run multiple tracks because they want everyone in the same room at the same time. It is an open meeting that allows for dialogue with every speaker. The panelists are questioned and the audience can relate the information back to their specific institutions. In 2007, almost 1,200 participants attended and the number grows annually.

One feature that was unique at this conference last year was live limb salvage cases. A vascular surgeon, Dr. Neville, did a bypass graft under a live closed circuit TV connection into the hotel. The endovascular surgeon did angioplasties. Dr. Steinberg performed bioengineered tissue grafting and tendon lengthening. Dr. Attinger did an amputation of a Charcot foot and the closure. The conference organizers tried to show a snapshot for those not in the operating room what really goes on there when they send patients to surgery. For those conference participants already working in the operating room, this feature allowed them to refine what they are doing and get new ideas. This live feature received universally good feedback.

## Veterans Affairs Healthcare System

The Veterans Affairs Healthcare System has been a leader in education, research, and treatment of the diabetic foot. It's well known and respected Preservation Amputation Care and Treatment (PACT) Program was first organized and implemented in 1989 by the VA to address the complex problems presented by the patient with diabetes and the comorbidities that affect the foot. The program was a success in preventing lower limb amputations but became even more successful in 1993 when performance measures were instituted. These measures included noting the patients hemoglobin A1c, a visual foot exam for identification of deformities, palpation of foot pulses, and a monofilament testing device exam. These measures helped to quantify the extent of the factors affecting the foot of the patient with diabetes. The VA has done well in its efforts to address the issues affecting the diabetic foot and is considered to be well ahead of the curve in this area.

## A Patient Registry

In their book, *Crossing the Quality Chasm,* The Institute of Medicine Committee on Quality Care in America says, "There are gaps in all levels of prevention that result in increased health systems costs and unnecessary human illness." One method to help close the gaps and lower the costs is a patient registry. This collection of data would be the repository of critical information concerning all aspects of the health of the patient with diabetes. Like the quote from Ed McMahon to Johnny Carson who played the character Carnac the Magnificent, "Everything you need to know is right here." It would be available to authorized physicians, other healthcare providers, and to you so that your diabetes history would be available for review and update guaranteeing the highest quality of care.

A patient registry for healthcare workers could include:

- Records on foot circulation
- Protective sensation test results
- Foot and deformities history
- Diabetic education, status of footgear, diabetic shoes, or insoles
- Lab results
- Vital signs
- Smoking status
- Nutritional goals and achievements

- Exercise status
- Blood glucose levels (random and A1c)
- Needs for ongoing professional foot, dental, and eye care
- Due dates for screenings and physicians' tests
- Reminder for patient follow-up
- Previous foot and leg surgeries
- Previous amputations

This registry would provide a document that ensures you get the best care from your primary care physician and the other members of your inter-disciplinary team—your posse. The repositories of human medical knowledge and those teachers with the skills to teach this knowledge could be found at every medical school in the world. This includes all schools of allopathic and osteopathic medicine, pharmacy, nursing, and all allied healthcare specialists.

## Healthcare Reform: Is Universal Healthcare Coverage the Answer?

Another area that needs to move in the right direction is that of healthcare coverage. I asked wound care specialist, Cynthia Fleck, RN, about whether or not she thought wound care services should be covered by private insurance, Medicare, Medicaid, or HMOs. Here is her response:

*Although I am not a reimbursement expert, I do know that most private insurance companies, HMOs and PPOs have some coverage for various wound care services and products. Centers for Medicare and Medicaid Services (CMS) are often dictated by prospective payment systems or a per diem rate to care for the patient based on their diagnostic codes and state by state regulations.*

*Healthcare reform in the U.S. needs to be addressed so that more people can access the benefits of wound care. I believe patients need to become major stakeholders in their own care. The current system is broken and in serious financial trouble. An educated patient who demonstrates prudent self-care and practices prevention and disease control will ultimately be our best weapon against sky-rocketing wound care costs and the need for reform and expense containment. Education is the name of the game!*

Recently, I saw Denis A. Cortese, MD, President and CEO, Mayo Clinic on public television discussing disease prevention and the U.S. Healthcare Industry. He favors universal healthcare as a solution to the issue of prevention because all patients will have health insurance that can be transferred between private and government insurers. It is theirs for a lifetime regardless of employment or age. In that way, patients will be assured access to healthcare and preventive healthcare and the costs will be equitably distributed among those entities that take the financial risks in healthcare.

He explained that younger patients, while practicing prevention, demonstrate meager cost savings to their current medical insurers. Healthcare insurance companies cannot make a financial profit by promoting health prevention. So their thinking must be, "Why should an insurer pay the costs of prevention in younger patients with limited financial return on their investment of healthcare dollars when they feel the ultimate beneficiary of a preventive healthcare system will be Medicare?"

> *If you start getting into coverage based on risk factors or risk levels, it might mean a higher risk patient gets coverage while someone who's a risk level zero does not. I think all diabetic patients should be covered since it is a progressive disease.*
> —Howard Green, DPM

According to Dr. Lee J. Sanders, patients with diabetes in the United States are not receiving the best available care. In his term as the president of healthcare and education for the American Diabetes Association, Dr. Sanders asked the Centers for Medicare and Medicaid Services to expand coverage of preventative foot care to patients with diabetes and PAD with loss of protective sensation. He helped to develop the national guidelines and the American Diabetes Association's position on third party reimbursement for DM education and supplies.[6]

1. The goal of medical care for people with diabetes is to optimize glycemic control and minimize complications.

2. An integral component of diabetes is self-management education delivered by an inter-disciplinary team.

3. Today, self-management education is understood to be such a critical part of diabetes care that medical

treatment of diabetes without systemic self-management education is regarded as inadequate.

4. Participants in self-management education programs have been found to decrease lower extremity amputation rates, reduce medication costs, and have fewer emergency room visits and hospitalizations.

5. As such, insurers must reimburse for diabetes-related medical treatment as well as for self-assessment education programs that have met accepted standards such as the American Diabetes Association's National Standards for Diabetes Self Management Education.

6. Because no single diabetes treatment is appropriate for all people with diabetes, providers and patients should have access to a broad array of medications and supplies to develop an effective treatment modality.

7. Diabetes management needs individualization. Therefore, it is not uncommon for practitioners to uniquely tailor treatment for their patients.

Dr. Jim Wrobel reports on patient access to care and what could be done to give people better access to foot care? Should it be universal insurance? He replied:

If you look at the amputation numbers over the country using CDC data, they seem to be somewhat level over the past two years. They haven't gone up, as they were until the late '90s. When we have a managed care environment with inter-disciplinary clinics like the VA system along with a well-run PACT program, we see the amputation rates actually decreasing.

The political wind has been about universal healthcare. That may be a good solution, especially when they're talking about having a medical care record system where there's personal communication between all providers in the system. When we get a new patient in our system, they've already got a problem, but we don't know what has been done to try to manage it. If a patient's history is in a universal medical record system before they come to us, we can identify problems before they emerge and possibly prevent them. Using the electronic medical record would give us a better, more inter-disciplinary approach. Better communication would make a big difference and would improve the care we are able to give our patients.

## It's Time for Insurance Companies to Pay Up for Prevention!

We should be removing the barriers to treatment and encouraging patients to use preventative education and behavior. Instead, most private insurance companies are hesitant to cover intervention that could prevent many deaths. The problem is worsening, with an ever-widening gap between those who have access to adequate medical care and those who do not.

Disease management companies that focus on diabetic care that lack programs for amputation prevention are considered "disease management light" when it comes to foot care. They use the phones to contact clients to remind them to take their medicines, to eat and exercise, but they do nothing to educate about foot health or encourage their clients to practice preventive foot care behaviors.

Payers seem to want evidence of clinical and financial outcomes to tell them where the money is. Our work in the VA system has shown reductions in the rates of amputations as well as decreases in costs. We do prevention by education, but healthcare companies do not understand the benefits of inter-disciplinary care, the tools, and the team.

One of the deficiencies of our medical healthcare system is that while touting prevention, payers rarely are willing to pay for it and have been slow to realize the benefits of prevention both to the patient and their bottom line, financially. So while bureaucrats discuss and actuaries calculate, people with diabetes continue to lose legs at an alarming rate. If a patient with diabetes were to see a podiatrist for no other reason except to have a foot evaluation for amputation prevention, it would not be a covered service or reimbursable by insurance. This paradigm must change.

Dr. David Armstrong responded to my question about whether or not insurance companies should pay for prevention. He replied thusly:

> Those who are paying for the problem, like insurance companies, don't think much about diabetes or diabetic foot problems because of the fact that they really are silent problems. Instead of preaching to one another—doctors preaching to patients, patients preaching to doctors—about why this is important, we need to actually get to the policymakers to help us

*make a difference. Part of that might be to give them something that they can care about—something like cancer. When most policy makers think about cancer, someone in their family had it. If you look at most of the complications of the diabetic foot or diabetes in the extremities, they're at least as bad as most high-grade cancers. We would never think of withholding therapy for someone with lung, colon, or prostate cancer, but it happens all the time in people with diabetes. The mortality rate is around 50 percent for most of these cancers and they have a survival rate of less than five years. If we can get this message to policymakers and help them to see that diabetes doesn't have to be as bad as cancer, then that's a big step in the right direction toward improvement in care.*

In an article titled "Periodic Medical Exams of Diabetics by Podiatric Physicians" in *Podiatry Management Online,* Ken Malkin, DPM, asks several good questions. Is screening medically necessary care? A patient with diabetes may develop any number of complications. But, how does the patient know when he or she is developing early retinopathy except by ophthalmology exam? How does one know if a patient has a loss of protective sensation unless given a medical exam that involves using the monofilament test or other similar modalities?

But, how does a doctor get paid for providing these tests if insurance companies, Medicare, and other payers are not willing to pay for preventative treatment or cover at-risk foot care? The companies must realize that these tests are a necessary part of a medical evaluation. Visits for prevention of diabetic complications to the foot should be a paid service by insurance companies.

The backward economics of the healthcare industry have been discussed in this year's presidential primaries and debates. Presidential candidates are passionate about better healthcare and the need for podiatric care. The candidates are asking a good question: Why do insurance companies pay for an expensive operation to amputate the foot of a diabetic, but won't reimburse for cheaper preventative visits to a podiatrist that could make surgery unnecessary? Insurance companies are paying for the wrong things. Instead of prevention, they are paying to have legs taken off. No one is paid to do prevention. Insurance companies are part of the problem rather than part of the solution.

"I've heard that the overall cost for amputation is over $37,000 per lower extremity amputation," says Dr. Malkin. "I think we're probably talking about at least a foot or below-the-knee amputation, and I don't think that includes prosthetics and aftercare. I think the incentives for wound healing are not aligned properly, either. For example, the in-home care industry does more aggressive things to heal because their financial incentives are aligned to heal the wound as soon as possible. They get a flat sum of money and make more money if they heal patients faster with fewer visits. It's an interesting dynamic to see them searching for anything to heal a wound as quickly as possible with the least amount of intervention. They're using things like hyperbaric oxygen, which does wonders with some of these wounds, and they are using the Wound VAC, which I think is another very good modality."

## Dr. Bob Frykberg on Access to Healthcare

In his podiatry practice in the southwestern part of the United States, Bob sees a lot of Hispanic and Native American folks with diabetes who do not have healthcare insurance and adequate patient services. I've asked him questions in an interview style to address this issue. Here is our conversation:

Bob: I think education or preventative measures are key. Most of the patients who have coverage, even some who don't have coverage (because we have a lot of illegals) they have access. They walk into an emergency room, but then they wait. It's not the most efficient way to provide care. I think more than access we have to focus on prevention and education constantly. PCPs have to focus on prevention even though they're busy. At the VA, we have access. People just go to their primary care and they get in. On the outside, it's not so easy. Many doctors' offices are very busy and they can't see everybody right away who needs to be seen unless they go to urgent health centers or emergency rooms. So we certainly need more providers, more clinics, more urgency clinics, more homeless or indigent clinics. Neighborhood health centers, I think, would be a great idea. I used to work in neighborhood health centers thirty years ago in Boston and provided access to local communities in the city. Houston, New York City...many cities have local neighborhood health centers, which would be a good idea if they could secure funding, but funding is always the problem. Dollars are always being taken away from the budget. One of the best ways to provide access is through a triage or primary care center that makes a diagnosis and refers the patient to a specialty center if there is a problem.

Mark: What do you think is the resistance in the insurance industry and the political climate to prevention? Why are we having such a tough time with prevention?

Bob: Our system is geared toward pay for service, and procedure, and not pay for condition. HMOs will pay for prevention, the VA will more or less pay for prevention, I think Kaiser ... most quota systems will pay for prevention, but Medicare ... I think now they pay for some educational services. They do pay for diabetic foot care for patients with the condition, but most private payers are not because it costs money and if there's not a disease or an ankle problem, they haven't realized that paying the short dollars in advance is going to prevent the large dollars that will be expended later on if these people get into trouble. It's reorientation of the way that these insurers think.

Mark: People who are served in inter- or multi-disciplinary clinics seem to do better. What can we do to stimulate more of those kinds of facilities and arrangements?

Bob: I think anybody who reads the literature realizes that's the way to go. That's why most diabetes centers have multi-disciplinary approaches. Joslin Clinic—one of the first models— had podiatry care back in the 1920s. They had their own surgeons, teaching nurses, and dressing nurses or what they called foot care nurses. Most HMOs or closed health plans have it now. A large proportion of practitioners in this country are private practitioners. They have their own small groups. They don't have a multi-disciplinary practice but they have a multi-disciplinary network that they refer to. Educating patients and providers to know who to go to at what point and to work together, especially in the hospital setting is very important. Things have certainly improved over where we were ten to fifteen years ago and will continue to improve as more literature suggests that's the way to go.

When we look at the issue of healthcare costs that are rising, prevention can be extremely cost effective with an eye to patient satisfaction. Patient education is the keystone of prevention. Education about diabetes is an area that most patients have poor or little knowledge. I'd like to recommend the idea of CPE: Continuing Patient Education. Just as I am required to obtain a certain amount of CME credits (Continuing Medical Education) for re-licensure, I believe that patients should also have the opportunity to receive ongoing education about their diabetes and its complications. In return for attending and learning about their diabetes, insurance companies could provide reductions in healthcare premiums or reduction in co-pays for office visits.

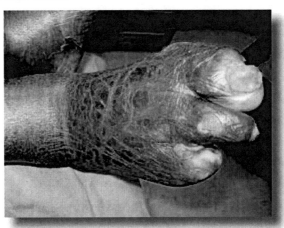

**End Stage Renal Disease Patient with Two Toes Amputated**

## Do I Really Need this Operation?

In the final analysis, if you have practiced preventive behaviors and followed your physician's recommendations for treating your wound or infection, and continue to have pain, a non-healing wound, or infection, you may have no choice except to lose a part of your foot or leg. It may be the best alternative to avoid an even worse situation. There are several scenarios that may leave a patient no choice except to lose a leg. For example, if you have had an angioplasty or bypass and your blood supply has been compromised to the point where the tissues are not viable and a portion of your body has died from gangrene, or if you have a non-healing wound or a bone infection that does not respond to conservative nonsurgical therapy that could lead to pain and a life-threatening situation, it may be better to remove the affected body part. Every patient undergoing an amputation should have the benefit of psychological counseling both pre and post operatively to discuss their fears or concerns.

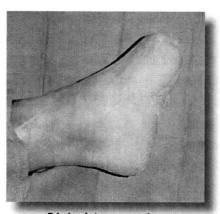

**Digital Amputation**

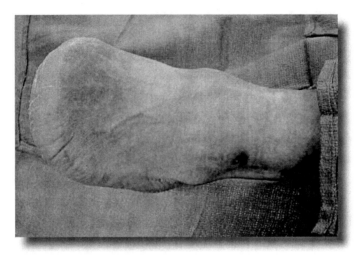

**Diabetic Foot with Trans Metatarsal Amputation**

## If Ya Gotta, Ya Gotta

In my interview with Dr. Chris Attinger, Medical Director of Wound Healing Clinic, and Professor of Plastic Surgery at Georgetown University Hospital, I asked him, "What if you must take off the leg?" To which, he answered:

*If you must take off the leg, it's not necessarily a bad thing. We have an amputee support group and 95 percent of them have told me, "Why did you try so hard? Why didn't you take the leg off sooner?" They found life with a prosthesis is fine. Getting over the fear of wearing a prosthesis is a big move so we have them see the prosthesis before they have an amputation. We also have them see a psychiatrist. Preparing them with those steps makes the transition much smoother.*

*Most people aren't able to have the benefits of a multi-disciplinary limb salvage team. Dr. Gayle Reiber's, MPH, PhD,* from the University of Washington, Seattle, work showed there was a nine-fold variation if a diabetic ended up in an emergency room whether he was going to lose his leg or not. The chances of him losing a leg was as high as one in four in certain places and as low as one in twenty in other places. It depended on where the patient went for care, so I think education is a big deal. People should be educated that legs can be salvaged. I'm sure the Podiatry Association and the Foot Medical Society are striving to get that message across.

Dr. Attinger continues, for each day that a patient is not walking, it takes them four days to recover. Whoever's planning the reconstruction has to have an intelligent plan that can be accomplished in a realistic time frame especially when dealing with elderly patients. If the patient is seventy-five or eighty years old and frail, they may be better off losing their leg and walking with a prosthesis within six weeks instead of keeping them in bed or a wheelchair for half a year. Salvage is great but you don't want it at the risk of losing the patient.

I am more and more conscious of what the patient can tolerate and what kind of foot I can leave him when I'm done. If I don't think I'm going to give him a good biomechanical foot, then I'm much more likely to consider amputation. I don't want to save the leg just to save the leg. I want it to be something that's not going to break down two years or in a year. You have to know potentially what will work, what won't work and decide accordingly.

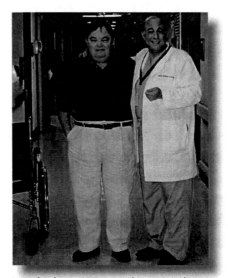

**Healed patient and Dr. Hinkes.**

This is a patient who came to me after he had the front of both feet (trans-metatarsal) amputated due to diabetes. He had ulcers and could not walk. I teased him about how my payback would be a walk down the hall with him after he healed. This picture commemorates that stroll.

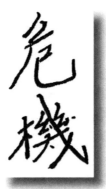

There is a famous Chinese symbol that has two meanings. One is danger and the other is opportunity. There surely can be no better description of the situation of the patient with diabetes. At this crossroad, patients can decide how they may want to live out their lives. Bad habits should become a thing of the past as they are presented with an opportunity to change their lives for better health. Recognizing that PAD is affecting all organs and system of their body, and it has contributed to the loss of their leg, they should move forward to preventing any further complication of PAD. Blood glucose control should be the first step followed by smoking cessation Developing an exercise program should be next. As we have said, the patient most likely to have an amputation is the patient who has already *had* an amputation. So the focus next should be on protecting and preventing any of the triggers from happening to the remaining foot that could lead to the loss of the other leg.

With a special focus on amputation prevention, the goal of this book is to be an educational resource and to present the issues and topics that affect the foot health of the patient with diabetes. I hope that after reading this book you have learned about how diabetes and the comorbidities of peripheral neuropathy, peripheral vascular disease, and immunopathy can affect your foot and how you can control those forces that could harm you.

You now know that amputation prevention is possible. By understanding the triggers that can lead to infection, ulceration, and amputation, you also know how to prevent and avoid them. At last, you have a strategy that works!

The secret of amputation prevention is a lifestyle modification and common sense approach to better foot health. This cannot be just a passing thought or part-time behavior; it must become a part of you and your daily activity. You may have to live with your diabetes, but you do not have to let diabetes control your health. All you have to do is take an active role in your health—especially your foot health—and apply what you have learned in this book.

If you want to prevent foot problems or deal with an existing foot problem, I encourage you to find a healthcare team (your posse), who can advise you on how to resolve your problem or prevent new problems.

Let's summarize and conclude the best ways for you to prevent an amputation:

1. Control your blood sugar levels
2. Stop smoking
3. Good nutrition
4. Exercise
5. Practice preventive foot behaviors
6. Recognize if you are depressed or have compliance issues and seek help
7. Form a partnership with your doctors

With these recommendations, you have everything you need to succeed and *Keep the Legs You Stand On.*

## Foot Notes: How to Reduce the Number of LE AMPS

Eighty-five percent of patients with diabetes who undergo amputations had a foot ulcer. Patients with diabetes account for sixty percent of all LE amps. Here are some things you can do to prevent a lower-extremity amputation:

1. Properly-fitted footgear to protect the foot from calluses and corns and ulcers.
2. Patient education
3. Professional foot exam
4. Appropriate foot hygiene
5. Good glycemic control

## How to Save a Limb

1. Early detection of peripheral arterial disease (PAD)
2. Know risks of PAD
    a. Smoking
    b. High cholesterol
    c. High blood pressure
    d. Physical inactivity
    e. Obesity
    f. Diabetes
3. Who might be affected? Those with:
    • Decreased or absent pulses
    • Claudication (muscle cramps due to lack of circulation)
    • Hypertension
    • Chest pain

# Appendix A

## Foot Care Guidelines

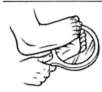

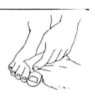

1. INSPECT your feet each day. Use your eyes, hands, and/or a mirror. Look for cracks, blisters scratches, redness, heat, color changes, ulcers or dry skin.

2. WASH your feet daily with warm water and mild soap, just like you wash your hands. Do not soak your feet.

3. DRY your feet well, especially between the toes. Pat with a soft towel to dry, instead of rubbing. Use unscented powder if needed.

4. FILE or trim your nails straight across. Ingrown nails and calluses should be treated by a health care provider. Never use razors or over-the-counter medications to treat corns or calluses.

5. APPLY lotion after bathing and at bedtime if your feet or legs are dry or scaly. Do not use it between your toes.

6. CHANGE daily into clean, white cotton or wool socks that are not too big, have no seams, and are not tight around the tops. If your feet get cold at night, wear socks to bed.

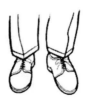

7. EXAMINE your shoes before putting them on. Feel inside with your hands for pebbles, nails, torn linings or anything which could rub against your feet.

8. WEAR shoes that fit. Leather shoes protect feet from injury and keep them warm and dry.

9. NEVER walk barefoot. Wear shoes or slippers indoors, even if just going to the bathroom.

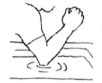 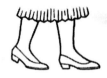

10. DON'T smoke. Smoking reduces the blood flow to your feet.

Nashville VAMC
Irh 5/99

11. CHECK the temperature of bath water with your elbow before bathing. Do not use hot water bottles or heating pads on your feet.

.2. BREAK IN new shoes slowly. Start by wearing them for one hour on the first day and increase by one hour each day. Plan ahead to purchase new shoes before your old ones wear out.

- Inspect your feet daily for cuts, blisters, redness, swelling or nail problems. Use a magnifying hand mirror to see the bottom of your feet. Call you doctor if you find anything unusual.
- Gently wash your feet in lukewarm (not hot) water—the temperature you would use on a newborn baby—using a soft cloth or sponge.
- Dry your feet carefully and thoroughly—especially between the toes.
- Moisturize daily to prevent itching or cracking. Do not use moisturizer between the toes since this could encourage infection.
- Cut your nails carefully, then file the edges smooth. Cut them straight across without clipping the corners which could cause the nail to become ingrown.
- Do not trim corns or calluses. Let your doctor do this for you.
- Wear clean, dry socks and change them daily. Wear the correct type of sock as we discussed in Chapter 12.

- Wear socks to bed so your feet do not get cold. Do not use a heating pad or hot water bottle on cold feet.
- Before putting on your shoes, shake them out to make sure there are no foreign objects inside. A small pebble or twig rubbing against your foot or toe could cause enough friction to create a blister.
- Avoid walking in rain or snow, and keep your feet warm. Always wear shoes outside. In fact, never walk barefoot, even in the house. You could step on something and injure your foot without knowing it if you have neuropathy.
- Get a foot exam on a regular basis to help prevent foot complications. A nationwide survey of over 1,200 people with type 2 diabetes reveals a low rate of preventive screening services. Seventy percent reported receiving an annual foot exam but only 50.3 percent of them reported having a monofilament exam—an essential diagnostic exam to identify loss of protective sensation that is linked to peripheral sensory neuropathy.
- Have an annual dilated eye exam.
- Have an annual dental exam

# Appendix B

## Ways to Quit Smoking

According to the American Heart Association, if you quit smoking you'll live longer and stay healthier. Smoking has been linked to 90 percent of all lung cancer cases and to over 430,000 smoking-related deaths every year. Chronic bronchitis and emphysema have been linked with smoking. Overall death rates from cancer are twice as high among smokers. Heavy smokers have death rates that are four times greater than non-smokers. Smoking causes vasoconstriction and further limits the circulation of fresh oxygenated blood necessary for normal body function. In the patient with diabetes, smoking can complicate an already bad situation by negatively affecting their circulation and thus their ability to heal a wound that can lead to amputation.

**New Ways to Quit Smoking:**

1. Nicotine replacement therapy can be supplied as a gum, skin patch, nasal spray, inhaler, or lozenges and can double your chances of quitting for good. These methods work by providing a replacement source of nicotine.

2. Non-Nicotine therapy pill is available by prescription that doesn't contain nicotine. It reduces the symptoms of nicotine withdrawal by acting on chemicals in the brain related to nicotine craving. Zyban or Wellbutrin are the prescription medications

3. Information about "going cold" on your own is available from multiple sources on quitting smoking without the use of nicotine substitutes or non-nicotine medications. There are books, audiotapes, and videotapes that can help you stop smoking.

4. There are support groups that can help, too. Stop smoking support groups can be found at hospitals and in the phone book under the title of "Smokers Information and Treatment Centers."

5. Web sites that have information you can use are:
www.cancer.org
www.cancer.gov
www.americanheart.org
www.lungsusa.org
www.cdc.gov/tobacco
www.ahcpr.gov/clinic
www.findhelp.com
www.quitnet.org
www.transformations.com
www.amputationprevention.com
http://surgeongeneral.gov/tobacco/quits.htm
www.diabetes-exercise.org

# Appendix C

## Recommended Reading

Many of the experts who contributed interviews, endorsements, quotations, and material for this book are also prolific writers. Many have literally published hundreds of articles. I will try to list the books they have written, but if I miss any, it was by mistake and certainly not intentional.

- *101 Foot Care Tips for People with Diabetes* by Jessie Ahroni ISBN-13: 978-1580400404.
- *A Practical Manual of Diabetic Foot Care* by Michael E. Edmonds, Alethea V. M. Foster, and Lee Sanders ISBN-13: 978-1405161473.
- *Atlas of Foot Disorders* by Larry Harkless ISBN-13: 9780721642918.
- *Clinical Care of the Diabetic Foot* by David G. Armstrong and Lawrence Lavery ISBN-13: 978-1580402231.
- *Death by Pedicure the Dirty Secrets of Nail Salons* by Dr. Robert Spalding. ISBN 978-0-9711068-2-6; Publisher Chattanooga Fu Fu Factory. Order from Dr. Robert Spalding, Area Podiatry Center, 1225 Taft Hwy., Signal Mt, TN 37377. Web site: www.justfortoenails.com

- *Diabesity: The Obesity-Diabetes Epidemic That Threatens America--And What We Must Do to Stop It* by Francine R. Kaufman, MD ISBN: 978-0-553-80384-6 (0-553-80384-0).
- *Diabetic Eye Disease: Lessons From A Diabetic Eye Doctor (How To Avoid Blindness and Get Great Eye Care)* by Dr. A. Paul Chous www.diabeticeyes.com/book.htm.
- *Handbook of Common Foot Problems* by Lawrence B. Harkless ISBN-13: 978-0443078293.
- *Pain Management : An Issue of Clinics in Podiatric Medicine and Surgery* by John S. Steinberg ISBN-13: 9781416063414.
- *Pain: The Gift Nobody Wants* by Philip Yancey and Paul Brand. ISBN 13: 978-0788163722.
- *•Peripheral Neuropathy: When the Numbness, Weakness, and Pain Won't Stop* by Norman Latov ISBN-13: 978-1932603590.
- *Primary Podiatric Medicine* by Jeffrey M. Robbins ISBN-13: 978-0721643632.
- *Right to Recover, Winning the Political and Religious Wars over Stem Cell Research in America* by Yvonne Perry ISBN 978-1-933449-41-8. Available at Nightengale Press www.nightengalepress.biz/.
- *The Foot in Diabetes* (Practical Diabetes) (Hardcover) by Andrew Boulton, Peter Cavanagh, and Gerry Ryman ISBN-13: 978-0470015049.
- *The Philatelic History of Diabetes* by Lee Sanders ISBN-13: 978-1580400848.

# Appendix D

## Other Helpful Resources

The International Working Group for the Diabetic Foot on classification system for the diabetic foot.

Executive Office
Avenue Emile de Mot, 19
B-1000 Brussels, Belguim
Telephone: +32-2-5385511
E-mail: info@idf.org
Web site: www.idf.org

### Web Sites for More Information on Diabetes

- **www.uptodateonline.com** Up-to-date clinical information covering diabetes.
- **www.emedicine.com**  eMedicine has clinical information on diabetes.
- **www.medscape.com**  Medscape offers clinical information on diabetes.
- **www.nlm.nih.gov** National Library of Medicine is the world's largest medical library.
- **www.pubmed.com** PubMed. National Library of Medicine

(NLM). Medical literature search site.

- **www.medlineplus.gov** Medline Plus. National Library of Medicine (NLM). Search engine for health topics, conditions and diseases.

- **http://content.nejm.org/collections** The New England Journal of Medicine. Source for clinical materials grouped by publisher.

- **www.clinicaltrials.gov** Clinical Trials.gov. National Institutes of Health (NIH). Listing of ongoing clinical trials.

- **www.nccam.nih.gov** National Center for Complementary and Alternative Medicine. National Institutes of Health (NIH). Site that reviews complementary and alternative medicine research, clinical trials and health information.

- **www.mdanderson.org/departments/cimer** MD Anderson Hospital Complementary/Integrative Medicine Education Resource.

- **www.amfoundation.org** Alternative Medicine Foundation.

- **www.omhrc.gov** The Department of Health and Human Services. The Office of Minority Health. Site focused on improving and protecting the health of racial and ethnic minority populations.

- **www.meharry.org/FL** Factline. National Library of Medicine (NLM) Meharry Medical College. Health disparities faced by women minority groups and the elderly.

- **www.cdc.gov/omhd** Office of Minority Health. Centers for Disease Control ad Prevention (CDC). Reference site.

- **www.ninds.nih.gov/disorders/disorder_index.htm** Information Page. National Institute of Neurological Disorders and Stroke (NINDS). Reference page with extensive links on many diseases including Alzheimer's Disease.

- **www.anemia.org** National Anemia Action Council. Resource for anemia patients and professionals.

- **www.vascularweb.org** Vascular Web. The Society for Vascular Surgery. Site with good clinical information for professionals and patients.

- **www.nlhep.org** National Lung Health Education Program. Educational site with resources on tobacco control, smoking cessation, lung cancer, and breathing tests.

- **www.clinicaltrials.gov** Clinical Trials.gov. National Institute of Health (NIH).

- **www.omhrc.gov** The Office of Minority Health (OMH) U.S. Department of Health and Human Services. Site dedicated to improve and protect the health of racial and ethnic minority populations.

- **www.hrsa.gov/culturalcompetence** Cultural Competence Resources for Health Care Providers. Health Resources and Services Administration. U.S. Department of Health and Human Services.

- **www.cdc.gov/omhd** Office of Minority Health. Centers for Disease Control and Prevention (CDC). Reference site.

- **www.nlm.nih.gov/medlineplus/diabetestype1.html** Diabetes Type 1 Medline Plus National Library of Medicine (NLM). Resource site.

- **www.nlm.nih.gov/medlineplus/diabetes.html** Diabetes Medline Plus. National Library of Medicine (NLM). Resource site.

- **http://diabetes.niddk.nih.gov/intro/index.htm** Introduction to Diabetes. National Diabetes Information Clearinghouse (NDIC) National Institute of Diabetes and Digestive and Kidney Diseases (NIDDK).

- **www.lww.com/product/?978-0-7817-2796-9** Joslin's Diabetes Mellitus, 2004 Lippincott Williams & Wilkins.

- **www.ndep.nih.gov** National Diabetes Education Program. National Institutes of Health (NIH).

- **www.eldercare.gov** Eldercare Locator. U.S. Department of Health and Human Services. Extensive Information on senior services.

- **www.usa.gov/Topics/Seniors.shtml** Senior Citizens' Resources. Extensive resources for seniors.

- **www.aoa.dhhs.gov** Administration on Aging. U.S. Department of Health and Human Services. Federal website on resources for older Americans.

- **www.eldercareteam.com** The Eldercare Team. Site for eldercare caregivers on questions and answers resources and support.

- **www.benefitscheckup.org** BenefitsCheckUp. The National Council on Aging. Resources for seniors to find benefit programs.

- **www.gilbertguide.com** Gilbert Guide. Resource of information on senior care facilities and resources.

- **www.hapnetwork.org** Health Assistance Partnership. Site to help Medicare beneficiaries with healthcare.

- **www.cardiab.com** Cardiovascular Diabetology. BioMed Central. Site the discusses diabetes and cardiovascular disease.

- **www.diabetes.org** La Diabetes y los Latinos. American Diabetes Association. Site in Spanish for patients with diabetes.

- **http://diabetes.niddk.nih.gov/spanish/pubs/ dictionary/index.htm** Diccionario de la Diabetes (NIDDK). Spanish dictionary for diabetes.

- **http://diabetes.niddk.nih.gov/spanish/index.asp** Informacion en Espanol-Diabetes (NIDDK).

- **www.pparx.org/Intro.php** Partnership for Prescription Assistance.

- **www.medicare.gov/spanish/overview.asp** Medicare in Spanish.

- **www.aarp.org/espanol** AARP in Spanish.

- **www.geriatricsandaging.ca/** Geriatrics and Aging. Educational site that addresses health concerns of older adults.

- **www.medscape.com/resource/geriatric** Geriatric Care Medscape. Site for geriatric resources.

- **www.aoa.gov** Administration of Aging (AOA) U.S. Department of Health and Human Services. Site with geriatric resources for professionals, patients and caregivers. Translations in German, Spanish, French, Italian, Korean, Japanese, Chinese and Portuguese.

- **www.lipid.org** National Lipid Association. Resource for clinical articles and education.

- **www.nhlbi.nih.gov/health/public/heart/hbp/dash** Lowering Your Blood Pressure with DASH (Dietary Approaches to Stop Hypertension) National Heart Lung and Blood Institute. Dietary guidelines for blood pressure reduction.

- **www.hypertensiononline.org** Hypertension Online. Baylor College of Medicine-Houston, Texas. Educational site for hypertension/blood pressure.

- **www.cdc.gov/ncidod/dhqp/index.html** Infection Control in Healthcare Settings. Centers for Disease Control and Prevention (CDC). Resource for Healthcare-Associated Infections, Protecting Patients, Protecting Healthcare Workers, and Infection Control Guidelines.

- **www.mdchoice.com** Medical Information Finder.

- **www.freemedicaljournals.com** Free Medical Journals. Access to online free and full text journals.

- **www.medicare.gov** Medicare U.S. Department of Health and Human Services. Comprehensive site for Medicare resources.

- www.nlm.nih.gov/medlineplus/ medicareprescriptiondrugplan.html Medicare Prescription Drug Plan. Medline Plus. National Library of Medicine (NLM). Resources on Medicare prescription drug coverage.

- www.ssa.gov/mediinfo.htm Medicare Social Security Online. Resources on Medicare.

- www.familiesusa.org/issues/medicare/medicare-central-home.html Medicare Central Families USA. Consumer health information on Medicare.

- www.medicarerights.org Medicare Rights Center. Information on Medicare.

- www.kidney.org National Kidney Foundation. Site for kidney information.

- www.nutrition.gov Nutrition.gov U.S. Department of Agriculture (USDA). Site for online access on information on nutrition.

- http://fnic.nal.usda.gov Food and Nutrition Information Center (FNIC). Extensive nutritional resources.

- www.mypyramid.gov U.S. Department of Agriculture (USDA) site with resources to help improve nutrition.

- www.cfsan.fda.gov Center for Food Safety and Applied Nutrition. U.S. Food and Drug Administration (FDA). Nutrition resource.

- www.kidshealth.org/parent/nutrition_fit/index.html Nutrition and Fitness, Kids Health, Nemours Foundation. Resource for parents on kids' nutrition and fitness.

- **www.kidsnutrition.org** Kid's Nutrition. Baylor College of Medicine- Houston, Texas. Resource for children's nutrition.
- **www.nlm.nih.gov/medlineplus/childnutrition.html** Child Nutrition. Medline Plus. National Library of Medicine (NLM.) Resource for child nutrition.
- **www.cdc.gov/nccdphp/dnpa/obesity** Overweight and Obesity. Centers for Disease Control and Prevention (CDC). Obesity review.
- **www.agingeye.net** The Eye Digest. The University of Illinois Eye and Ear Infirmary Chicago, Illinois. Review of diabetic retinopathy.
- **www.unos.org** United Network for Organ Sharing (UNOS).
- **www.shareyourlife.org** Coalition on Donation-Donate Life.
- **www.medscape.com/resource/painmgmt** Advanced Approaches to Chronic Pain Management. Medscape. Site dedicated to managing intractable pain.
- **www.npaf.org** National Patient Advocate Foundation. Site for National Network for Healthcare Access and patient advocacy information.
- **www.quackwatch.org** QuackWatch. A guide to quackery health fraud and intelligent decisions.
- **www.ckdinsights.com** Searchfor educational materials on renal disease, peritoneal dialysis, drug interactions and dialysis of drugs.

- **www.rxmed.com** RxMed. Reference site for pharmaceutical information and herbal and dietary supplements.

- **www.nlm.nih.gov/medlineplus/druginformation.html** Drugs, supplements and herbal information. National Library of Medicine (NLM).

- **www.pparx.org/Intro.php** Partnership for Prescription Assistance for patients, caregivers, and professionals.

- **www.needymeds.com** Needy Meds. Resource for prescription medicine assistance.

- **www.rxhope.com** RxHope. Online patient assistance portal to locate patient pharmaceutical assistance programs.

- **www.ssa.gov/prescriptionhelp** Helping with Prescription Drug Costs. Social Security Online. Resource for Medicare beneficiaries who may qualify for prescription assistance if they have limited income and resources.

- **www.medicare.gov/spap.asp** State Pharmaceutical Assistance Programs. Medicare. Resource by state for prescription assistance resources.

- **www.rxassist.org** RxAssist. Resource of patient assistance programs on free and low-cost medications.

- **www.apha.org** Public Health Links. American Public Health Association. Resources under Programs and Resources.

- **www.nysmokefree.com/newweb/default.aspx** The New York State Smoker's Quitsite. Smoking cessation.

- **www.quitnet.com** QuitNet. Boston University Smoking cessation site.

- **www.nlm.nih.gov/medlineplus/smokingcessation. html** Smoking Cessation. Medline plus National Library of Medicine (NLM).

- **www.smokefree.gov** Resource for smoking cessation.

- **www.thestretchinghandbook.com** Site with Stretching Exercises.

- **www.authentichappiness.sas.upenn.edu** Authentic Happiness. University of Pennsylvania- Philadelphia, Pennsylvania. A site focused on the study of positive motions, strength-based character and healthy institutions.

- **www.aath.org** Association for Applied & Therapeutic Humor.

- **www.nlm.nih.gov/medlineplus/weightcontrol.html** Weight Control Medline Plus National Library of Medicine (NLM). Resources for weight management.

- **http://health.nih.gov/result.asp/725** Weight loss/ dieting. U.S. Department of Health and Human Services/ National Institutes of Health (NIH).

## Internet Sites for More Information on Prevention

www.amputationprevention.com
www.diabetes.org
www.apma.org
www.webmd.com
www.prevention.com
www.padcoalition.org/wp
www.ampa.org
www.webmd.com
www.emedicinehealth.com
www.diabetesnet.com/diabetes
www.podiatrychannel.com

## Herbal and Dietary Supplements

www.itmonline.org/arts/diabherb.htm
www.diabetesmellitus-information.com/diabetes_herbs.htm
www.heartspring.net/diabetes_cinnamon.html
www.nutritionexpress.com
www.gymnema.net/
www.endocrinologist.com/herbs.html

## Food and Nutrition
www.healingwithnutrition.com/ddisease/diabetes/diabetes.
html

## Diabetes Educators

www.diabeteseducator.org/

## Kidney Disease
Diabetes is the leading cause of new cases of end-stage renal disease, accounting for about 40 percent of new cases.www. vapodiatry.com/Medical_info.html.

## Blindness
Diabetes is the leading cause of new cases of blindness in adults 20 to 74 years of age. Each year 12,000 to 24,000 people lose their sight because of diabetes.
www.vapodiatry.com/Medical_info.html.

## Statistics
Statistics from CLEAR
www.diabeticfootonline.com/CLEAR/Patients.html.

- "Diabetes affects 21 million people in the US and 189 million people worldwide. By the year 2025 the prevalence of diabetes is expected to rise by 72 percent to 324 million people globally." ~ American Diabetes Association
- "Sixty to seventy percent of those with diabetes will develop peripheral neuropathy, or lose sensation in their feet.' ~ Dyck et al. Diabetic Neuropathy 1999
- "Up to 25 percent of those with diabetes will develop a foot ulcer." ~ Singh, Armstrong, Lipsky. J American Medical Association 2005
- "More than half of all foot ulcers (wounds) will become infected, requiring hospitalization and 1 in 5 will require an amputation." ~ Lavery, Armstrong, et al. Diabetes Care 2006

- Diabetes is attributed to about 80 percent of the 120,000 non-traumatic amputations performed yearly in the United States. ~ Armstrong et al. Amer Fam Phys 1998
- "Every thirty seconds, somewhere in the world, a limb is lost as a consequence of diabetes." ~ The Lancet (cover), Nov. 2005
- "After a major amputation, 50 percent of patients will have their other limb amputated within two years." Goldner. Diabetes 1960 ~ Armstrong, et al, J American Podiatric Medical Association, 1997
- Rule of 15 by Peter Sheehan: 15 percent of people with diabetes develop ulcers, 15 percent of ulcers develop osteomyelitis, and 15 percent of ulcers result in amputation.

# INDEX

# E

# F

# G

## L
Laser surgery, 266-268
Lasix, 230
Lavery, Lawrence, Dr., 108, 193, 270, 362, 376, 436-438,
      440-441
Lewi, Maurice, Dr., 98
Loss of protective sensation (LOPS). *See* Protective sensation
Lower extremity amputation. *See* Amputation

## M
Macroangiopathy, 215-217
Magnetic Resonance Angiogram (MRA), 236-237
Malkin, Ken, DPM, 466-467
Mallet toe, 156, 201
Massage, 408
Matrix tissue, 168-171, 174
McLeod, Margaret, 109
Measuring the foot, 357-358
Mechanical injuries, 202-203
Medicaid, 460-470
Medical College Admission Test (MCAT), 99-100
Medication, 174-175, 206-2067, 294-300, 408-410, 431-433
Medicare, 112, 330-332, 460-470
Microangiopathy, 216-217
Misdiagnosis, 117-120
Monofilament testing, 190-193
Morton, D.J., 142
Motor neuropathy, 201-202
Multi-disciplinary treatment, 115-117, 126-128, 433-436,
      447-449, 450-454, 469

## N

## O

of diabetes, 136-137, 359-368, 394-398, 406-407
of treatment, 207, 428-436

## Q, R
Radicular pain, 165, 185
Rehabilitation, 388, 391
Research, 446-450
Re-ulceration, 268-269
Risk, 50, 78-84, 89-92, 106-107, 231
Risk factors
  for amputation, 68-84
  for diabetes, 45-51
Robbins, Jeffrey, DPM, 105-108
Roehrick, Laura, RN, 376-381
Rogers, Lee, Dr., 82
Root, Merton, 142
Russia, 101

## S
St. Vincent declaration, 443-444
Sanders, Lee, DPM, 108, 374-375, 462-463
Secondary diseases. *See* comorbidities
Sedentary lifestyle, 46, 49
Self-care, 88-90, 96-97, 478-480
Sensory neuropathy, 159-161, 202-204, 226-229, 246-247
Shoes, 249, 318-358
  custom-molded, 326-328
  Crocs, 328-329
  extra-depth, 326
  surgical shoes, 325

## V

## W

## X, Y

## Z

# End Notes

## Introduction:

1. "Lower-Leg Amputations Are Increasing." <u>Wallstreet Journal</u>, Feb. 23, 2005.

## Chapter 1:

1. "Deaths-Leading Causes." <u>National Center for Health Statistics</u>. Accessed 30 April 2008. <http://www.cdc.gov/nchs/FASTATS/lcod.htm>.

2. "24 million Americans have diabetes." <u>MSNBC.com</u>. Accessed 30 April 2008. <http://www.msnbc.msn.com/id/25350702/>.

3. "Amputations Linked to Diabetes." International Review of Patient Care. September 1, 2005. <http://www.hospitalmanagement.net/features/feature627/>.

4. "Noncommunicable Diseases." <u>World Health Organization Regional Office for Europe</u>. Accessed 28 April 2008. <http://www.euro.who.int/noncommunicable/diseases/20050629_15>.

5. "Diabetes Data/Statistics." <u>The Office of Minority Health.</u> Accessed 22 April 2008. <ttp://www.omhrc.gov/templates/browse.aspx?lvl=3&lvlid=5>.

6. "The History of Diabetes." <u>Canadian Diabetes Association</u>. Accessed 30 April 2008. <http://www.diabetes.ca/Section_About/timeline.asp>.

7. "Denial." <u>American Diabetes Association</u>. Accessed 1 July 2008. <http://www.diabetes.org/gestational-diabetes/denial.jsp>.

8. Nebergall, PhD, Peter J. "Diabetes and Denial." Accessed 1 July 2008. <http://nfb.org/legacy/vodold/vspr9805.htm.>

**Chapter 2:**

1. "Deaths-Leading Causes." <u>National Center for Health Statistics</u>. Accessed 30 April 2008. <http://www.cdc.gov/nchs/FASTATS/lcod.htm>.

2. "The Diabetic Foot: Amputations Are Preventable." <u>International Diabetes Federation</u>. May 2005. Accessed 1 July 2008. <http://www.idf.org/home/index.cfm?node=1408>.

3. "Facts on Diabetes and the Foot." VA Podiatry.com. Accessed 1 July 2008. <http://www.vapodiatry.com/Medical_info.html>.

4. "Responding to the Diabetes Epidemic in Latin America: Helping Diabetics Help Themselves" Disease Control Priority Projects. Accessed 1 July 2008. <http://www.dcp2.org/features/19>.

5. "Arterial Leg Disease May Be More Common in Blacks." XagenaMedicinenews.net. Accessed 22 April, 2008. http://www.xagena.it/news/medicinenews_net_news/431cfe4bd4a84b68398e14af4be0bdc3.html

6. Cyr, Ruth Ann RN. "Talking with Elders about Diabetes." Accessed 22 April 2008. <http://www.niichro.com/Diabetes/Dia4.html>.

7. "Diabetes Data/Statistics." The Office of Minority Health. U.S. Department of Health & Human Services. Accessed 22 April, 2008. <http://www.omhrc.gov/templates/browse.aspx?lvl=3&lvlid=5>.

8. "Health Insurance Coverage: 2006." The U.S. Census Bureau. Accessed 1 July 2008. <http://www.census.gov/hhes/www/hlthins/hlthin06/hlth06asc.html>.

9. "24 Million Americans Have Diabetes." MSNBC.com. Accessed 1 July 2008. <http://www.msnbc.msn.com/id/25350702/>.

## Chapter 3:

1. "Five Foot Problems That Shouldn't Be Ignored." Asia's Best Doctors.com. Accessed 2 July 2008. <http://www.asiasbestdoctors.com/story_1385.html>.

## Chapter 5:

1. "What is the Average Number of Miles a Person Walks in Their Life?" Ask.Yahoo.com. 3 October 2006. Accessed 2 July 2008. <http://ask.yahoo.com/20061003.html>.

2. Schwartz, Ann V. "Diabetes Related Complications, Glycemic Control and Falls in Older Adults." Diabetes Care Vol. 31 #3 March 2008. Accessed online 2 July 2008. <http://tinyurl.com/3tr85q>.

Chapter 7:

1. "Treatment of Diabetic Foot Ulcers." Advances in Skin and Foot Care. April 2006.

2. GOAL A1c study group, ADA 63rd Scientific Sessions 2003 Glycemic Optomization with Algorithims and Labs At Point of Care.

Chapter 8:

1. APMA News, November/December 2006.

Chapter 9:

1. "Amputations Linked to Diabetes." HospitalManagement.net. Accessed 10 July 2008. <http://www.hospitalmanagement.net/features/feature627/>.

2. Schaper, Nicolass MD. "Clinical Care of the Diabetic Foot." Virginia: American Diabetes Association, 2005. p. 45.

3. "The Site Matters." Diabetes Care. Volume 30, Number 8, August 2007.

4. Boulton, MD, FRCP, Andrew JM. "An Integrated Health Care Approach is Needed: The Global Burden of Diabetic Foot Disease." Accessed 9 July 2008. <http://www.diabeticmctoday.com/HtmlPages/DMC0106/DMC0106_Boulton.html>.

5. Konig, et al. "Enzymatic Versus Autolytic Debridement of Chronic Leg Ulcers; a Prospective Randomized Trial." Journal of Wound Care; 14(7), July 2005.

6. Journal of Wound Care; 14(9), October 2005.

7. Paustian C. Debridement rates with activated polyacrylate dressings. Ostomy Wound Management 2003; 49(Suppl 1):2. Journal of Wound Care; 14(9), October 2005.)

**Chapter 10:**

1. Johnson, Linda A. "N.J. company revives honey as a dressing for wounds." Associated Press. 31 December 2007. <http://www.firerescue1.com/fire-products/ems-supplies/articles/331252->.

2. "Use of Honey." APMA News. September 2005, p. 65, 68.

3. Percival SL, Bowler PG, Russell D. Bacterial resistance to silver in wound care. Journal of Hospital Infections. 2005, p. 60, 1-7.

4. Markowitz, L, et al. "Digital Planimetry Software Provides Accurate Wound Measurements Including Areas by Tissue Type, a Summary of abstracts." The Center for Palliative Wound Care, Calvary Hospital, Bronx New York.

**Chapter 11:**

1. "The Truth About Your Immune System, a Special Health Report from Harvard Medical School." 2007. The President and Fellows of Harvard College.

2. Fleck CA, Chakravarthy D. "Understanding the Mechanisms of Collagen Dressings." Advances in Skin and Wound Care.

May 2007;20(5):256-259.

3.  Ibid.

**Chapter 13:**

1.  "Otzi The Iceman." Crystallinks.com. Accessed 9 July 2008. <http://www.crystalinks.com/oetzi.html>.

2.  "Testimonials." Crocs.com. Accessed 9 July 2008. <http://www.crocs.com/community/testimonials/>.

3.  "Therapeutic Shoe Bill." Atlas International. Accessed 9 July 2008. <http://www.atlasortho.com/tsb/shoebill.html>.

4.  Albert, Stephen, DPM. "Permission to Use Quote." Email on 6 August, 2008.

5.  "Podiatry, Shoes, and Contemporary Pedorthics." Podiatry Management, October 2003, p. 134.

**Chapter 14:**

1.  Rubin, Richard R. "Psychotherapy and Counseling in Diabetes Mellitus." Psychology in Diabetes Care. John Wiley & Sons, Ltd. 2000.

**Chapter 15:**

1.  Harkless, Larry. "The 3-Ms of Prevention." From author's notes taken at San Diego DefCon meeting. March 2008.

2.  "Diabetes Statistics." Health Insite.com Accessed 9 July 2008. <http://www.healthinsite.gov.au/topics/diabetes_statistics>.

3.  "The Multidisciplinary Footcare Team: Safe in the Hands of the NHS?" BNet.com. Accessed 9 July 2008. <http://

findarticles.com/p/articles/mi_m0MDQ/is_2_10/ai_
n19393465>.

4. Reduction in Diabetes-related Lower-Extremity Amputations
   in the Netherlands: 1991-2000." PubMed.com. Accessed 9 July
   2008. <http://www.ncbi.nlm.nih.gov/pubmed/15111518>.

5. International Journal of Epidemiology 2002;31:234-239
   International Epidemiological Association 2002. Accessed
   July 2008. <http://ije.oxfordjournals.org/cgi/content/
   abstract/31/1/234>.

Chapter 16:

1. "Amputations Linked to Diabetes." HospitalManagement.net.
   Accessed 10 July 2008. <http://www.hospitalmanagement.
   net/features/feature627/>.

2. "The Economic Imperative to Conquer Diabetes." Diabetes
   Care. Volume 31, Number 3, March 2008. P 624.

3. "Economic Costs of Diabetes in the U.S. in 2007." Diabetes
   Care. Volume 31, Number 3, March 2008. P 596.

Chapter 17:

1. "Meeting Marks 10th Anniversary of NIH Acupuncture
   Conference." CAM at the NIH. Accessed 10 July 2008.
   <http://nccam.nih.gov/news/newsletter/2008_april/
   acupuncturecon.htm#ncdc >.

2. Richard Salcido, MD. "Viagra and Wound Healing: The NO
   Connection." Advances in Skin & Wound Care. Vol. 21, No. 3.

3. Boykin, Joseph V, and Chris Baylis. "Hyperbaric Oxygen
   Therapy Mediates Increase Nitric Oxide Production Associated

with Wound Healing: A Preliminary Study." <u>Advances in Skin & Wound Care</u>. Vol. 20, No. 7 p 382.

4. Kalani, M. et al. "Hyperbaric oxygen (HBO) therapy in treatment of diabetic foot ulcers. Long-term follow-up." Accessed 10 July 2008. <u>PubMed.gov.</u> <http://www.ncbi.nlm.nih.gov/pubmed/12039398?ordinalpos=1&itool=EntrezSystem2.PEntrez.Pubmed.Pubmed_ResultsPanel.Pubmed_RVAbstractPlus>.

5. "Sugary Beverages Fuel the Obesity Epidemic." <u>Harvard Health Letter</u>. October 2006. Accessed 10 July 2008. <http://www.health.harvard.edu/press_releases/sugar-and-obesity.htm>.

6. "Dietary Supplement Fact Sheet: Vitamin A and Carotenoids." Office of Dietary Supplements Accessed 10 July 2008. <http://ods.od.nih.gov/factsheets/vitamina.asp>.

7. "Study: Vegan Diet Might Reverse Diabetes Symptoms." <u>ABC News online</u>. 27 July 2006. Accessed 10 July 2008. <http://abclocal.go.com/wls/story?section=news/health&id=4406968>.

8. "Alcohol, Wine and Cardiovascular Disease." <u>American Heart Association</u>. Accessed 10 July 2008. <http://www.americanheart.org/presenter.jhtml?identifier=4422>.

**Chapter 18:**

1. Kravitz, Steve, DPM. <u>Journal of Family Practice</u>. 1998:47.

2. Lavery, Lawrence A. Personal interview on 23 June 2008.

3. <u>Visionaries.org</u> Accessed 30 July 2008. <http://www.visionaries.org/episode_listings/season_07/index.php>.

4. Crossing the Quality Chasm. The Institute of Medicine Committee on Quality Care in America. Washington, D.C., National Academy Press, 2001.

5. "Dr. Driver Discussed Therapeutic Angiogenesis." APMA Daily eNews. July 29, 2008.

6. American Diabetes Association: Standards of Medical Care for Patients with Diabetes Mellitus (Position Statement). Diabetes Care 25(Suppl. 1):S33-S50, 2002.

# Bibliography

"2005 World Diabetes Day on Diabetic Foot Care."
International Working Group on the Diabetic Foot.
Accessed 29 January 2008. <http://www.iwgdf.
org/index.php?Itemid=52&id=35&option=com_
content&task=view>.

"24 Million Americans Have Diabetes." MSNBC.com.
Accessed 30 April 2008. <http://www.msnbc.msn.com/
id/25350702/>.

"A News Brief About Bypass Surgery and Amputations."
<http://www.diabetes.org/diabetesnewsarticle.
jsp?storyId=17680178&filename=20080523/
reuters20080523health00000013reutershealthewEDIT.
xml>.

"Alcohol, Wine, and Cardiovascular Disease."
American Heart Association. Accessed 10 <July
2008. http://www.americanheart.org/presenter.
jhtml?identifier=4422>.

"Amputations Linked to Diabetes." HospitalManagement.
net. Accessed 10 July 2008. <http://www.
hospitalmanagement.net/features/feature627/>.

"An Abnormality of Hemoglobin Synthesis." 30 June
2008. <http://www.nlm.nih.gov/medlineplus/ency/
article/001208.htm>.

"Arterial Leg Disease May Be More Common In Blacks."
Xagena Medicine. Center for the Advancement of
Health, 2005. Accessed 22 April, 2008. <http://
www.xagena.it/news/medicinenews_net_news/
431cfe4bd4a84b68398e14af4be0bdc3.html>.

"Consensus Statement: A Practical Guide for Managing
Pressure Ulcers with Negative Pressure Wound Therapy
Utilizing Vacuum-Assisted Closure- Understanding the
Treatment Algorithm." Advances in Skin & Wound Care,
Volume 21, Supplement. 1 January 2008.

"Consensus Statement: A Practical Guide for Managing
Pressure Ulcers with Negative Pressure Wound Therapy
Utilizing Vacuum-Assisted Closure- Understanding the
Treatment Algorithm." Advances in Skin & Wound Care.
Volume 21, Supplement 1 January 2008.

"Custom-Molded Footwear—One Size Only." Podiatry
Management, October 2004.

"Deaths-Leading Causes." National Center for Health
Statistics. Accessed 30 April 2008. <http://www.cdc.
gov/nchs/FASTATS/lcod.htm>.

"Denial and Avoidance." Janine's Diabetes and Insulin
Pump Web page. Accessed 30 July 2008. <http://
www3.telus.net/public/camojo/denial.html>.

"Denial." American Diabetes Association. Accessed 1 July
2008. <http://www.diabetes.org/gestational-diabetes/
denial.jsp>.

"Depression Can Trigger Diabetes, Study Suggests."
Reuters. 17 June 2008. Accessed 9 July 2008. <http://
www.msnbc.msn.com/id/25217007/>.

"Diabetes Data/Statistics." The Office of Minority Health.

Accessed 22 April, 2008. <http://www.omhrc.gov/templates/browse.aspx?lvl=3&lvlid=5>.

"Diabetes Data/Statistics." The Office of Minority Health. U.S. Department of Health & Human Services. Accessed 22 April, 2008. <http://www.omhrc.gov/templates/browse.aspx?lvl=3&lvlid=5>.

"Diabetes Statistics." Health Insite.com Accessed 9 July 2008. <http://www.healthinsite.gov.au/topics/diabetes_statistics>.

"Diabetes, Depression and Death." Diabetes Care. Vol 30, Number 12, December 07) pp 3005-3110.

"Diabetes: Foot Care." Familydoctor.org. Accessed 22 April 2008. <http://familydoctor.org/online/famdocen/home/common/diabetes/living/352.html>.

"Diabetic Foot Infections; Microbiology Made Modern?" Diabetes Care, Volume 30 Number 8, pp. 2171-2172. August 2007.

"Diabetic Foot." Wikipedia.com. Accessed 23 April 2008. <http://en.wikipedia.org/wiki/Diabetic_foot>.

"Dietary Supplement Fact Sheet: Vitamin A and Carotenoids." Accessed 10 July 2008. <http://ods.od.nih.gov/factsheets/vitamina.asp>.

"Dr. Driver Discussed Therapeutic Angiogenesis." APMA Daily eNews. July 29, 2008.

"Economic Costs of Diabetes in the U.S. in 2007." Diabetes Care. Volume 31, Number 3, March 2008. P.596.

"Evaluation of the Self-Administered Indicator Plaster Neuropad for the Diagnosis of Neuropathy in Diabetes." Diabetes Care, The American Diabetes Association. November 19, 2007. Accessed 24 April

2008. <http://care.diabetesjournals.org/cgi/content/ abstract/31/2/236>.

"Facts on Diabetes and the Foot." VA Podiatry.com. Accessed 1 July 2008. <http://www.vapodiatry.com/ Medical_info.html>.

"Five Foot Problems That Shouldn't Be Ignored." Asia's Best Doctors.com. Accessed 2 July 2008. <http://www. asiasbestdoctors.com/story_1385.html>.

"Health Insurance Coverage: 2006." The U.S. Census Bureau. Accessed 1 July 2008. <http://www.census. gov/hhes/www/hlthins/hlthin06/hlth06asc.html>.

"How Americans 18 Years of Age or Older Treated Selected Foot Problems During the Past Twelve Months-2000." American Podiatric Medical Association.

"Indicator Plaster Neuropad Is Key In Early Diabetic Neuropathy Detection." Battle Diabetes. 22 March 2008. Accessed 21 April 2008. <http://www. battlediabetes.com/diabetic-neuropathy-neuropad/>.

"Items for the Week: Inadequate Footwear Triples Risk For Diabetes Amputation Risk." DiabetesinControl.com. Accessed 13 May 2008. <http://www.diabetesincontrol. com/modules.php?name=News&file=article&sid=2227>.

"Lower-Leg Amputations Are Increasing." Wallstreet Journal, Feb. 23, 2005.

"Meeting Marks 10th Anniversary of NIH Acupuncture Conference." CAM at the NIH. Accessed 10 July 2008. <http://nccam.nih.gov/news/newsletter/2008_april/ acupuncturecon.htm#ncdc >.

"Methacillin Resistant Staphylococcus Aureus Diabetic Foot Infections; Microbiology Made Modern?" Diabetes Care,

Volume 30 Number 8. August 2007 pp 2171-2172.

"Multi-year Data Shows PAD Treatment Prevents Amputation." From Science Daily. March 20, 2007. Accessed 24 May 2007. http//:www.sciencedaily.com/releases/2007/03.

"Noncommunicable Diseases." World Health Organization Regional Office for Europe. Accessed 28 April 2008. <http://www.euro.who.int/noncommunicable/diseases/20050629_15>.

"Otzi The Iceman." Crystallinks.com. Accessed 9 July 2008. <http://www.crystalinks.com/oetzi.html>.

"Paul Brand." Wikipedia.org. 31 July 2008. <http://en.wikipedia.org/wiki/Paul_Wilson_Brand>.

"Peripheral arterial disease is on the Rise." DOC News. Clinical News. January 2008, page 7.

"Podiatry, Shoes, and Contemporary Pedorthics." Podiatry Management, October 2003, p. 134.

"Preventing Diabetic Amputations" Bio on Lee J. Sanders DPM. U.S. Medicine. August 2003. Accessed on 31 July 2008. <http://www.usmedicine.com/article.cfm?articleID=714&issueID=53>.

"Reduction in Diabetes-related Lower-Extremity Amputations in the Netherlands: 1991-2000." PubMed.com. Accessed 9 July 2008. <http://www.ncbi.nlm.nih.gov/pubmed/15111518>.

"Responding to the Diabetes Epidemic in Latin America: Helping Diabetics Help Themselves" Disease Control Priority Projects. Accessed 1 July 2008. <http://www.dcp2.org/features/19>.

"Risk Factors for Recurrent Diabetic Foot Ulcers. The Site Matters." Diabetes Care, Volume 30, Number 8, August 2007.

"Senior Health Costs Projected to Soar, Number of Elderly Will Double by 2030; CDC Says Key Is Preventing Disease." MSNBC.com. Accessed March. 8, 2007. <http://www.msnbc.msn.com/id/17518459/print/1/displaymode/1098/>.

"Shoes and Orthotics." American Orthopaedic Foot & Ankle Society. Accessed 23 April 2008. <http://www.aofas.org/i4a/pages/index.cfm?pageid=3320>.

"St Vincent Declaration Diabetes Mellitus in Europe: A Problem at All Ages in All Countries." Patient UK. Accessed 30 July 2008. <http://www.patient.co.uk/showdoc/40002292/>.

"St. Vincent's Declaration." International Diabetes Federation. Accessed 30 July 2008. <http://www.idf.org/home/index.cfm?node=839>.

"Statistics by Country for Diabetes." CureReasearch.com. Accessed 30 June, 2008. <http://www.cureresearch.com/d/diabetes/stats-country.htm>.

"Study: Vegan Diet Might Reverse Diabetes Symptoms." ABC News online. 27 July 2006. Accessed 10 July 2008. <http://abclocal.go.com/wls/story?section=news/health&id=4406968>.

"Sugary Beverages Fuel the Obesity Epidemic." Harvard Health Letter. October 2006. Accessed 10 July 2008. <http://www.health.harvard.edu/press_releases/sugar-and-obesity.htm>.

"Testimonials." Crocs.com. Accessed 9 July 2008. <http://www.crocs.com/community/testimonials/>.

"The Diabetes Epidemic Among American Indians and Alaska Natives." National Diabetes Education Program. Accessed April 22, 2008. <www.ndep.nih.gov>.

"The Diabetic Foot: Amputations Are Preventable." International Diabetes Federation. May 2005. Accessed 1 July 2008. <http://www.idf.org/home/index.cfm?node=1408>.

"The Diabetic Foot: Amputations Are Preventable." IWGDF. May 2005. Accessed 16 April 2007. <http://www.idf.org/home/index.cfm?node=1408>.

"The Economic Imperative to Conquer Diabetes." Diabetes Care. Volume 31, Number 3, March 2008. P. 624.

"The History of Diabetes." Canadian Diabetes Association. Accessed 30 April 2008.

"The Multidisciplinary Footcare Team: Safe in the Hands of the NHS?" BNet.com. Accessed 9 July 2008. <http://findarticles.com/p/articles/mi_m0MDQ/is_2_10/ai_n19393465>.

"The Site Matters." Diabetes Care. Volume 30, Number 8, August 2007.

"The Super Foods that Heal." DiabeticDietSecrets.com. Accessed 30 July 2008. <http://diabetic-diet-secrets.com/members/super-foods-that-heal.html>.

"The Truth About Your Immune System, a Special Health Report from Harvard Medical School." 2007. The President and Fellows of Harvard College.

"Therapeutic Shoe Bill." Atlas International. Accessed 9 July 2008. <http://www.atlasortho.com/tsb/shoebill.html>.

"Treatment of Diabetic Foot Ulcers." <u>Advances in Skin and Foot Care.</u> April 2006.

"Use of Honey." <u>APMA News</u>. From advertisement sheet on VPT's September 2005, p. 65, 68 "The Journal of Family Practice," June 2005, Vol. 54, No. 6.

"What are mg/dl and mmol/l? How to convert? Glucose? Cholesterol?" <u>FAQs.org</u>. Accessed 24 April 2008. <http://www.faqs.org/faqs/diabetes/faq/part1/section-9.html>.

"What is the Average Number of Miles a Person Walks in Their Life?" <u>Ask.Yahoo.com</u>. 3 October 2006. Accessed 2 July 2008. <http://ask.yahoo.com/20061003.html>.

American Diabetes Association: Standards of Medical Care for Patients with Diabetes Mellitus (Position Statement). <u>Diabetes Care</u> 25(Suppl. 1):S33-S50, 2002.

Armstrong, David and Lavery, Lawrence, eds., "Clinical Care of the Diabetic Foot." <u>Virginia: American Diabetes Association</u>, 2005, p. 45.

Armstrong, David G. et al. "Preventing Foot Ulcers in Patients With Diabetes." <u>Journal of the American Medical Association.</u> Vol. 293 No. 2, January 12, 2005. Accessed 24 April 2008. <http://jama.ama-assn.org/cgi/content/full/293/2/217>.

Armstrong, David. Phone Interview with Author. 9 June 2008.

Attinger, Christopher. Phone Interview with Author. 24 June 2008.

Bakker, Dr. Karel. "World Diabetes Day." <u>International Working Group on the Diabetic Foot</u>. 2005. Accessed 29 January 2008.

Barclay, Eliza. "Responding to the Diabetes Epidemic in Latin America: Helping Diabetics Help Themselves." Disease Control Priorities Projects. November 1, 2006. Accessed 30 July 2008. <http://www.dcp2.org/features/19/responding-to-the-diabetes-epidemic-in-latin-america-helping-diabetics-help-themselves>.

Bell, Ronny et al, eds. "Diabetic Foot Self-care Practices in a Rural, Triethnic Population." The Diabetes Educator. Vol. 31, Number 1. January/February 2005, p. 75.

Boulton Dr. Andrew JM, et al. "The global burden of diabetic foot disease." Lancet. 366;1719-1724.

Boulton, Dr. Andrew JM. "An Integrated Healthcare Approach is Needed: The Global Burden of Diabetic Foot Disease." Diabetic MC Today. Accessed 22 April 2008. <http://www.diabeticmctoday.com/HtmlPages/DMC0106/DMC0106_Boulton.html>.

Bouton, Andrew, JM, MD, FRCP. "The Global Burden of Diabetic Foot Disease." Diabetic Microsasular Complication Today. Jan/Feb 2006 pp 23-29.

Boykin, Joseph V, and Chris Baylis. "Hyperbaric Oxygen Therapy Mediates Increase Nitric Oxide Production Associated with Wound Healing: A Preliminary Study." Advances in Skin & Wound Care. Vol. 20, No. 7 p 382.

Crossing the Quality Chasm. The Institute of Medicine Committee on Quality Care in America. Washington, D.C., National Academy Press, 2001.

Cyr, RN Ruth Ann. "Talking with Elders about Diabetes." Accessed 12 April 2008. <http://www.niichro.com/Diabetes/Dia4.html>.

Deeb, Dr. Larry, MD. Professional Section Quarterly for ADA

News Summer 2006.
Fleck, C.A. "Differentiating MMPs, Biofilm, Endotoxins, Exotoxins, and Cytokines." Advances in Skin and Wound Care 2006; 19(2):77-81).
Fleck, C.A. "Identifying Infection in Chronic Wounds." Advances in Skin and Wound Care. January/February 2006, p. 19.
Fleck, C.A. and D. McCord. "The Dawn of Advanced Skin Care." Extended Care Product News; 95(5): 32, 34-39, September 2004.
Fleck, Cynthia. Phone Interview with Author. 6 May 2008.
Frykberg, Bob, DPM. Phone Interview with Author. 2 May 2008.
Green, Howard, DPM. Phone Interview with Author. 27 April 2008.
Groom, M. "Decreasing the Incidence of Skin Tears in the Extended Care Setting with the Use of a New Line of Advanced Skin Care Products Containing Olivamine." Presented at the 18th Annual Symposium on Advances in Skin and Wound Care and 15th Annual Medical Research Forum on Wound Repair in San Diego, CA, 21-24 April 2005.
Halperin, Linda, MD. Personal interview. 1 May 2008.
Harkless, Larry. "The 3 Ms of Prevention." From notes taken at Los Angeles DF Con meeting. March 2008
Hunter, Ken. "Diabetics See Dramatic Increase in Lower Limb Amputations." Accessed 1 July, 2008. <http://www.eurekalert.org/pub_releases/2006-09/p-dsd091306.php.>
International Journal of Epidemiology 2002; 31:234-239 International Epidemiological Association 2002.

Accessed 9 July 2008. <http://ije.oxfordjournals.org/
cgi/content/abstract/31/1/234>.

Janisse, Dennis J., C. Ped., Phone Interview with Author. 4
May 2008.

Johnson, Linda A. "N.J. Company Revives Honey as a
Dressing for Wounds." Associated Press. 31 December
2007. <http://www.firerescue1.com/fire-products/
ems-supplies/articles/331252->.

Kahn, Richard PhD. "A New Name and Numbers Game for
A1c." DOC news. May 1, 2007 Volume 4 Number 5 p. 3,
American Diabetes Association Services. Accessed 24
April 2008. <http://docnews.diabetesjournals.org/cgi/
content/full/4/5/3>.

Kalani, M. et al. "Hyperbaric Oxygen (HBO) Therapy
in Treatment of Diabetic Foot Ulcers. Long-term
follow-up." Accessed 10 July 2008. PubMed.
gov. <http://www.ncbi.nlm.nih.gov/pubmed/
12039398?ordinalpos=1&itool=EntrezSystem2.
PEntrez.Pubmed.Pubmed_ResultsPanel.Pubmed_
RVAbstractPlus>.

Kent, DJ. "The Presence of an Instructional Pamphlet on a
Wound Dressing." Peer review.

Kidney Disease Article. 30 June 2008. <http://
kidneydiseases.about.com/od/symptomsof/a/uremia.
htm>.

King, RE Aubert and WH Herman. "Global Burden Of
Diabetes, 1995-2025: Prevalence, Numerical Estimates,
and Projections." American Diabetes Association.
Diabetes Care, Vol. 21, Issue 9, pp. 1414-1431.

Konig, et al. "Enzymatic Versus Autolytic Debridement of
Chronic Leg Ulcers; a Prospective Randomized Trial."

Journal of Wound Care; 14(7), July 2005.

Kravitz, Steve, DPM. Journal of Family Practice. 1998:47.

Lavery, Lawrence A.,DPM., Phone Interview with Author. 23 June 2008.

Lee, Steve, DO. Review provided by VeriMed Healthcare Network. 6/18/2007.

Markowitz, L, et al. "Digital Planimetry Software Provides Accurate Wound Measurements Including Areas by Tissue Type, a Summary of abstracts." The Center for Palliative Wound Care, Calvary Hospital, Bronx New York.

Mathur, Dr. Ruchi and William C. Shiel, Jr. "Hemoglobin A1c Test." DOC news. May 2007. Accessed 24 April 2008. <http://www.medicinenet.com/hemoglobin_a1c_test/article.htm>.

McLeod, Elaine, CDE. Personal interview. 1 April 2008.

Nebergall, PhD, Peter J. "Diabetes and Denial." Accessed 1 July 2008. <http://nfb.org/legacy/vodold/vspr9805.htm>.

Paustian C. Debridement Rates with Activated Polyacrylate Dressings. Ostomy Wound Management 2003; 49(Suppl 1):2. Journal of Wound Care; 14(9), October 2005.)

Percival SL, Bowler PG, Russell D. Bacterial Resistance to Silver in Wound Care. Journal of Hospital Infections. 2005, p. 60, 1-7.

Powers, James, MD, Phone Interview with Author. 24 June 2008

Robbins, Jeffrey, DPM. Phone Interview with Author. 1 April 2008.

Robbins, Jessica M. et al. "Nutritionist Visits, Diabetes Classes, and Hostpitaliztion Rates and Charges." The

Urban Diabetes Study, Diabetes Care, Vol. 31, Number 4, April 2008.

Roehrick, Laura, RN. Phone Interview with Yvonne Perry on Behalf of Author. 26 March 2008.

Rubin, Richard R. "Psychotherapy and Counseling in Diabetes Mellitus." Psychology in Diabetes Care. John Wiley & Sons, Ltd. 2000.

Salcido, Richard, MD. "Viagra and Wound Healing: The NO Connection." Advances in Skin & Wound Care, Vol. 21, No. 3.

Schaper, Nicholas, MD. "Clinical Care of the Diabetic Foot." Virginia: American Diabetes Association, 2005. p. 45.

Schwartz, Ann V, MD. "Diabetes Related Complications, Glycemic Control and Falls in Older Adults." Diabetes Care Vol. 31 #3. March 2008. Accessed Online 2 July 2008. <http://tinyurl.com/3tr85q>.

Shor, Robert, I, DPM, C.Ped, " Preventive Footwear for Recurrent Diabetic Foot Ulcers." Podiatry Management. October 2004, pp. 117-123.

Spalding, Robert, DPM Death by Pedicure The Dirty Secret of Nail Salons. Publisher Chattanooga Fu Fu Factory. September 2006.

Steinberg, John, DPM. Phone Interview with Author. 5 June 2008.

Thompson, Patricia et al. "Advances in Skin & Wound Care." Woundcarejournal.com Vol. 20, No. 11, p 586. November 2007.

Udell, DPM Elliot. Responses/Comments (Non-Clinical) Active Part 2 PM News. August 06, 2008 #3,316.

Podiatry Management. Accessed online 7 August 2008.
<http://www.podiatrym.com/search3.cfm?id=21131>.
Vinik, Aaron, I, MD. "Lower Extremity Disease More
Prevalent in Diabetic Population" Diabetic Microsasular
Complication Today. Jan/Feb 2006 pp 23-29.
Visionaries.org Accessed 30 July 2008. <http://www.
visionaries.org/episode_listings/season_07/index.php>.
Wrobel, James, DPM. Phone Interview with Author. 25 June
2008
Zamorano, Ruben. Phone Interview with Author. 1 May
2008.
Zhu, Chongbin. Phone Interview with Author. 12 April 2008.

## Photo Credits:

Most photos in this book were taken by Mark Hinkes, DPM, with the permission of the patients photographed. Other graphics and photos are from http://www.podiatrychannel.com and http://itre.cis.upenn.edu.

534

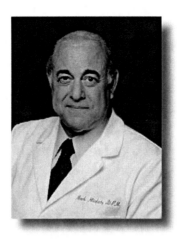

## About the Author

Dr. Mark Hinkes is a Doctor of Podiatric Medicine at the Veterans Affairs Medical Center in Nashville, Tennessee (Tennessee Valley Healthcare System) where he serves as the Chief of Podiatry Services and Director of Podiatric Medical Education. He is responsible for providing the full spectrum of foot health services including primary podiatric care, pedal biomechanical evaluation, orthotic/prosthetic services, preventive foot care for at-risk limbs, and foot surgery services. He also provides consultation services for primary care, emergency care services, and specialty service clinics.

Before moving to Nashville, Dr. Hinkes was the Chief of the Podiatry Service at the Veterans Affairs Medical Center in Salem, Virginia. He served as National Field Advisor for Quality Assurance for Podiatric Medicine for the Veterans Administration. He has been the Chairman of the Preservation Amputation Care and Treatment (PACT) Program over the past ten years, five years at each of the VA Hospitals.

Dr. Hinkes has been a consultant for hospitals, extended care facilities, and corporations. He has served on multiple hospital committees, lectured internationally and nationally for community groups and schools, and has published peer-reviewed journal articles. Dr. Hinkes participated in teaching podiatric medicine at the graduate level at Barry University in Miami, Florida from 1987 to 1998 as Adjunct Associate Professor of Podiatric Medicine. He is bilingual, English-Spanish, and has been a consultant to the electronic and print media in both languages and been President of the Dade County (Florida) Podiatric Medical Association. He has served as a clinical investigator for Novartis Pharmaceuticals.

Dr. Hinkes started his podiatric medical career in Miami, Florida where he completed his American Podiatric Medical Association-approved medical/surgical residency training at Westchester General Hospital from 1976-1977 under the direction of Keith B. Kashuk, DPM. Between 1977 and 1998, he held clinical, medical, and surgical privileges at Westchester General Hospital, South Miami Hospital, Baptist Hospital, and Kendall Regional Medical Center in Miami. He has participated in podiatric residency training as a clinician/clinical instructor and provided office rotations for students. He has provided clinical instruction in office and hospital operating room settings on foot pathology and foot surgery. He has lectured on various topics including hallux abducto valgus, digital deformities, nerve entrapment syndromes, nail pathology, functional biomechanics and orthotics, diabetic foot care, managed healthcare, and practice management.

Dr. Hinkes graduated in May 1976 from Ohio College of Podiatric Medicine in Cleveland as a member of Phi Alpha Pi Professional Fraternity. In January 1973, he obtained his Bachelor of Science in Psychology from Loyola University of Chicago, Illinois. His post-graduate training was conducted at Westchester General Hospital in Miami, Florida. His teaching at post-graduate level includes Vanderbilt University School of Nursing and Geriatric Medicine in Nashville where he taught issues in common foot problems and foot health, the diabetic foot ulcer and amputation prevention in the at-risk patient.

Dr. Hinkes is certified by the American Board of Podiatric Surgery and the American Professional Wound Care Association. He is a diplomat of the American College of Foot & Ankle Surgeons. His professional memberships include the American Podiatric Medical Association, the Federal Services Podiatric Medical Association, and the American Diabetes Association. He is the founder of Amputation Prevention Partners, LLC.

In his leisure time, Dr. Hinkes enjoys gardening, traveling, and creating stained glass art.

Dr. Hinkes is available for speaking engagements and clinical instruction in foot care clinics. He may be contacted on his Web site at www.amputationprevention.com.

*Etter Dee@ SBC Global.Net*

156-157 pictures of toes
181-182 text

$ 759.79

Gerard
J Gerald Mann

service King

widflower

CK# 7326
April 26, 2019

Del of mc

2) V dau = Con
fun

Stephen & Don:

LaVergne, TN USA
09 November 2009
163549LV00004B/7/P